A Modern Approach to Veterinary Medicine

A Modern Approach to Veterinary Medicine

Editor: Gerardo Bailey

STATES
ACADEMIC PRESS
www.statesacademicpress.com

States Academic Press,
109 South 5th Street,
Brooklyn, NY 11249, USA

Visit us on the World Wide Web at:
www.statesacademicpress.com

ISBN: 978-1-63989-007-1 (Hardback)

Cataloging-in-Publication Data

A modern approach to veterinary medicine / edited by Gerardo Bailey.
p. cm.
Includes bibliographical references and index.
ISBN 978-1-63989-007-1
1. Veterinary medicine. 2. Animals--Diseases. 3. Animal health. I. Bailey, Gerardo.
SF745 .M63 2022
636.089--dc23

Table of Contents

Preface

The branch of medicine that is concerned with the diagnosis, prevention and treatment of disease, disorder and injury in animals is called veterinary medicine. Its domain ranges from domesticated animals to wild animals. Different species of animals suffer from different diseases which can be treated by using a wide spectrum of veterinary medicines. Its main aim is to keep the animals healthy and safe. This field also maintains food supply through monitoring the health of livestock. Research in this domain is focused on wildlife and ecosystem health, human-animal interfaces and zoonotic diseases. This book traces the progress of this field and highlights some of its key concepts and applications. For all readers who are interested in veterinary medicine, the case studies included in this book will serve as an excellent guide to develop a comprehensive understanding. This book aims to shed light on some of the unexplored aspects of veterinary medicine and the recent researches in this field.

The researches compiled throughout the book are authentic and of high quality, combining several disciplines and from very diverse regions from around the world. Drawing on the contributions of many researchers from diverse countries, the book's objective is to provide the readers with the latest achievements in the area of research. This book will surely be a source of knowledge to all interested and researching the field.

In the end, I would like to express my deep sense of gratitude to all the authors for meeting the set deadlines in completing and submitting their research chapters. I would also like to thank the publisher for the support offered to us throughout the course of the book. Finally, I extend my sincere thanks to my family for being a constant source of inspiration and encouragement.

Editor

1

A systematic review of clinical audit in companion animal veterinary medicine

Nicole Rose[1], Lorraine Toews[2] and Daniel S. J. Pang[3,4*]

Abstract

Background: Clinical audit is a quality improvement process with the goal of continuously improving quality of patient care as assessed by explicit criteria. In human medicine clinical audit has become an integral and required component of the standard of care. In contrast, in veterinary medicine there appear to have been a limited number of clinical audits published, indicating that while clinical audit is recognised, its adoption in veterinary medicine is still in its infancy. A systematic review was designed to report and evaluate the veterinary literature on clinical audit in companion animal species (dog, cat, horse). A systematic search of English and French articles using Proquest Dissertations and Theses database (February 6, 2014), CAB Abstracts (March 21, 2014 and April 4, 2014), Scopus (March 21, 2014), Web of Science Citation index (March 21, 2014) and OVID Medline (March 21, 2014) was performed. Included articles were those either discussing clinical audit (such as review articles and editorials) or reporting parts of, or complete, audit cycles.

Results: The majority of articles describing clinical audit were reviews. From 89 articles identified, twenty-one articles were included and available for review. Twelve articles were reviews of clinical audit in veterinary medicine, five articles included at least one veterinary clinical audit, one thesis was identified, one report was of a veterinary clinical audit website and two articles reported incomplete clinical audits. There was no indication of an increase in the number of published clinical audits since the first report in 1998. However, there was evidence of article misclassification, with studies fulfilling the criteria of clinical audit not appropriately recognised. Quality of study design and reporting of findings varied considerably, with information missing on key components, including duration of study, changes in practice implemented between audits, development of explicit criteria and appropriate statistical analyses.

Conclusions: Available evidence suggests the application and reporting of clinical audit in veterinary medicine is sporadic despite the potential to improve patient care, though the true incidence of clinical audit reporting is likely to be underestimated due to incorrect indexing. Reporting standards of clinical audits are highly variable, limiting evaluation, application and repeatability of published work.

Keywords: Clinical audit, Systematic review, Veterinary, Audit

Background

Clinical audit is a quality improvement tool that facilitates the evaluation and improvement of care [1, 2]. In human medicine, it has become a standard of care required by some national governing bodies [3] and its implementation has yielded measurable improvements in clinical care [4–8]. Furthermore, the absence of clinical audit has been identified in allowing persistent poor performance, resulting in failures of care [9]. In veterinary medicine, national level audit with explicit criteria and reporting standards set by governing bodies does not currently exist. The only nationally mandated audit the authors are aware of is the requirement that clinics participating in the Royal College of Veterinary Surgeons Practice Standards Scheme perform audits to evaluate clinical outcomes (with the implication that these are limited to individual clinics) [10], though many veterinary clinics do perform informal audits through practices such as mortality and morbidity rounds. A formal clinical audit, first described in veterinary

* Correspondence: dsjpang@ucalgary.ca
[3]Veterinary Clinical and Diagnostic Sciences, Faculty of Veterinary Medicine, University of Calgary, Calgary, AB, Canada
[4]Hotchkiss Brain Institute, University of Calgary, Calgary, AB, Canada
Full list of author information is available at the end of the article

medicine by Mosedale [2], is centred around a structured audit cycle. In its simplest form, a clinical audit can be described by a 4 step process: Plan-Do-Study-Act (PDSA) [11–14]. This process is cyclical in nature to allow for continuous monitoring of performance and improvement [1, 11–14]. In the "Plan" step, a clear problem is identified [14]. The problem can be an outcome, such as anesthetic mortality rate, or a process associated with achieving an outcome, such as the number of patients receiving a physical examination prior to general anesthesia. When a clinical audit focuses on an outcome or process it may be described as an "outcome [clinical] audit" or "process [clinical] audit", respectively. The "Do" step is the process of data collection [1, 11–14]. Following data collection, the "Study" step is analysis of the data followed by comparison of results to a predetermined set of standards ("explicit criteria") [11, 14–16]. Finally, the "Act" step is the development of recommendations based upon the outcome of "Study". These recommendations are then implemented and additional audit cycles performed [1, 11–14]. In summary, clinical audit compares a current standard of care against clearly defined criteria and uses this information to drive change with the goal of improvement in patient care [1, 14]. The process should be cyclical, with regular re-evaluation to achieve the goal of continual improvement [1, 12, 14, 17].

The key principles of clinical audit are the selection of explicit criteria and its cyclical nature. Selected criteria should be easily measured, relevant to the process/outcome of interest, based on available evidence and clearly defined ("explicit"). Where there is insufficient evidence to identify criteria, clinical audit allows for performance comparison with other institutions ("benchmarking"). The tracking of performance through regular audit creates an "audit cycle", resulting in a continuous cycle of improvement [1, 17]. Absence of a cyclical process, as is common with traditional audit (audit of clinical practice), results in a limited ability to generate continuous improvement [18]. This is an important distinction; due to the absence of explicit criteria (as defined above) and a cyclical evaluation of performance an audit of clinical practice often takes the form of a simple survey of practice and lacks the ability to drive and monitor improvement through a cyclical process.

Clinical audit has been variably defined in veterinary and human medicine [1, 11, 12, 19, 20]. Burgess [11] defines clinical audit as "a quality improvement process that seeks to improve patient care and outcomes through systematic review of care against explicit criteria and the implementation of change" [11]. Since an initial description in 1998 [2], it is unclear to what extent clinical audit is being reported in the veterinary literature and how closely reported studies adhere to the principles of an audit cycle. The purpose of this study was to perform a systematic review of the reporting of clinical audit in the veterinary literature related to companion animals (dogs, cats and horses).

Methods

A systematic review was performed in accordance with the Preferred Reporting Items for Systematic Reviews and Meta-Analyses (PRISMA) guidelines [21]. The Cochrane Collaboration's Cochrane Handbook of Systematic Reviews of Interventions (version 5.1.0) 2011, which is widely recognized as the gold standard for conducting systematic reviews, was used to guide our processes, along with guidance from the Centre for Reviews and Dissemination [22, 23].

Key search concepts and synonyms were developed by the review team (NR, DP). A health sciences librarian (LT) refined the search strategy by conducting iterative database queries. To ensure a high degree of search sensitivity, a combination of subject headings and text words were used and the search strategy was adapted to the search interface and indexing conventions of each database.

The following electronic databases were searched to identify journal literature and conference papers: OVID CAB Abstracts 1910 to 2014 (searched March 21, 2014 and April 4, 2014), OVID MEDLINE 1946–2014 (searched March 21, 2014), Scopus 1960 to 2014 (searched March 21, 2014) and Web of Science 1899 to 2014 (searched March 21, 2014). Search results for all databases were limited to studies published in English or French. No study design, publication type or publication date limits were applied to the search results.

As veterinary conference papers and proceedings are very selectively indexed in research databases (not all papers may be indexed for a given year, nor is indexing consistent from year to year), and relevant full-text conference proceedings are often not available (library subscriptions are prioritised to peer-reviewed journals), to identify additional unpublished studies we also searched the International Veterinary Information Service (IVIS) website tables of contents for the Annual American Association of Equine Practitioners and the British Equine Veterinary Association conference proceedings, using the terms: "audit", "governance", "event" and "incident". The IVIS website did not provide access to abstracts for any of the relevant small animal conferences. The ProQuest Dissertations and Theses database was searched from 1861 to February 6th, 2014.

The full search strategy is documented in Table 1 and Additional file 1. Search results were downloaded into a commercial reference management software program (EndNote version X6, Thomson Reuters, New York, NY, USA) and duplicates were removed manually. Reference lists of included studies were scanned to identify additional sources.

Table 1 Electronic database search strategy for OVID CAB Abstracts <1910 to 2014 Week 12>

1. (critical event[a] review[a] or critical event[a] report[a] or critical event[a] audit[a] or critical event meeting[a] criticalinciden[a] review[a] or critical inciden[a] report[a] or critical inciden[a] audit[a] or critical inciden[a] meeting[a] significantevent[a] review[a] or significant event[a] report[a] or significant event[a] audit[a] or significant event[a] meeting[a]).af.
2. (chart audit or chart audits or chart auditing or clinical audit or clinical audits or clinical auditing orclinical governance or medical record[a] audit[a] or medical audit[a] or outcome[a] audit[a] or process audit[a] or prescription[a] audit[a] or medicines audit[a] or liability audit[a]).af.
3. auditing[b]
4. 1 or 2 or 3
5. exp veterinary practice[b]
6. exp veterinary services[b]
7. exp veterinary science[b]or veterinary medicine[b]or veterinarians[b]or veterinary profession[b]
8. (veterinary or veterinarian[a] or small animal practice[a] or large animal practice[a] or equine practice[a] or bovinepractice[a] or dairy practice[a] or beef cattle practice[a] or mixed practice[a]).af.
9. 5 or 6 or 7 or 8
10. 4 and 9
11 limit 10 to ((english or french) and (conference or journal))

"exp" denotes that the search term was exploded; [a]indicates that the word stem and all variant endings were retrieved. "[b]"identifies the preceding words as a subject heading indexing term. The same search strategy was conducted in all databases, adapted to the search syntax and conventions of each database (see Additional file 1)

Two authors (NR, DP) independently screened all abstracts for inclusion and any disagreement resolved through discussion to reach consensus. For the purposes of this review, clinical audit as defined by Burgess [11] ("clinical audit is a quality improvement process that seeks to improve patient care and outcomes through systematic review of care against explicit criteria and the implementation of change") was applied as the criterion standard [11]. Inclusion criteria for the final review were: 1. Articles reporting at least two of the four components of the clinical audit cycle (data collection, review of data against defined criteria, implementing change, re-auditing) and 2. Articles that discussed the process or benefits of clinical audit in veterinary medicine. Following identification of included articles, each article was read by two authors (NR, DP) and the following information extracted to facilitate critical appraisal: aim, explicit criteria, study population, collected data, analysis performed, intervention(s) implemented.

Exclusion criteria were 1. Non-veterinary studies and, 2. Clinical audit not related to individual companion animal care.

Results

The initial database literature research yielded 89 potential original articles (Fig. 1). Of these, 19 articles were disqualified because they were limited to the human medical literature. This resulted in 70 veterinary articles, of which 49 were excluded as they did not discuss clinical audit in companion animal care (11 food safety/biosecurity, 11 herd health, 21 business in veterinary medicine, 3 lab animal/wildlife related, 2 incidence of disease, and 1 disaster response). Initial search terms included large animal practice (Table 1 and Additional file 1) in case any clinical audits were performed where these species were treated as companion animals. With the exception of equine practice, none were identified. This resulted in 21 articles included in the analysis. The minority (n = 6) of these described the full audit cycle, and were therefore correctly classified as clinical audit (Table 2). These six articles described 10 separate clinical audits, the majority of which were focused on outcomes ("outcome audit", n = 8) [2, 14, 20, 24, 25]. There were two clinical audits assessing the process(es) which might contribute to change ("process audit") [20, 26]. Two articles simply described audits, without documented completion of the clinical audit cycle, such as implementation of change or re-audit [27, 28].

The majority (n = 13) of the identified articles were reviews of clinical audit and its application to clinical practice (Table 3). The publication dates of clinical audits and reviews are sporadic with no clear pattern of increase in recent years (Fig. 2).

Sample size calculations

The most prevalent form of data analysis was descriptive, in the form of summary data (e.g. total number of affected cases) or percentages [2, 14, 20, 24, 26]. Where percentages were reported, none of the identified studies applied suitable statistical analyses to evaluate the reported percentage changes, such as Chi squared test or Fisher's exact test. Analysis (Fisher's exact test) of published data revealed that the description by Viner [24] of an increased implementation of arterial blood pressure recording was the only clinical audit to show a statistically significant improvement (p < 0.0001; note that an assumption was made that the sample size of the second audit equalled that of the first, as this information was not provided) [24].

In contrast, analysis of reports by Mosedale [2], Dunn and Dunn [26] and Viner [14] did not support the claimed improvements (under the following assumptions: two-tailed test with alpha and beta levels of 0.05 and 0.8, respectively) [2, 14, 26].

A documented reduction in post-operative infection rates was not statistically significant (p = 0.41, Fisher's exact test); sample sizes of approximately 370 surgeries (sample sizes of 147 and 236 were collected) would be required to identify a 25 % change in infection rates [2]. The sample size during the second audit (n = 6) of Dunn and Dunn [26] was only sufficient to detect a change in antibiotic use of 75 %. The difference between audits had

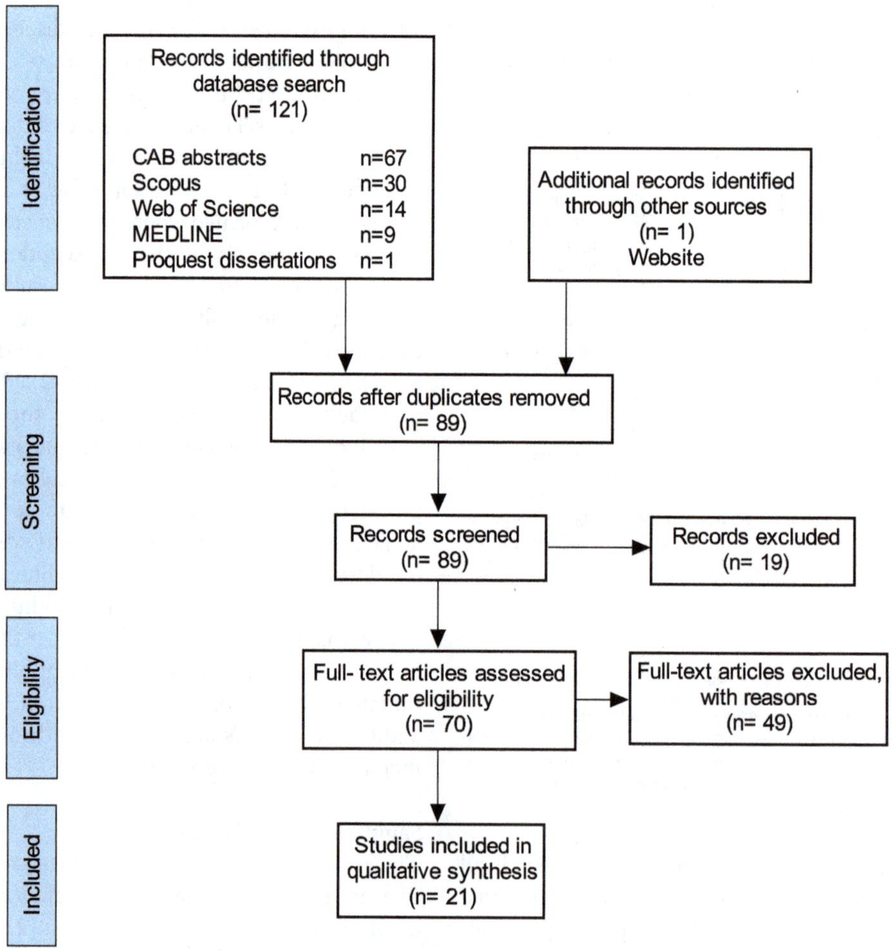

Fig. 1 PRISMA diagram summarising literature screening process

a *p* value of 0.65 (Fisher's exact test) and a sample size of 60 would have been required to detect a change of 25 %. Analysis (Fisher's exact test with Bonferroni's correction) of an effort to improve peri-anaesthetic mortality rates in rabbits as a result of an unspecified change in anaesthetic protocol revealed *p* values ranging from 0.51-1.00 for pairwise comparisons between the three audits performed [14].

Discussion

We applied the definition of Burgess [11], that "clinical audit is a quality improvement process that seeks to improve patient care and outcomes through systematic review of care against explicit criteria and the implementation of change" [11], to analyse the identified studies (Table 2). We focused specifically on study design, quality of reporting, evidence of a cyclical process and implementation of change, definition and application of explicit criteria, and systematic review of care including the use of appropriate statistical testing.

Overall, the majority of identified audits suffered from weaknesses in study design and reporting, with resultant limitations on the possibility of identifying real improvement and the repeatability of audits.

Study design

The most common study design employed was a retrospective audit of clinical practice followed by an intervention and prospective audit (Table 2) [14, 20, 24, 26]. The reliance on retrospective data collection is limited by a dependence on record quality; the accuracy and completeness of records specific to the clinical audit subject as well as essential supporting information such as the population of animals presented to a clinic (a necessary denominator for study assessment). Many of the clinical audits identified relied on searches of computerised records to identify cases for audit. This has the considerable advantage of speed but the disadvantage of relying on accuracy in entering the appropriate key word(s) associated with the audit subject. It is likely that accuracy of tagging case records in a clinic and the type of computerised billing or

Table 2 Characteristics of articles reporting clinical audits

Reference	Audit subject	Aim	Explicit criteria	Population	Data	Data presentation & analysis	Full audit 2cycle (Y/N)	Outcome(s)/ Intervention(s)	Article type
[a]Mosedale, 1998 [2]	1. Client waiting times	75 % of clients seen within 10 min of appointment time	Standard agreed within clinic	Not reported	Waiting times	Descriptive	N	1. 77.2 % on time, 83.1 % within 5 min, 93.1 % within 10 min, 13.8 % arrived late	Clinical audit – prospective design
	2. Anesthetic death	100 % survival	Published anesthetic mortality (0.14 %) rates	2282 anesthetics (species not reported)	Patient & staff id, procedure, drugs	Descriptive	N	2. 0.13 % mortality	
	3. Surgical infection	Minimal infection	Published surgical infection rates (2.5 % for clean procedures)	389 surgeries (species not reported); 241 audit 1, 148 audit 2	Dog and cat neuters, incl culture of suspected infections	Descriptive & identification of infections by surgery type/ surgeon	Y	9 suspected infections (241 surgeries), with 5 (2.1 %) positive culture. Following re-training in aseptic technique, re-audit showed 0.67 % (148 surgeries) infection rate (positive culture)	
[a]Viner, 2005 [14]	Rabbit anesthesia	Reduction in anesthetic mortality rate	Not specified	158 rabbits over 3 years (year 1, 41 cases; year 2, 59 cases; year 3, 58 cases)	Anaesthetic mortality rate	Descriptive	Y	Update of anesthetic protocol – details not provided4 % (100 cases) mortality before update, 0 % (58 cases) after, over 1 year	Clinical audit – combination of retrospective and prospective
[a]Viner, 2006 [20]	1. Diagnosis of congestive heart failure	Increased thoracic radiograph use to aid diagnosis of congestive heart failure	Expert opinion and published criteria	25 dogs	Computer records were used in all audits for an initial retrospective evaluation followed by prospective follow-up	Descriptive	Y	Radiography use increased from 84 % ($n = 19$) - 100 % ($n = 6$), through increased client communication & education	Clinical audit - Thesis (Doctorate in professional studies)Mix of retrospective and prospective study design
	2. Pruritis management	Standardised diagnosis of pruritis	Consensus discussion within clinic as well as expert opinion and published criteria. Structured approach to achieve definitive diagnosis	174 dogs	As above	Descriptive	Y	Definitive diagnosis rate increased from 56 % ($n = 24$) to 82 % ($n = 75$). Practice guidelines for establishing diagnoses established.	As above

Table 2 Characteristics of articles reporting clinical audits *(Continued)*

	3. Feline hypertension screening	Improve detection of hypertension in at-risk patients	Mean arterial blood pressure (ABP) > 220 mmHg with clinical signs or mean ABP > 180 mmHg with signs (blindness, retinal haemorrhage, seizure, tachycardia)	99 cats	As above	Descriptive	Y	Use of blood pressure measurement increased from 5-83 cats over 6 months. Implemented changes unclear.	As above
	4. Renal disease management	Improve management of feline chronic renal disease	Expert opinion and published criteria. Specific diet, ACE inhibitor, regular blood work	4 cats	As above	Descriptive	N	Failed due to insufficient cases ($n = 4$)	As above
	5. Performance of obesity clinic	Improve owner compliance in attending weight loss clinic for pets and meeting targets	75 % of referred animals attend weight loss clinic and 90 % of animals achieving weight loss target	Unclear	As above	Descriptive	Y	Failed to achieve criteria (52 % attendance). Workflow to refer patients to obesity clinic described.	As above
	6. Complications following neutering	Reduce post-operative complications	Consensus discussion within clinic. Complication defined as deviation from uneventful recovery	90 dogs, 149 cats	As above	Descriptive	Y	Reduction in post-operative complications from 47-36 % (bitch spay), 8.3-1.8 % (cat spay). Increase in complications from 26-29 % (dog castration). 0 % complications (cat castration. Log books available to record audit data.	As above
[a]Viner, 2010 [24]	Use of blood pressure measurement in cats	Improve identification of hypertension in cats	Not specified – targeted at "high risk" cases (chronic nephritis, hyperthyroidism, cardiomyopathy)	79 cats over 3 x 2 month periods (month 1, 6 cases; month 2, 22 cases; month 3, 51 cases)	Number of blood pressure measurements billed	Descriptive	Y	First 2 months: 6 blood pressure measurements, 2nd 6 months: 22 measurements, 3rd 2 months: 51 measurements	Clinical audit – retrospective and prospective
Dunn and Dunn, 2012 [26]	Antibiotic use in small animal clinic	Appropriate prescribing of fluoroquinolone antibiotics	Published guidelines for antibiotic use: clinical evidence of infection, culture and sensitivity testing with tailored therapy	89 cases (cats and dogs; 72 cases over 12 months [audit 1], 17 cases over 3 months [audit 2])	Computer records search for antibiotic prescription	Descriptive	Y	Clinic meeting – discuss rationale for antibiotic use guidelines and adherence to policy. Re-audit showed improvement amongst permanent staff and poor performance from a locum veterinarian unaware of practice policy	Clinical audit – retrospective and prospective

Table 2 Characteristics of articles reporting clinical audits *(Continued)*

Elliston et al., 2012 [27]	Post-operative wound healing in small animal clinic	Identify suspected wound infections associated with different suture materials	None described	115 dogs, 170 cats undergoing ovariohyste-rectomy	Case records	Risk ratio, Chi square and Fisher's exact tests	N	Identified increased risk of wound infection when catgut used for subcutaneous or muscle closure (RR 3.8 and 7.6, respectively)	Audit – retrospective cohort study
Akinrinmade and Adekunle, 2012 [28]	Perioperative antibiotic use in veterinary teaching hospital.	Evaluate compliance of prophylactic use of antibiotics for surgery	General recommendations for perioperative antibiotic use	108 small animals (species not specified)	Case records – minimum data set required described	Descriptive	N	Justification of antibiotic use in only 35 % of cases. Antibiotics administered for clean procedures without justification. Rationale for antibiotic type and duration of use unclear. Many records did not meet requirement for minimum data set	Audit - restrospective
Proot and Corr, 2013 [25]	Surgical complication rate associated with learning a stifle surgical procedure	To apply quality control analysis (cumulative summation) to assess surgeon performance	Published criteria for surgical complication rates used to set limits for analysis. Criteria redefined (more stringent) as training progressed	122 dogs (167 stifle surgeries)	Consecutive records, 6 months follow up, defined of retrospective complications	Control chart (cumulative summation curve)	Y	Performance improved after 22 procedures (failure rate was acceptable during these procedures) and remained acceptable (more stringent criteria) for the remaining 145 procedures	Clinical audit - retrospective

A full clinical audit cycle is defined as an initial audit (comparing measures of interest against defined criteria), followed by data analysis and proposed intervention(s), and at least one follow-up audit to assess impact of intervention(s). Articles not fulfilling the definition of clinical audit are identified as "audit". Interventions are changes implemented during the audit cycle with the aim of improving care. Criteria are standards against which collected data are compared. [a]Article includes both a review and an example of clinical audit (article only included in Table 2). ***NA*****, Not applicable**

Table 3 Characteristics of articles describing or reviewing the application of clinical audit in veterinary medicine (without reporting clinical audit data)

Reference	Summary	Article type
Rayment, 2002 [12]	Discusses clinical audit in human and veterinary medicine	Review
Moore et al., 2003 [47]	Discusses the use of clinical audit and role of continuing education in improving performance	Review
Viner et al., 2005 [17]	Describes implementation of audit in human medicine as a framework for widespread adoption in veterinary medicine	Review
SPVS/PDF MSc veterinary clinical audit group, 2005 [48]	Provides tools and education for veterinarians to perform clinical audit and contribute to national audit	Website
Mair et al., 2005 [49]	Discusses creating a colic database to help create guidelines for performing clinical audit	Editorial
Mair, 2006 [50]	Update on clinical audit in equine practice and role of evidence based medicine in determining standards	Editorial
Mair et al., 2008 [51]	Results from a survey of large animal surgeons to assess the feasibility of creating a national colic database	Survey
Godsall, 2008 [52]	Discusses the benefits of clinical governance and clinical audit in veterinary medicine	News article
Mair, 2009 [19]	Review of clinical governance and clinical audit and proposal for an international equine colic database	Review
Viner, 2009 [53]	Review of clinical audit and its role in clinical governance	Review
Dunn, 2012 [40]	Discusses clinical audit in human and veterinary medicine	Review
Viner, 2012 [54]	Discusses role of clinical governance in veterinary medicine	Book Chapter
O'Neill, 2012 [55]	Describes an electronic database (VetCompass) and a potential role in developing a national level resource for clinical audit	Review

Though the definition of clinical audit was not consistent between papers, they share the common theme of describing a key component of an audit cycle: sustained and ongoing improvement of care

database software employed [20]. Additionally, a key word search could lead to a single animal/case being counted numerous times if the procedure being studied was performed multiple times in the same animal [20, 24]. One approach employed to deal with this issue was to focus the clinical audit on the performance of a procedure, such as number of arterial blood pressure measurements performed, rather than the number of unique cases handled [20, 24]. When working with computerised records, a prospective clinical audit design provides the potential for educating staff in the importance of consistent and accurate records, allowing a more accurate comparison of different audit periods. Where computerised search (retrospective) for the initial audit preceded a prospective audit, it is difficult to identify inaccuracies in computerised data recording without some comparison of case numbers [20]. This problem is compounded when the subject of the clinical audit occurs uncommonly during the study period e.g. chronic kidney disease in cats [20].

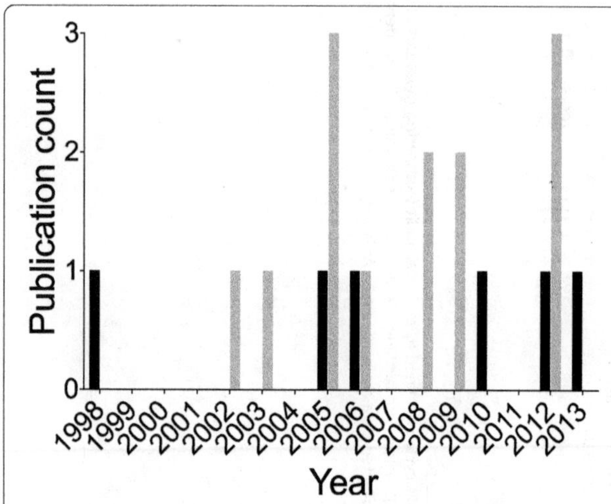

Fig. 2 Histogram showing the sporadic publication rate of clinical audits in veterinary medicine (from studies reported in Table 2 [black bars] and 3 [grey bars]). Literature searches conducted between February – April, 2014

Several of the identified studies reported a prospective study design, commonly using a simple handwritten log, with the advantage of focused data collection [2, 20, 25]. Ideally, though often limited by labour costs, data collection would be performed by an independent observer to avoid selective reporting. In prospective studies, a possible confound of participants knowing they are being observed should be considered, as being under observation may change behaviour in a way that influences outcome (Hawthorne effect) [29]. The occurrence and impact of behavioural changes will be easier to track if the clinical audit focuses on the process(es) of care ("process audit") rather than an outcome measure ("outcome audit"). Where retrospective and prospective approaches are included within the same clinical audit [14, 20, 24, 26], unless processes are clearly described in both retrospective and prospective arms, it is difficult to evaluate the impact of the Hawthorne effect and interpret the results.

The majority of identified clinical audits were outcome-based. While it is tempting to focus on outcome (e.g. return of spontaneous circulation following cardiac arrest), as it is the ultimate measure of failure/success, unless the steps (processes) of clinical care are described and recorded (e.g. frequency of chest compressions) it is impossible to compare clinical audits, replicate studies and maximise learning [20, 25]. Furthermore, where the key process(es) associated with a successful outcome are unknown, limiting focus to outcomes limits evaluation of the clinical audit when an improvement in outcome is not achieved. Conversely, when an outcome audit achieves improvement, unclear documentation of processes inhibits identification of potentially contributing processes [14]. Though clinical audits are not designed to establish a causal relationship, accurate reporting will help identify areas for further improvement and research.

Quality of reporting

In general, reporting quality was highly variable between studies with deviations from expected standards in scientific reports. These limitations make it difficult, if not impossible, to evaluate results, compare findings between clinical audits or replicate clinical audits. Reporting deficits ranged from not identifying the species studied, not describing the criteria/methods of case selection (including omission of the number of eligible cases versus those collected), neglecting a detailed description of the changes implemented during the clinical audit cycle or intervening time between audits [2, 14, 20, 24–26]. Those audits that formed the focus of a paper, rather than being included in a general review, tended to follow a higher standard of reporting [25, 26].

As a result of the limitations described above, as well the limited power of many of the identified audits (see Systematic review of care, below), it is difficult to evaluate the claimed improvements in care. Where failure to achieve improvements were identified common causes included poor owner compliance, selection of an uncommon disease, and limited statistical power [20].

Cyclical process and implementation of change

Of the 15 audits reported in 8 publications, five audits (33 %) failed to demonstrate that a cyclical process had been followed [2, 20, 27, 28]. Furthermore, in 2 (20 %) of the audits that included a cyclical process it was unclear which interventions or changes were implemented between audit cycles [14, 20]. Claimed improvements were made by four of the published audits, though further analysis revealed that only one may have had sufficient power [24]. In contrast to a patient-centred approach, Proot and Corr [25] focused on documenting an improvement in individual performance, using a statistical process control chart approach to track performance (see Systematic review of care, below) [25].

Explicit criteria

The role of identifying explicit criteria as a standard of care allows comparison of performance [1].

Sources of explicit criteria vary depending on the availability of high quality evidence or peer-reviewed consensus guidelines. The identified studies report 3 broad types of criteria: those resulting from consensus discussion within a clinic [2], those based on published guidelines or evidence [2, 25, 26] and criteria based on a combination of these latter approaches [20]. Where explicit criteria were not applied or reported [14, 24, 27, 28], improvements in performance can still be demonstrated but may be misleading if they are below published standards. Conversely, performance exceeding published standards that goes unrecognised limits the opportunity to learn from, or apply, successful practice. Ideally, explicit criteria should be based on available high quality evidence. In the face of the limited evidence available in many areas of veterinary medicine, consensus guidelines combining available evidence with expert interpretation produced by professional bodies can be used [30–33]. In contrast, guidelines developed within a single clinic are likely to be limited by the smaller pool of experience and expertise available.

Systematic review of care

Review of care was limited by over-interpretation of percentage changes without appropriate statistical analyses. In particular, the reporting of percentages in the presence of small sample sizes is misleading as a small change in numbers will have a dramatic effect on the resultant percentage [20, 24, 26]. Subsequent analyses revealed that only one of the identified clinical audits resulted in a statistically significant change [24].

Additionally, while it is tempting to select an easily measurable and emotionally-charged outcome, such as anaesthetic death, as the subject of a clinical audit, where such events are rare it is difficult to achieve an appropriate sample size within a single centre.

Despite the sample size limitations some audits were successful in identifying several potential areas of improvement within each clinic: Mosedale [2] and Dunn and Dunn [26] both recognised the potential for individual performance to have a negative impact on clinical practice through poor aseptic technique, adherence to clinical guidelines and communication (Table 2) [2, 14].

Viner's [20] doctoral thesis clearly reported the cyclical clinical audit process and iterative approach which was often used to achieve improvements in performance [20]. This body of work is particularly instructive in highlighting factors contributing to unsuccessful clinical audits, including client communication and compliance (clinical audit of a weight loss clinic), case identification and recruitment (clinical audit of feline chronic renal disease management), loosely defined criteria of care (clinical audit of post-operative complications). These failures, as with negative study results in biomedical research, are seldom reported in the literature but have a role to play in learning the pitfalls of conducting clinical audit [34].

One study applied a statistical process control chart to evaluate performance [25]. Such an approach is relatively novel in human and veterinary medicine and originates from quality control procedures for production systems [35]. This, and similar statistical techniques, allows very rapid feedback on performance and can be applied to document the learning curve associated with a new technique, the consistent performance of a skill and as a means to facilitate early identification of poor performance as a result of dramatic failures in care [36, 37].

Failure and success of clinical audits

There were two instances of clinical audit failure recorded in the studies identified; management of chronic kidney disease in cats and performance of a weight loss clinic [20]. These highlighted two different pitfalls: selection of a feasible subject and achieving change in complex systems. In the former, subject selection can be guided by either a pilot study or examination of retrospective data to identify feasibility [1, 11, 38]. When the selected subject is part of a complex system, the risk of failure can be minimised by identifying the processes associated with the outcome of interest [1, 11]. Additionally, an early realisation that changes in human behaviour may be necessary, though hard to achieve, can help design a feasible study. Behavioural barriers, staff communication and record keeping were identified by Viner during evaluation of the clinical audit of the weight loss clinic [20].

Rayment [12] identified the following benefits to implementing clinical audit in veterinary medicine: a reduction of clinical error, the promotion of high standards of care, a gain in the confidence of clients and the promotion of team building amongst staff members [12]. Many of these benefits were described in the identified audits [2, 14, 20, 24, 26]. From these, several important lessons can be learned.

Objective data collection was essential in both identifying sub-standard care and assessing the effect on outcomes when changes were implemented [2, 14, 20, 24, 26]. Without data collection identification of deficits requires marked deviation from normal practice. Such deviation may be difficult to identify when a clinic is assessed as a whole, where the performance of individuals within the group may not be obvious [2, 26]. Furthermore, clinical audit introduces objectivity in recording data, eliminating the inherent risks of relying on memory and confirmation bias [2]. The collected data can form the basis for discussion at staff meetings and allow for input from various parties regarding how care can be improved [26]. Successful clinical audit is predicated on a supportive environment and staff involvement at all levels [39]. This is reflected by the association between a multidisciplinary approach (not limited to veterinarians) and improved practice [2, 14, 20, 24, 40]. Where staff changes occur, audit can confirm that acceptable standards are being maintained, avoiding the assumption that clinic policies will be followed [26]. Where current practice meets acceptable standards, clinical audit can serve as positive reinforcement at a team or individual level [17, 26].

Maintaining the audit cycle over the long term can be difficult. Of the identified studies, a minority were performed for longer than a few months [14, 20, 25]. However, as evident from large-scale audits in production animals, with appropriate support sustained improvement is achievable [41, 42].

Future of clinical audit

Though clinical audit is clearly recognized and implemented in veterinary medicine, the small number of published studies limits firm conclusions regarding the adoption and application of clinical audit from being drawn (Fig. 2). Additionally, the publication dates of identified articles (Fig. 2), do not show a clear pattern of increasing clinical audit publications. However, these data should be evaluated cautiously as it is not possible to know to what extent clinical audit occurs without dissemination in the form of an accessible publication, and in performing this systematic review it was apparent that articles fulfilling the criteria of clinical audit were not identified by the search strategies employed. These potential omissions reflect the well-recognised limitations of article indexing, affecting medicine and veterinary medicine, as well as the poor recognition of clinical audit in veterinary medicine [43]. Accurate article indexing is critical to identification of relevant articles through a structured search strategy. Indexing is based on words included in the title, abstract and key words of an article, and it is likely that many authors are not fully aware of the implications of omitting certain terms (such as "clinical audit") on the visibility of their article. Related to this, the misuse of the term "clinical audit" adds to confusion regarding its definition [27].

Several recent examples highlight the issue of indexing [44–46]. Hofmeister et al. [46] performed a study fulfilling the criteria of clinical audit [46]. In a prospective, observational pre-post intervention study design they performed an initial audit of anesthesia patient safety incidents measured against explicit criteria (from available literature), implemented changes (related to misinjection, performance of endotracheal intubation and anesthesia machine check), and re-audited, with the outcome of creating a successful decrease in patient safety incidents (from 3.6 % to 1.4 % over the course of over 4000 anesthetic procedures, $p < 0.0001$). Furthermore, this study exemplified several of the supporting measures discussed above e.g. involvement of several levels of clinic staff (veterinarians and AHTs), prospective data collection and changes in human behavior. This study clearly fulfills the definition of clinical audit, though it was not identified through our search strategy. Broadening the search sufficiently to identify such articles would have prevented a systematic review of the literature as the resultant search would be overwhelmingly broad and unstructured, without guaranteeing that results were complete or reproducible, the cornerstone of systematic review. The solution to this problem is the correct and accurate indexing of articles through education of authors, reviewers and editors [42].

Conclusion

Clinical audits have the potential to generate a measurable improvement in clinical practice and add to evidence-based veterinary medicine. Healthcare, in both human and veterinary medicine, is constantly evolving, indicating an increasing role for clinical audits in the future. By performing audit cycles, the quality of care offered can be monitored, evaluated and continually improved [12]. The number of clearly identifiable clinical audits in the scientific literature remains small, though the number of publications identified is an underestimation due to inaccurate article indexing.

Unfortunately, the majority of published audits failed to generate an improvement in quality as a result of weak study design. Frequent departures from recognised reporting standards limited opportunities to learn from the work performed.

Competing interests
The authors declare that they have no competing interests.

Authors' contributions
NR and DP conceived of the study and analysed data, NR and LT collected data, all authors contributed to drafting of the manuscript. All authors read and approved the final manuscript.

Acknowledgments
The authors wish to thank the anonymous reviewers for their constructive comments and Dr Grace Kwong (Faculty of Veterinary Medicine, University of Calgary) for statistical support.

Author details
[1]Western Veterinary Specialist and Emergency Centre, Calgary, AB, Canada. [2]Health Sciences Library, University of Calgary, Calgary, AB, Canada. [3]Veterinary Clinical and Diagnostic Sciences, Faculty of Veterinary Medicine, University of Calgary, Calgary, AB, Canada. [4]Hotchkiss Brain Institute, University of Calgary, Calgary, AB, Canada.

References

1. Langley G, Moen R, Nolan K, Nolan T, Norman C, Provost L. The improvement guide: a practical approach to enhancing organizational performance, 2nd edn. San Francisco, CA, USA: Jossey-Bass; 2009
2. Mosedale P. Introducing clinical audit to veterinary practice. Practice. 1998;20(1):40–2.
3. Good medical practice [http://www.gmc-uk.org/guidance/good_medical_practice.asp]. Accessed 15 Feb 2015.
4. Patel NK, Sarraf KM, Joseph S, Lee C, Middleton FR. Implementing the National Hip Fracture Database: An audit of care. Injury. 2013;44(12):1934–9.
5. Audit NP. Impact of NICE guidance on rates of haemorrhage after tonsillectomy: an evaluation of guidance issued during an ongoing national tonsillectomy audit. Qual Saf Health Care. 2008;17(4):264–8.
6. Haynes AB, Weiser TG, Berry WR, Lipsitz SR, Breizat AH, Dellinger EP, et al. Changes in safety attitude and relationship to decreased postoperative morbidity and mortality following implementation of a checklist-based surgical safety intervention. BMJ Qual Safety. 2011;20(1):102–7.
7. Pronovost P, Needham D, Berenholtz S, Sinopoli D, Chu H, Cosgrove S, et al. An intervention to decrease catheter-related bloodstream infections in the ICU. New Engl J Med. 2006;355(26):2725–32.
8. Shonfeld A, Riyat A, Kotecha A, Sacks M. Critical care transfers: using audit to make a difference. Anaesthesia. 2011;66(10):946–7.
9. The Stationary Office. Learning from Bristol: the report of the public inquiry into children's heart surgery at the Bristol Royal Infirmary 1984–1995. London: The Stationary Office; 2001.
10. Royal College of Veterinary Surgeons. Practice standards scheme manual. London: Royal College of Veterinary Surgeons; 2014. [http://www.rcvs.org.uk/document-library/pss-review-2015-small-animal-draft-modules/]. Accessed 8 Jan 2014.
11. Burgess R. New Principles of Best Practice in Clinical Audit. 2nd ed. Oxford: Radcliffe Publishing; 2011.
12. Rayment K. Clinical audit - A means of evaluating 'quality'. Practice. 2002; 24(8):481–4.
13. The Royal College of Anaesthetists. Raising the Standard: a compendium of audit recipes for continous quality improvement in anaesthesia. London: The Royal College of Anaesthetists; 2012.
14. Viner B. Clinical audit in veterinary practice - the story so far. Practice. 2005; 27(4):215–8.
15. Weissman N, Allison J, Kiefe C, Farmer R, Weaver M, Williams O, et al. Achievable benchmarks of care: the ABCs of benchmarking. J Eval Clin Pract. 1999;5(3):269–81.
16. Hall R, Khan F, Bayley M, Asllani E, Lindsay P, Hill M, et al. Benchmarks for acute stroke care delivery. Int J Qual Heath C. 2013;25(6):710–8.
17. Viner B, Jenner C. Clinical audit - learning from the medical profession. Vet Rec. 2005;157(22):695–6.
18. Farrell C, Hill D. Time for change: traditional audit or continuous improvement? Anaesthesia. 2012;67(7):699–702.
19. Mair TS. Clinical governance, clinical audit, and the potential value of a database of equine colic surgery (Special Issue: New perspectives in equine colic). Vet Clin N Am-Equine. 2009;25(2):193–8.
20. Viner B. Introducing clinical audit into veterinary practice. *Msc(VetGP)*. London, UK: Middlesex University; 2006.
21. Liberati A, Altman DG, Tetzlaff J, Mulrow C, Gotzsche PC, Ioannidis JP, et al. The PRISMA statement for reporting systematic reviews and meta-analyses of studies that evaluate health care interventions: explanation and elaboration. PLoS Med. 2009;6(7), e1000100.
22. Centre for Reviews and Dissemination [http://www.york.ac.uk/inst/crd/pdf/Systematic_Reviews.pdf]. Accessed 5 July 2014.
23. Cochrane Handbook for Systematic Reviews of Interventions Version 5.1.0 [http://handbook.cochrane.org/]. Accessed 15 Feb 2015.

24. Viner B. Clinical effectiveness. What does it mean for practitioners - and cats? J Feline Med Surg. 2010;12(7):561–8.
25. Proot JL, Corr SA. Clinical audit for the tibial tuberosity advancement procedure: establishing the learning curve and monitoring ongoing performance for the tibial tuberosity advancement procedure using the cumulative summation technique. Vet Comp Orthopaed. 2013;26(4):280–4.
26. Dunn F, Dunn J. Clinical audit: application in small animal practice. In Practice. 2012;34(4):243–5.
27. Elliston R, Heayns B, Fish C. A clinical audit to identify factors contributing to surgical wound healing complications. Veterinary Nurse. 2012;3(3):188-95.
28. Akinrinmade JF, Adekunle OM. An audit of surgical antibiotic prophylaxis at the Veterinary Teaching Hospital, Ibadan. Niger Vet J. 2012;33(4):609–16.
29. Parsons HM. What happened at Hawthorne? Science. 1974;183(4128):922–32.
30. Harold D, Jensen T, Johnson A, Knowles P, Meyer R, Rucinsky R, et al. 2013 AAHA/AAFP fluid therapy guidelines for dogs and cats. J Am Anim Hosp Assoc. 2013;49(3):149–59.
31. Behrend E, Kooistra H, Nelson R, Reusch C, Scott-Moncrief J. Diagnosis of spontaneous canine hyperadrenocorticism: 2012 ACVIM Consensus Statement (Small Animal). J Vet Intern Med. 2013;27:1292–304.
32. Brainard B, Boller M, Fletcher D. RECOVER evidence and knowledge gap analysis on veterinary CPR. Part 5: monitoring. J Vet Emerg Crit Car. 2012; 22(S1):S65–84.
33. Hearnshaw H, Harker R, Cheater F, Baker R, Grimshaw G. Expert consensus on the desirable characteristics of review criteria for the improvement of healthcare quality. Qual Health Care. 2001;10(3):173–8.
34. Dwan K, Altman D, Arnaiz J, Bloom J, Chan A-W, Cronin E, et al. Systematic review of the empirical evidence of study publication bias and outcome reporting bias. Plos One. 2008;3(8):1–31.
35. Biau D, Williams S, Schlup M, Nizard R, Porcher R. Quantitative and individualized assessment of the learning curve using LC-CUSUM. Brit J Surg. 2008;95:925–9.
36. Campbell R, Hecker K, Biau D, Pang D. Student attainment of proficiency in a clinical skill: the asssessment of individual learning curves. PLoS One. 2014;9(2).
37. Spiegelhalter D, Grigg O, Kinsman R, Treasure T. Risk-adjusted sequential probability ratio tests: applications to Bristol, Shipman and adult cardiac surgery. Int J Qual Health C. 2003;15(1):7–13.
38. Dixon N. Good practice in clinical audit. 1996. A summary of selected literature to support criteria for clinical audit National Centre for Clinical Audit.
39. Johnston G, Crombie IK, Davies HT, Alder EM, Millard A. Reviewing audit: barriers and facilitating factors for effective clinical audit. Qual Health Care. 2000;9(1):23–36.
40. Dunn J. Clinical audit: A tool in the defence of clinical standards. Practice. 2012;34(3):167–9.
41. Grandin T. Effect of animal welfare audits of slaughter plants by a major fast food company on cattle handling and stunning practices. J Am Vet Med Assoc. 2000;216:848–51.
42. Grandin T. Maintenance of good animal welfare standards in beef slaughter plants by use of auditing programs. J Am Vet Med A. 2005;226(3):370–3.
43. Dickersin K, Scherer R, Lefebvre C. Systematic Reviews: Identifying relevant studies for systematic reviews. Brit Med J. 1994;309(6964):1286–91.
44. Bille C, Auvigne V, Bomassi E, Durieux P, Libermann S, Rattez E. An evidence-based medicine approach to small animal anaesthetic mortality in a referral practice: the influence of initiating three recommendations on subsequent anaesthetic deaths. Vet Anesth Analg. 2014;41:249–58.
45. Bille C, Auvigne V, Libermann S, Bomassi E, Durieux P, Rattez E. Risk of anaesthetic mortality in dogs and cats: an observational cohort study of 3546 cases. Vet Anesth Analg. 2012;39:59–68.
46. Hofmeister E, Quandt J, Braun C, Shepard M. Development, implementation and impact of simple patient safety interventions in a university teaching hospital. Vet Anesth Analg. 2014;41:243–8.
47. Moore DA, Klingborg DJ. Using clinical audits to identify practitioner learning needs. J Vet Med Educ. 2003;30(1):57–61.
48. Clinical Audit Group Strategy [http://www.vetaudit.co.uk/]. Accessed 10 April 2015.
49. Mair TS, White NA. Improving quality of care in colic surgery: Time for international audit? Equine Vet J. 2005;37(4):287–8.
50. Mair TS. Evidence-based medicine and clinical audit: what progress in equine practice? Equine Vet Educ. 2006;18(1):2–4.
51. Mair TS, White NA. The creation of an international audit and database of equine colic surgery: survey of attitudes of surgeons (Special issue: colic). Equine Vet J. 2008;40(4):400–4.
52. Godsall S. Using clinical audits as tools for positive change in practice. Vet Times. 2008;38(17):8.
53. Viner B. Using audit to improve clinical effectiveness. Practice. 2009; 31(5):240–3.
54. Viner B. Clinical governance. In: Clarke C, Chapman M, editors. BSAVA Manual of Small Animal Practice Management and Development. Quedgeley: British Small Animal Veterinary Association; 2012. p. 501–20.
55. O'Neill D. VetCompass clinical data points the way forward. Vet Ir J. 2012;2(7):353–6.

2

Characterization of endocannabinoids and related acylethanolamides in the synovial fluid of dogs with osteoarthritis

Carmela Valastro[1*], Debora Campanile[1], Mariarosaria Marinaro[2], Delia Franchini[1], Fabiana Piscitelli[3], Roberta Verde[3], Vincenzo Di Marzo[3] and Antonio Di Bello[1]

Abstract

Background: Cannabis-based drugs have been shown to be effective in inflammatory diseases. A number of endocannabinoids including N- arachidonoylethanolamide (anandamide, AEA) and 2-arachidonyl glycerol (2-AG) with activity at the cannabinoid receptors (CBR) CBR1 and CBR2, have been identified. Other structurally related endogenous fatty acid compounds such as oleoylethanolamide (OEA) and palmitoyl ethanolamide (PEA) have been identified in biological tissues. These compounds do not bind to CBR but might be involved in facilitating the actions of directly acting endocannabinoids and thus are commonly termed "entourage" compounds due to their ability to modulate the endocannabinoid system. The aim of this study was to evaluate the presence of endocannabinoids and entourage compounds in the synovial fluid of dogs with osteoarthritis subjected to arthrotomy of the knee joint. Cytokines and cytology were studied as well.

Results: AEA, 2-AG, OEA and PEA were all present in the synovial fluid of arthritic knees and in the contralateral joints; in addition, a significant increase of OEA and 2AG levels were noted in SF from OA knees when compared to the contralateral joints.

Conclusion: The identification and quantification of endocannabinoids and entourage compounds levels in synovial fluids from dogs with OA of the knee is reported for the first time. Our data are instrumental for future studies involving a greater number of dogs. Cannabinoids represent an emerging and innovative pharmacological tool for the treatment of OA and further studies are warranted to evaluate the effectiveness of cannabinoids in veterinary medicine.

Keywords: Endocannabinoid system, Entourage compounds, Synovial fluid, Osteoarthritis, Dog

Background

Osteoarthritis (OA), also known as degenerative joint disease (DJD), is characterized by a gradual loss of cartilage and results in the development of bony spurs and cysts at the margins of the joints [1]. The articular cartilage is damaged by a complex interplay of genetic, metabolic, biochemical and biomechanical factors followed by activation of inflammatory responses involving the cartilage, subchondral bone and synovium [2]. Pro-inflammatory cytokines and chemokines are abundant in OA [3, 4]. OA is one of the most common chronic musculoskeletal diseases in dogs and it is a significant cause of pain and disability [5].

Non steroidal anti-inflammatory drugs do not always provide adequate pain relief and may have severe side effects [6]. Thus, there is an urgent need for the development of treatments for arthritis. Over the last two decades a new biochemical/physiological signaling system, the endocannabinoid system (ECS), composed of two cannabinoid receptors and their ligands has been described [7].

* Correspondence: carmela.valastro@uniba.it
[1]Department of Veterinary Medicine, University of Bari "Aldo Moro", SP. Casamassima km 3, 70010 Bari, Valenzano, Italy
Full list of author information is available at the end of the article

The ECS has been implicated in a wide range of physiological and pathophysiological processes [8]. Cannabinoid receptor activation can modulate inflammation and nociception in animal models of joint inflammation [9, 10]. To date two cannabinoid receptors, have been cloned [cannabinoid receptor type 1 (CBR1) and cannabinoid receptor type 2 (CBR2)], and the two major endogenous endocannabinoids have been identified as arachidonoyl ethanolamide [anandamide (AEA)] and 2-arachidonoylglycerol (2-AG) [11].

Other structurally related endogenous fatty acid compounds such as oleoylethanolamide (OEA) and palmitoylethanolamide (PEA) have been identified in biological tissues. These compounds do not bind to cannabinoid receptors but may facilitate the action of endocannabinoids and are termed "entourage" compounds due to their ability to modulate the ECS [12, 13]. However, OEA and PEA can directly activate other receptors, in particular the peroxisome proliferator-activated receptor-α [14], which is involved in the control of inflammation and pain [15]. Cannabinoids are synthesized on demand, and in the central nervous system they are produced mainly postsynaptically to act as retrograde messengers regulating the release of a variety of neurotransmitters at the presynaptic level [16].

The ECS can be exploited as a potential therapeutic option for OA. Indeed, some studies have demonstrated the anti-nociceptive effects of CBR agonists in rodent models of OA [17]. Moreover, the presence of CBRs on chondrocytes [18] and bone [19] suggest a possible role of cannabinoids in cartilage alteration and bone remodeling occurring in OA. Nonetheless, only few studies have investigated the endocannabinoid tone during OA. In humans, AEA and 2-AG were elevated in patients with OA whereas they were not detected in synovial fluids from patients with no joint symptoms. Furthermore, CBR1 and CBR2 were present in the synovia of these patients [6]. A recent study showed that levels of 2-AG were significantly elevated in the synovial fluid of patients who experienced higher postoperative pain after total knee arthroplasty and that the levels of PEA correlated with functional disability in OA [20].

Due to the lack of data on dogs, the aim of the present study was to measure ECs and related compounds in the synovial fluid of dogs with OA. In addition, the degree of inflammation and the level of some proinflammatory cytokines were studied as well.

Methods

Ten dogs were enrolled in the study. They were subjected to arthrotomy of the knee joint for monolateral reconstruction of the anterior cruciate ligament.

Surgery was conducted at the Department of Veterinary Medicine, Section of Surgery and Obstetrics of the University of Bari.

Four dogs were mixed breed, two chow chow, 1 labrador, 1 kurzhaar, 1 rottweiler and 1 pomeranian; there were 7 females and 3 males and their age was between 5 and 13 years. Dogs weighted between 8 and 40 Kg. Dogs were considered to be healthy based on physical examination, packed cell volume (PCV) and total solids (TS).

All dogs showed radiological signs of OA when subjected to X-ray examinations of the knee joint while no signs of OA were observed in the contralateral knee joints.

Radiographic examinations were routinely performed and assessed by a team of radiologists from Department of Veterinary Medicine.

The same anaesthesiological protocol was used for all dogs.

After premedication with dexmedetomidine (1 mcg/Kg IM) and methadone (0,2 mg/Kg IM), anesthesia was induced with propofol (to effect EV) and maintained with isofluorane delivered in oxygen.

Aspirates of synovial fluid were obtained from arthritic joints using a 26 gauge needle attached to a 2,5 ml syringe after the exposure of the joint capsule and before its cut.

The synovial fluid of the contralateral knee was collected with the owner's written consent.

After surgery, all dogs received adequate antibiotic and analgesic therapies.

In all cases, the postoperative course was normal.

Synovial fluids were collected for cytokines quantification, cytology and measurement of ECs.

The Ethical Committee of the Department of Veterinary Medicine – University of Bari approved the procedures (approval n. 6/2016).

Quantification of inflammatory cytokines in synovial fluids

Tumor necrosis factor (TNF)-alpha and interleukin (IL)-1beta levels in synovial fluids were measured using two commercially available ELISA kits specific for dog cytokines (Kingfisher Biotech, Inc., St. Paul, MN, USA) according to the manufacturer's instructions.

Measurement of ECs and related N-acylethanolamines in synovial fluids

The extraction, purification, and quantification of ECs from synovial fluid was performed as previously described for plasma [21]. Briefly, synovial fluids were dounce-homogenized and extracted with chloroform/methanol/Tris–HCl 50 mmol/l pH 7.5 (2:1:1, vol/vol) containing internal standards ($[^2H]_8$ AEA 5 pmol; $[^2H]_5$ 2-AG, $[^2H]_5$ PEA and $[^2H]_4$ OEA 50 pmol each). The lipid-containing organic phase was dried down, weighed, and pre-purified by open-bed chromatography on silica gel. Fractions were obtained by eluting the column with 99:1, 90:10 and 50:50 (*v*/v) chloroform/methanol. The 90:10 fraction was used for AEA, 2-AG, PEA and OEA quantification by liquid chromatography–atmospheric pressure chemical ionization–mass spectrometry by using a Shimadzu high-performance liquid chromatography apparatus (LC-10ADVP) coupled to a Shimadzu (LCMS-2020) quadrupole mass spectrometry via a Shimadzu atmospheric pressure chemical ionization interface as previously described [22]. The amount of ECs, quantified by isotope dilution with the above mentioned deuterated standards, was expressed as pmol per ml (of synovial fluid volume) or pmol per milligram (of lipid extract weight).

Statistical analysis

All data depicted in Figs. 1 and 2 are reported as arithmetic mean ± SEM. Differences between OA and "healthy" SFs were compared by Student's t-test. A p value ≤0.05 was considered significant.

Results

Cytological examination of the SFs was performed and it showed an increased number of inflammatory cells in SFs from the OA knees. In fact, an increased percentage of neutrophils, ranging from 18% to 38% (average 26,2% ± SD 6,67%), was observed in OA SFs when compared to contralateral joints (all SFs contained <10% neutrophils). In addition, a high percentage of mononuclear cells, including lymphocytes, ranging from 65% to 81% (average 76,6% ± SD 4,43%) was observed in OA SFs only. In one case, the presence of clusters of synovial cells, which appear in the hyperplasia of the synovial membrane, was found.

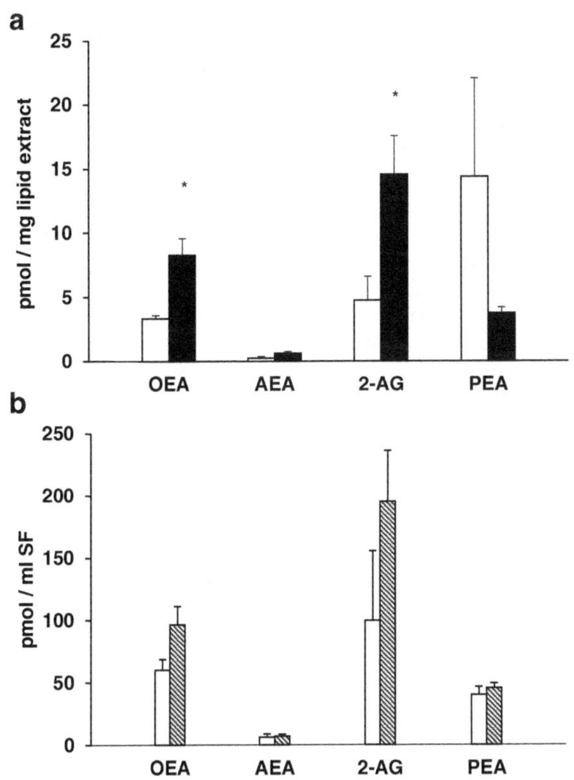

Fig. 1 Levels of ECs measured in SFs from contralateral (white histograms) and OA (black histograms) joints. Data are expressed as pmol/mg of lipid extract (**a**) or pmol/ml of SF (**b**) and are reported as arithmetic mean ± SEM. Differences were compared by the Student's t test and asterisks indicate significant differences (OA vs healthy joints; $p < 0.05$)

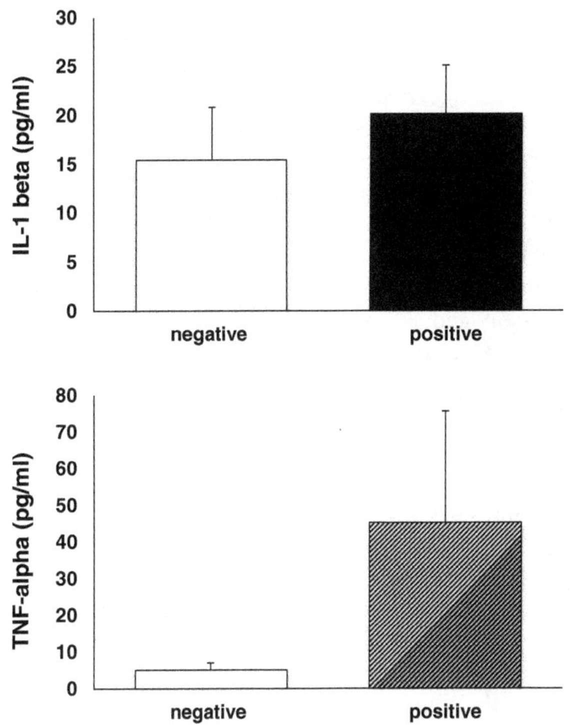

Fig. 2 IL-1 beta and TNF-alpha levels were measured in SFs from contralateral (white histograms) and OA (black/grey histograms) joints by ELISA. Data are reported as arithmetic mean ± SEM

The concentration of AEA, 2-AG, OEA and PEA were measured in all SFs and results are reported in Fig. 1a and b. There was a significant increase in 2-AG and OEA levels in OA SFs when compared to the contralateral samples (Fig. 1a).

The results of the levels of two inflammatory cytokines are reported in Fig. 2. Although there was an increased level of TNF-alpha in SFs from OA joints, it was not significantly different from the level observed in the SFs from contralateral knees ($p > 0.05$). Similar levels of IL-1 beta were observed in synovial fluids from OA versus contralateral joints ($p > 0.05$).

Discussion

In the present study, the identification and quantification of ECs (and related acylethanolamides) in SFs from dogs with OA of the knee is reported.

In particular, AEA, 2-AG, OEA and PEA were all measurable in the SFs from OA knees and in the SFs from contralateral joints and a significant increase of OEA and 2-AG levels was noted in SFs from OA knees when compared to those from contralateral joints. To our knowledge, this is the first report showing detectable levels of ECs, and related compounds, in SFs from OA and contralateral joints of dogs.

The detection of PEA, although at similar levels in OA and "healthy" SFs, is of particular interest because of its known anti-inflammatory activity [23] via nuclear peroxisome proliferator activating receptor-α (PPAR-α) activation and EC entourage effects. In addition, these effects can also be exerted by OEA, often with higher potency [14].

Endocannabinoids are synthesized on demand by several cell types, including immune cells, such as macrophages and T cells, which are present in human OA joints [24].

Endocannabinoids are rapidly produced "on-demand" from their cellular precursors. Once synthesized, they are rapidly released in the extracellular space and bind receptors present either on the same cells (the ones who have produced them) or on neighbour cells.

Since their biological activity is very rapid, specific and occurs in a limited anatomical space, it is very unlikely their diffusion in the bloodstream. Therefore the presence in the contralateral joint is unlikely due to a simple passive diffusion from other sites (including the systemic source).

Endothelial cells can also synthesize ECs [25, 26] and thus contribute to their accumulation. Vascular elements are important in the progression of the DJD since neovascularization is one of the early changes in the synovium and it is thought to be linked to bone and cartilage destruction [27].

The main elements of the EC signaling system, including CBR1 and CBR2 mRNA and proteins, were found in synovial biopsies from patients with advanced osteoarthritis and rheumatoid arthritis [6]. Both AEA and 2-AG were detected in the SF of these patients, but not in healthy volunteers. This latter finding is different from the data reported here. Some animals included in the study were aged with probable bilateral OA of the knee and with no clinical sign of lameness in one knee. Therefore, an early and/or undiagnosed arthritic change in the contralateral knee considered "healthy", cannot be ruled out, nor it can be excluded that the altered load could induce inflammation in the contralateral non-arthritic knee. This could explain the presence of AEA, 2-AG, OEA and PEA also in the clinical healthy contralateral joints.

Indeed, the presence of similar levels of IL-1β and TNF-α in SFs from both OA and contralateral joints could have the same explanation. Levels of cytokines in OA are very variable due to the variable degree of synovial hypertrophy, synovial effusions, subchondral bone marrow oedema and presence of inflammatory cells in the sub-lining tissues [28]. The inflammatory component is therefore variable. It must be underlined that the activation of CBR2 is associated with decreases in immune cell function, including attenuated cytokine release [29, 30].

Conclusions

We have demonstrated the presence of AEA, 2-AG, OEA and PEA in the SF of dogs with OA.

We have found these same mediators in the SF obtained from contralateral knees. Our data open the avenue to future studies involving a higher number of dogs and aimed at defining the role played by these compounds in OA of the dogs.

Both plant-derived and synthetic agonists of CBRs represent an emerging and innovative pharmacological tool for the treatment of OA. Pharmacological studies have showed the anti-nociceptive effects of these compounds in rodent models of this pathology and compelling evidence suggests an active role of the ECS in the pathophysiology of this disease.

The potential effect of cannabinoids in slowing OA disease progression in veterinary clinical practice still remains to be explored. Further studies are therefore needed to evaluate the effectiveness of cannabinoids as an innovative treatment in veterinary medicine.

Abbreviations

2-AG: 2-arachidonyl glycerol; AEA: N- arachidonoylethanolamide, anandamide; CBR: Cannabinoid receptor; DJD: Degenerative joint disease; EC: Endocannabinoid; ECS: Endocannabinoid system; IL: Interleukin; OA: Osteoarthritis; OEA: Oleoylethanolamide; PCV: Packed cell volume; PEA: Palmitoyl ethanolamihave; SF: Synovial fluid; TNF: Tumor necrosis factor; TS: Total solids

Acknowledgements

Not applicable

Funding

No specific funding was received for this study.

Authors' contributions

CV, DC and MM contributed equally to this work. CV and DC designed and performed the study, recruited patients and drafted the manuscript. MM performed the cytokine analysis, performed the statistics and contributed to writing and revising the manuscript. FP, RV and VDM performed the endocannabinoids analysis, analyzed the data and reviewed the manuscript. DF was involved in postoperative course of patients and reviewed the manuscript. ADB supervised the research project from the clinical point of view, performed the surgery and reviewed the paper. All authors critically read and approved the final version of the manuscript.

Consent for publication
Not applicable

Competing interests
The authors declare that they have no competing interests.

Author details
[1]Department of Veterinary Medicine, University of Bari "Aldo Moro", SP. Casamassima km 3, 70010 Bari, Valenzano, Italy. [2]Department of Infectious Diseases, Istituto Superiore di Sanità, Viale Regina Elena 299, 00161 Rome, Italy. [3]Endocannabinoid Research Group (ERG), Institute of Biomolecular Chemistry (ICB), Consiglio Nazionale delle Ricerche (CNR), Via Campi Flegrei 34, 80078 Pozzuoli, Napoli, Italy.

References

1. La Porta C, Bura SA, Negrete R, Maldonado R. Involvement of the endocannabinoid system in osteoarthritis pain. Eur J Neurosci. 2014;39:485–500.
2. Haseeb A, Haqqi TM. Immunopathogenesis of osteoarthritis. Clin Immunol. 2013;146:185–96.
3. Feldmann M, Brennan FM, Maini RN. Role of cytokines in rheumatoid arthtritis. Ann Rev Immunol. 1996;14:397–440.
4. Sutton S, Clutterbuck A, Harris P, Gent T, Freeman S, Foster N, Barrett-Jolley R, Mobasheri A. The contribution of the synovium, synovial derived inflammatory cytokines and neuropeptides to the pathogenesis of osteoarthritis. Vet J. 2009;179:10–24.
5. Johnston SA. Ostheoarthritis, joint anatomy, physiology, and pathobiology. Vet Cli North Am Small Anim Pract. 1997;27:699–723.
6. Richardson D, Pearson RG, Kurian N, Latif ML, Garle MJ, Barrett DA, Kendall DA, Scammell BE, Reeve AJ, Chapman V. Characterisation of the cannabinoid receptor system in synovial tissue and fluid in patients with osteoarthritis and rheumatoid arthritis. Arthritis Res Ther. 2008;10:43.
7. Mc Partland JM, Duncan M, Di Marzo V, Pertwee RG. Are cannabidiol and Δ^9 -tetrahydrocannabivarin negative modulators of the endocannabinoid sustem? A systemic review. Brit J Pharmacol. 2015;172:737–53.
8. Mackie K. Cannabinoid receptors as therapeutic targets. Annu Rev Pharmacol Toxicol. 2006;46:101–22.
9. Elmes SJR, Jhaveri MD, Smart D, Kendall DA, Chapman V. Activation of CB_1 and CB_2 receptors attenuates the induction and maintenance of inflammatory pain in rat. Pain. 2005;118:327–35.
10. Smith FL, Fujimori K, Lowe J, Welch SP. Characterization of Δ^9-tetrahydrocannabinol and anandamide antinociception in nonarthritic and arthritic rats. Pharmacol Biochem Behav. 1998;60:183–91.
11. Mc Partland JM, Guy GW, Di Marzo V. Care and feeding of the endocannabinoid system: a systematic review of potential clinical interventions that upregulate the endocannabinoid system. PLoS One. 2014;9:1–21.
12. Lambert DM, Di Marzo V. The palmitoylethanolamide and oleamide enigmas: are those two fatty acid amides cannabimimetic? Curr Med Chem. 1999;6:757–73.
13. Mechoulam R, Fride E, Di Marzo V. Endocannabinoids. Eur J Pharmacol. 1998;359:1–18.
14. O'Sullivan SE. Cannabinoids go nuclear: evidence for activation of peroxisome proliferator-activate receptors. Brit J Pharmacol. 2007;152:576–82.
15. Capasso R, Hoareau L, Monteleone P, Izzo AA, Di Marzo V. Role and regulation of acylethanolamides in energy balance: focus on adipocytes and β-cells. Brit J Pharmacol. 2007;152:676–90.
16. Wilson RI, Nicoll RA. Endocannabinoid signaling in the brain. Science. 2002; 296:678–82.
17. Schuelert N, McDougall JJ. Cannabinoid-mediated antinociception is enhanced in rat osteoarthritic knees. Arthritis Rheum. 2008;58:145–53.
18. Mbvundula EC, Bunning RA, Rainsford KD. Arthritis and cannabinoids: HU-210 and Win-55,212-2 prevent IL-1alpha-induced matrix degradation in bovine articular chondrocytes in-vitro. J Pharm Pharmacol. 2006;58:351–8.
19. Idris AI, Ralston SH. Role of cannabinoids in regulation of bone remodeling. Front Endocrinol. 2012;3:136.
20. Azim S, Nicholson J, Rebecchi M, Galbavy W, Feng T, Reinsel R, Volkow ND, Benveniste H, Kaczocha M, et al. Endocannabinoids and acute pain following total knee arthroplasty. Pain. 2015;156:341–7.
21. Berge K, Piscitelli F, Hoem N, Silvestri C, Meyer I, Banni S, Di Marzo V. Chronic treatment with krill powder reduces plasma triglyceride and anandamide levels in mildly obese man. Lipids Health Dis. 2013;12:78.
22. Matias I, Petrosino S, Racioppi A, Capasso R, Izzo AA, Di Marzo V. Dysregulation of peripheral endocannabinoid levels in hyperglycemia and obesity: effect of high fat diets. Mol Cell Endocrinol. 2008;286:66–78.
23. Lambert DM, Vsndevoorde S, Jonsson KO, Fowler CJ. The palmitoylethanolamide family: a new class of anti-inflammatory agents? Curr Med Chem. 2002;9:663–74.
24. Haynes MK, Hume EL, Smith JB. Phenotypic characterization of inflammatory cells from osteoarthritic synovium and synovial fluids. Clin Immunol. 2002; 105:315–25.
25. Deutsch DG, Goligorsky MS, Schmid PC, Krebsbach RJ, Schmid HH, Das SK, Dey SK, Arreaza G, Thorup C, Stefano G, Moore LC. Production and physiological actions of anandamide in the vasculature of the rat kidney. J Clin Invest. 1997;100:1538–46.
26. Sugiura T, Kodaka T, Nakane S, Kishimoto S, Kondo S, Waku K. Detection of an endogenous cannabimimetic molecule, 2-Arachidonoylglycerol, and cannabinoid CB_1receptor mRNAin human vascular cells: is 2-Arachidonoylglycerol a possible vasomodulator? Biochem Biophys Res Commun. 1998;243:838–43.
27. Maruotti N, Cantatore FP, Crivellato E, Vacca A, Ribatti D. Angiogenesis in rheumatoid arthritis. Histol Histopathol. 2006;21:557–66.
28. Schaible HG, Richter F, Ebersberger A, Boettger MK, Vanegas H, Natura G, Vazquez E, von Banchet Segond G. Joint pain. Exp Brain Res. 2009;196:153–62.
29. Croxford JL, Yamamura T. Cannabinoids and the immune system: potential for the treatment of inflammatory disease? J Neuroimmunol. 2005;166:3–18.
30. Klein TW. Cannabinoid-based drugs as anti-inflammatory therapeutics. Nat Rev Immunol. 2005;5:400–11.

3

Omental adipose tissue is a more suitable source of canine Mesenchymal stem cells

Francisca Bahamondes[1,2*], Estefania Flores[2], Gino Cattaneo[2], Flavia Bruna[1] and Paulette Conget[1]

Abstract

Background: Mesenchymal Stem Cells (MSCs) are a promising therapeutic tool in veterinary medicine. Currently the subcutaneous adipose tissue is the leading source of MSCs in dogs. MSCs derived from distinct fat depots have shown dissimilarities in their accessibility and therapeutic potential. The aims of our work were to determine the suitability of omental adipose tissue as a source of MSCs, according to sampling success, cell yield and paracrine properties of isolated cells, and compared to subcutaneous adipose tissue.

Results: While sampling success of omental adipose tissue was 100% (14 collections from14 donors) for subcutaneous adipose tissue it was 71% (10 collections from 14 donors). MSCs could be isolated from both sources. Cell yield was significantly higher for omental than for subcutaneous adipose tissue (38 ± 1 vs. 30 ± 1 CFU-F/g tissue, $p < 0.0001$). No differences were observed between sources regarding cell proliferation potential (73 ± 1 vs. 74 ± 1 CDPL) and cell senescence (at passage 10, both cultures presented enlarged cells with cytoplasmic vacuoles and cellular debris). Omental- and subcutaneous-derived MSCs expressed at the same level bFGF, PDGF, HGF, VEGF, ANG1 and IL-10. Irrespective of the source, isolated MSCs induced proliferation, migration and vascularization of target cells, and inhibited the activation of T lymphocytes.

Conclusion: Compared to subcutaneous adipose tissue, omental adipose tissue is a more suitable source of MSCs in dogs. Since it can be procured from donors with any body condition, its collection procedure is always feasible, its cell yield is high and the MSCs isolated from it have desirable differentiation and paracrine potentials.

Keywords: Mesenchymal stem cell, Source, Adipose tissue, Omentum, Canine, Dog

Background

Mesenchymal stem cells (MSCs) are non-hematopoietic precursor cells that can be differentiated, among others, into chondrocytes, osteocytes and adipocytes [1]. Together, MSCs secrete trophic, vasculogenic and immunomodulatory factors that have a paracrine effect on tissue resident cells [2–4]. Hence, MSCs are a promissory therapeutic tool for regenerative medicine [5].

The leading source of MSCs is the bone marrow. In 2001, they were isolated for the first time from adipose tissue [6]. When compared to bone marrow, adipose tissue appeared as a superior source of MSCs due to the fact that a less invasive procedure is required to procure it [7–9].

In veterinary medicine, it has been proven that the administration of adipose-derived MSCs have therapeutic effects in small animal patients, particularly in cats and dogs [10–13]. Adult dogs have adipose tissue locates mainly in subcutaneous and visceral depots. Thus, adipose tissue may be procured through minimally invasive procedures from arms, thighs and abdomen (subcutaneous), or from omentum, kidney and liver (visceral) [14, 15]. While the abundance of subcutaneous adipose tissue depends on the body condition, the extent of omentum is relatively constant [16, 17]. It has been demonstrated that there are MSCs in the omentum of both dogs [10, 18] and humans [19, 20]. Omental-derived MSCs are similar to subcutaneous-derived MSCs according to their proliferation and surface antigen expression [18]. Up to our knowledge, no data are available regarding the abundance and paracrine potential of omental-derived MSCs. Since previous studies showed that adipose-derived MSC properties vary from depot to

* Correspondence: fbahamondesg@ug.uchile.cl
[1]Centro de Medicina Regenerativa, Facultad de Medicina, Clínica Alemana - Universidad del Desarrollo, Av. Las Condes 12,438, Lo Barnechea, Santiago 7710162, Chile
[2]Departamento de Ciencias Clínicas, Facultad de Ciencias Veterinarias y Pecuarias, Universidad de Chile, Av. Santa Rosa 11,735, Santiago, Chile

depot [21], it will be also interesting to compare MSCs isolated form omentum with those isolated from subcutaneous fat, the leading adipose source of MSCs.

The aims of our work were to determine the suitability of omental adipose tissue as a source of MSCs, according to sampling success, cell yield and paracrine properties of isolated cells, and compared to subcutaneous adipose tissue.

Methods

Collection of adipose tissue

Fourteen female dogs of different breeds, 6–12 months old, with normal corporal condition, clinically healthy and having elective ovariohysterectomies were enrolled in the study, after client-owned provided written informed consent. Animals were pre-anesthetized with 0.04 mg/Kg Acepromazine (Holliday-Scott S.A, Buenos Aires, Argentina). General anesthesia was induced with 3 mg/Kg Propofol (Fresenius Kabi, Spain) and maintained with Isofluorane (Baxter Healthcare Corporation, Deerfield, IL). Approximately $3cm^3$ (5-10 g) of omental and subcutaneous adipose tissue were procured from greater omentum and abdominal region, respectively. Subsequently, an ovariohysterectomy was performed. Muscular and skin incisions were sutured with a simple, interrupted pattern. Up to three days post-surgery animals received 1 mg/Kg/24 h Ketoprofen (Merial Laboratorios, Argentina).

Study was approved by Ethic Committee Facultad de Ciencias Veterinarias y Pecuarias, Universidad de Chile (No. 03–2014).

Isolation, ex vivo expansion and characterization of MSCs

Adipose tissue samples were weighed, washed with phosphate buffered saline (PBS. Sigma, St. Louis, MO, USA) containing 80 μg/mL gentamycin (Sanderson Laboratory, Santiago, Chile), minced with scissors and scalpels, and digested in PBS containing 1 mg/mL collagenase type II (Gibco, Grand Island, NY, USA), at 37 °C, overnight. Enzyme activity was neutralized with alpha-MEM (Gibco, Auckland, NZ) supplemented with 10% fetal bovine serum (Gibco, Auckland, NZ) and 80 μg/mL gentamicin (Sanderson Laboratory, Santiago, Chile) (here after expansion medium), and centrifuged at 400×g for 10 min. Pelleted cells were resuspended in expansion medium and plated at a density of 50,000 nucleated cells/cm^2 and cultured under an atmosphere with 5% CO_2, at 37 °C. Fourty eight hours later, nonadherent cells were removed by media change. When 80% confluence was achieved, adherent cells were detached with 0.25% trypsin and 2.65 mM EDTA, centrifuged and subcultured at 5000 cells/cm^2. After two subcultures, adherent cells were characterized according to their adipogenic [21], chondrogenic [22] and osteogenic differentiation potential [23]. Although there are currently no consensus markers for canine MSCs as there are for human MSCs [1], immunophenotyping was performed by flow cytometry analysis after labeling with monoclonal antibodies against: $CD45^{FITC}$, $CD11b^{PE\text{-}Cy5}$, $CD44^{APC}$ and $CD90^{PE}$ or their respective isotype controls (rat $IgG2b^{FITC}$, rat $IgG2b^{PE\text{-}Cy5}$, rat $IgG2b^{APC}$ or rat $IgG2b^{PE}$; eBioscience, San Diego, CA).

Fibroblast-like Colony forming unit (CFU-F) assay

CFU-F assay was performed on freshly isolated cells as previously described [24]. Briefly, 500 mononuclear cells/cm^2 were cultured in expansion medium. At day 7, cells were fixed with 4% paraformaldehyde for 10 min and stained with 0.5% crystal violet (Sigma-Aldrich, St. Louis, MO) in 10% methanol for 20 min. Plates were observed under light microscope (Leica DM2000). Clusters containing more than 50 cells were scored as CFU-Fs and counted. Results were expressed as CFU-F per gram of tissue (CFU-F/g tissue).

Assays were performed in triplicate.

Evaluation of cumulative population doubling level (CPDL) and senescence

One thousand cells/cm^2 were seeded and cultured with expansion medium. The medium was changed every three days and cells were subcultured when reaching 80% confluence. The population doubling (PD) at each subculture was calculated according to the formula $PD = \ln (N_f/N_i) / \ln 2$, where N_i and N_f are initial and final cell numbers, respectively. The PDs of continuous subcultures were added to obtain CPDL [10].

Senescence was assessed looking for changes in cell morphology such as cell enlargement, accumulation of vacuoles and presence of cellular debris [25].

Assays were performed in triplicate.

RT-qPCR

RNA was extracted from cells using Tryzol (*Invitrogen*, Carlsbad, CA, USA) and treated with DNAse (*Invitrogen*, Carlsbad, CA, USA) following the manufacturer's instructions. One μg of RNA was reverse-transcribed using oligo-dT primers and Moloney murine leukemia virus reverse transcriptase. The abundance of mRNA was determined by qPCR using SYBR Green Technology and canine-specific primers for bFGF, PDGF HGF, VEGF, ANG1, IDO, IL-10 and 18S (Additional file 1: Table S1). Cycling condition were: 1 cycle, 94 °C for 10 min; 30–35 cycles, 94 °C for 10 min; optimal annealing temperature for 5 min; 72 °C for 4 min; 1 cycle, 64 °C for 10 min; 1 cycle, 40 °C for 30 min. The qPCR products were separated by electrophoresis on 2% agarose gel, stained with 1% ethidium bromide and visualized under UV light. Digital images were captured with

Alpha imagen software. Values were normalized to 18S mRNA levels. Relative gene expression was quantified with the $2^{-\Delta\Delta Ct}$ method [26].

Proliferation assay

Human fibroblasts were seeded at 4000 cells/cm^2 and cultivated with alpha-MEM (control) or alpha-MEM conditioned by MSCs for 24 h. The medium was changed every 3 days. Three, six, nine and 12 days later, cells were stained with 0.5% crystal violet in 10% methanol for 20 min. After four washes, crystal violet incorporated into the cells were solubilized with 50% methanol in PBS and quantified spectrophotometrically (absorbance at 570 nm) [24].

Assays were performed in triplicate.

Scratch assay

Human fibroblasts were seeded at 8000 cells/cm^2. After 24 h, a line in the monolayer was performed with a sterile p200 pipette tip and medium was changed by alpha-MEM (control) or alpha-MEM conditioned by MSCs for 24 h. Zero, six, and 12 h after scratching images were captured under a light microscope (Leica DM2000) with a digital camera (Leica DFC 295). Image J software (http://rsbweb.nih.gov/ij/) was used to quantify the scratch area [27].

Assays were performed in triplicate.

Tube formation assay

Human umbilical vein endothelial cells (HUVECs) were seeded at 3000 cells/cm^2 on 10 mg/mL growth factor-reduced Matrigel (BD Biosciences, Boston, MA, USA) and exposed to alpha-MEM (control), alpha-MEM conditioned by MSCs for 24 h or endothelial growth medium (Lonza, Walkersville, MD, USA) (positive control) [28]. Five hours later, images were captured under a light microscope using a digital camera. WimTube program (Wimasis GmbH, Munich, Germany) was used to quantify i) total tube length, ii) total branching point, iii) total loops.

Assays were performed in triplicate.

T lymphocyte proliferation assay

Canine peripheral blood mononuclear cells were labeled with carboxyfluorescein succinimidyl ester (Invitrogen/Molecular Probes, Eugene, OR) and cultivated with alpha-MEM (control) or alpha-MEM conditioned by MSCs for 24 h, supplemented with 4 uL (1:10) phytohaemaglutinin (Gibco, Invitrogen, Corporation, Scotland, UK). Five days later, cells were stained with monoclonal antibody against CD4^{PE} (Serotec, Kidlington, Oxford, United Kingdom) and analyzed by flow cytometry [29].

Assays were performed in triplicate.

Statistical analysis

Data are presented as mean ± S.E.M. To determine the statistical significance of intergroup differences a one-way ANOVA test was used to compare mean values among all groups and Student's unpaired *t*-test or Mann-Whitney test (non parametric) was used to compare mean values between two groups. $p < 0.05$ was considered as statistically significant.

Results

Omental adipose tissue has higher sampling success than subcutaneous adipose tissue

The age and weight of donor dogs were 10 ± 3 months and 12 ± 6 Kg (Table 1). Omental samples were procured from the 14 donors and subcutaneous samples were procured from 10 of them. Thus, the success sampling rates were 100% (14 of 14) for omental adipose tissue and 71% (10 of 14) for subcutaneous adipose tissue (Table 1). The average weight of the procured samples was 5.2 ± 4.5 g for omental and 2.4 ± 3.4 g for subcutaneal adipose tissue (Table 1).

Further characterization of adipose-derived MSCs was performed for samples obtained from the 10 donors in whom it was possible to obtain both omental and subcutaneous adipose tissues.

Omental adipose tissue and subcutaneous adipose tissue have MSCs

Cells isolated from both sources adhered to plastic and showed fibroblast-like morphology (Fig. 1a). Together, they were negative for hematopoietic markers (CD45 and CD11b) and positive for MSC markers (CD90 and CD44) (Fig. 1b). When exposed to adipogenic stimulus, cells differentiated into adipocytes that accumulate lipid droplets throughout the cytoplasm as confirmed by Oil Red O staining (Fig. 1c). After 21 days under chondrogenic induction, sulfated glycosaminoglycans were present in the matrix as revealed by Safranin O staining (Fig. 1c). Cell osteogenic differentiation was confirmed due to the appearance, 3 weeks after exposure to osteogenic medium, of calcium deposits that stained with Alizarin Red (Fig. 1c).

Omental adipose tissue has higher abundance of MSCs than subcutaneous adipose tissue

The relative abundance of MSCs in omental adipose tissue was 38 ± 1 CFU-F/g tissue and in subcutaneous adipose tissue was 30 ± 1 CFU-F/g tissue, $p < 0.0001$ (Fig. 2a-2b).

MSCs derived from omental and subcutaneous adipose tissues have a similar expansion potential

No statistical difference was observed bewteen omental- and subcutaneous-derived MSCs regarding

Table 1 Enrolled animals and procured samples characteristics

Donor (identifier)	Age (months)	Weight (kilograms)	Subcutaneous (grams)	Omental (grams)
B001	8	8	not available	6.3
P002	12	15	4.8	8.1
L003	7	11	4.6	9.8
P004	8	12	not available	3.1
K005	12	15	1.9	2.3
L006	7	12	4.5	8.4
P007	8	10	3.2	4.5
C008	12	16	3.1	7.1
C009	11	6	not available	3.2
S010	8	15	5.8	5.9
O011	8	7	not available	3.7
C012	12	10	1.5	3.0
P013	10	6	2.3	4.8
S014	10	18	3.3	3.2
TOTAL	10 ± 3	12 ± 6	2.4 ± 3.4	5.2 ± 4.5

their proliferation potential up to passage 12 (73 ± 1 vs. 74 ± 1 CDPL) (Fig. 2c). Senescence characteristics such as cell enlargement, generation of vacuoles and presence of cellular debris were seen from passage 10 in both MSCs (Fig. 2d).

MSCs derived from omental and subcutaneous adipose tissues have similar trophic properties

Both adipose-derived MSCs expressed at the same level the trophic factors bFGF, PDGF and HGF (Fig. 3a). Accordingly, no differences were observed in their potential

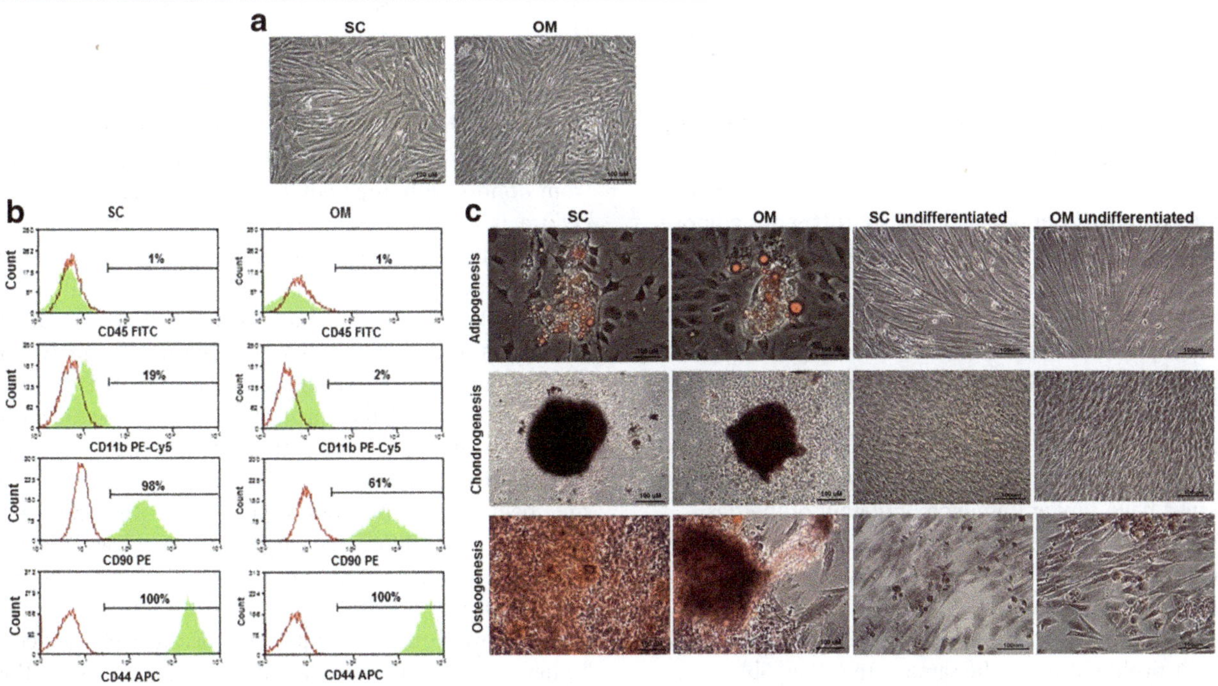

Fig. 1 Omental adipose tissue and subcutaneous adipose tissue have MSCs. **a** Representative photomicrographs of primary culture of subcutaneous- and omental-derived cells. **b** Flow cytometry analysis after immunostaining with monoclonal antibodies against CD45, CD11b, CD90 and CD44 (*green lines*) or isotype controls (*red lines*). **c** Representative photomicrographs of MSCs stained with Oil Red O (adipogenesis), Safranin O (chondrogenesis) or Alizarin Red (osteogenesis) 3 weeks after differentiation induction. Control undifferentiated cells are also shown. Abbreviations: SC: subcutaneous adipose tissue; OM: omental adipose tissue

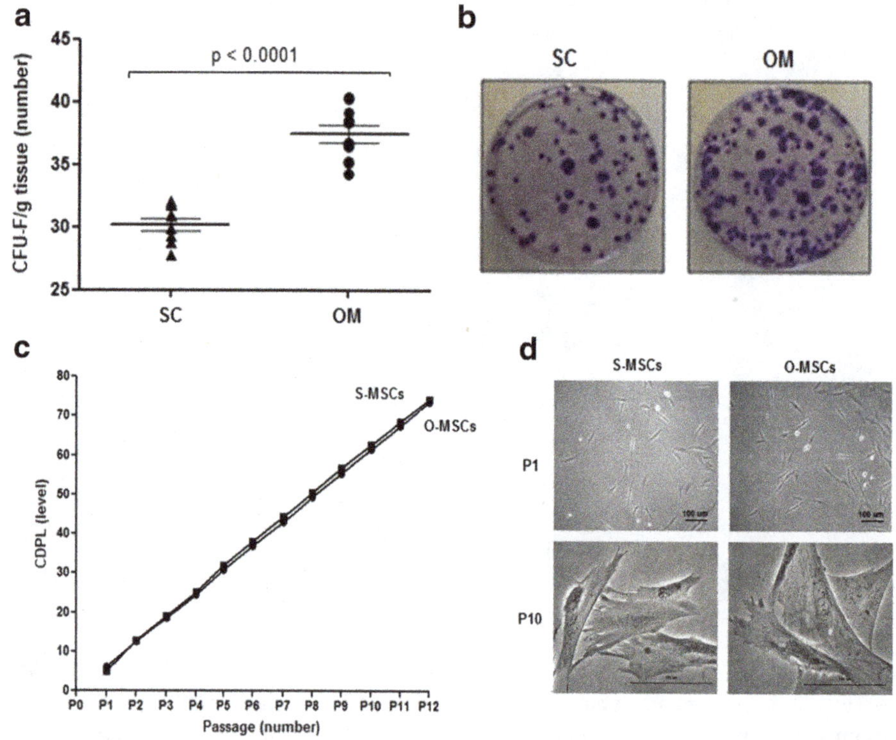

Fig. 2 Omental adipose tissue has higher abundance of MSCs than subcutaneous adipose tissue. **a** Quantitative analysis of CFU-Fs per gram of tissue sampled. **b** Representative photographs of plates stained with crystal violet 7 days after seeding of nucleated cells from tissue samples. **c** Quantitative analysis of CPDL up to passage 12. **d** Representative photomicrographs of S-MSCs and O-MSCs at passages 1 (P1) and 10 (P10). Abbreviations: SC: subcutaneous adipose tissue; OM: omental adipose tissue; CFU-F/g tissue: colony forming units per grams of tissue; S-MSCs: mesenchymal stem cells derived from subcutaneous adipose tissue; O-MSCs: mesenchymal stem cells derived from omental adipose tissue; CDPL: cumulative population doubling level

to promote human fibroblast proliferation and migration (Fig. 3b, c and d).

MSCs derived from omental and subcutaneous adipose tissues have similar vasculogenic properties

Irrespective of their origin, adipose-derived MSCs expressed VEGF and ANG1 (Fig. 4a). Consequently, they equally promote tube formation of HUVEC (total tube length, total branching point and total loops) (Fig. 4b and c).

MSCs derived from omental and subcutaneous adipose tissues have similar immunomodulatory properties

The gene expression level of IDO was significantly lower in omental MSCs than in subcutaneous cells ($p < 0.05$. Fig. 5a). The level of IL-10 did not differ significantly between them. Both adipose-derived MSCs prevent CD4+ T cell-proliferation at the same extent (Fig. 5b).

Discussion

A major challenge associated with MSC-based therapies is the selection of the source [14]. Here we showed in young and healthy female dogs that, compared to subcutaneous adipose tissue, omental adipose tissue is a more suitable source of MSCs. Since it can be procured from donors with any body condition, its collection procedure is always feasible, its cell yield is high and the MSCs isolated from it have desirable differentiation and paracrine potentials.

The fact that omental but not subcutaneous adipose tissue was always procurable may be attributed to volume variability of fat depots as well as to the expertise of the professional that procures them. In a study with 1265 dogs, it was shown that the size of collected samples was determined by the location of the adipose tissue, being visceral samples bigger than subcutaneous ones [12]. This difference might be critical when donor should be an emaciated patient due to either a chronic or a nutritional disease.

We showed that omental adipose tissue yielded a higher number of viable MSCs per gram of tissue than subcutaneous adipose tissue. These results are in agreement with other studies showing the same differences in humans [14] and dogs [10, 15].

Consistent with the results reported for human MSCs, canine MSCs isolated either from omental or

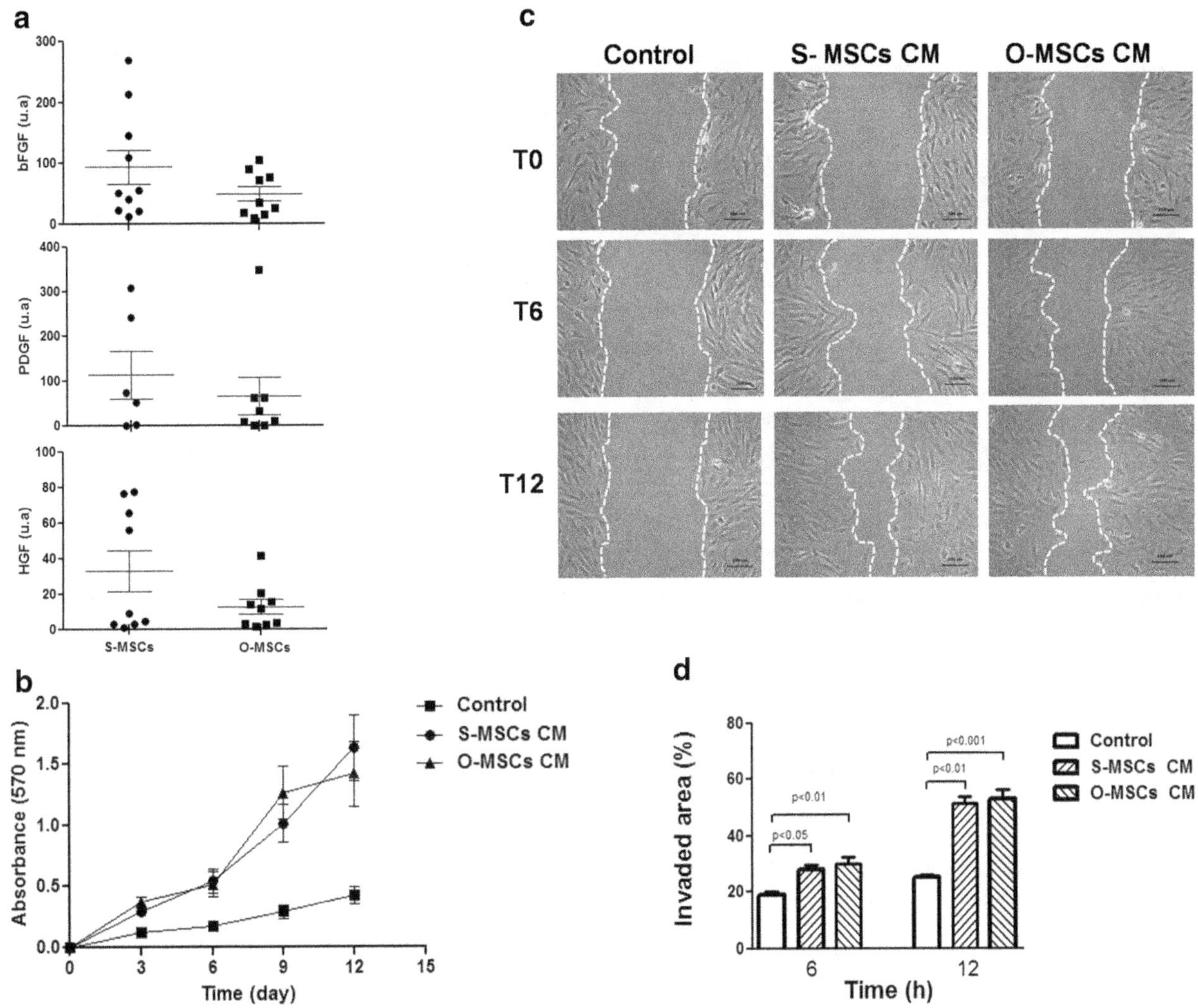

Fig. 3 MSCs derived from omental and subcutaneous adipose tissues have similar trophic properties. **a** Quantitative analysis of mRNA levels of trophic factors. **b** Quantitative analysis of proliferation kinetic of human fibroblast cultivated with S-MSCs CM or O-MSCs CM evaluated during 12 days. **c** Representative photomicrographs of invaded area at 0 (T0), six (T6) and 12 (T12) hours post exposure to CMs. **d** Quantitative analysis of invaded area evaluated as the percentage of area free of cells at 6 or 12 h post exposure to CM with respect to 0 h. Abbreviations: S-MSCs: mesenchymal stem cells derived from subcutaneous adipose tissue; O-MSCs: mesenchymal stem cells derived from omental adipose tissue; CM: conditioned medium; **bFGF**: basic fibroblast growth factor; **PDGF**: platelet-derived growth factor; **HGF**: hepatocyte growth factor

subcutaneous adipose tissue followed a lineal trend of proliferation up to passage 12 and senescence characteristics appeared at passage 10 [23, 30]. Thus, our data support a significant but limited expansion potential of canine MSCs. Hence, the feasibility to be procured and the cell richness of the sample take higher relevance in order to choose the best source of canine MSCs.

The secretory activity of MSCs favors a regenerative microenvironment [31, 32]. The trophic properties of MSCs depend on the secretion of growth factors that induce cell proliferation and migration [33–35]. We showed that canine MSCs isolated from omental or subcutaneous tissues express bFGF, PDGF and HGF. Both bFGF and PDGF elicit target cell proliferation after ligand-binding induction of receptor oligomerization, activation of intrinsic receptor tyrosine kinase and phosphorylation of specific residues in the cytoplasmic region [36–39]. HGF is a pleiotropic factor displaying mitogenic, motogenic, morphogenetic, and antiapoptotic activities in different target cells [40]. Indeed, HGF promotes hepatocytes, keratinocytes, renal tubule cell and endothelial cell proliferation, dissociation of epithelial cell colonies, cell motility, and invasion through extracellular matrix. More recently, it has been shown that bFGF, PDGF and HGF can induce biological responses also on MSCs [41–43]. Our functional studies showed that, irrespective of the source, canine MSCs secrete active mitogenic and motogenic factors.

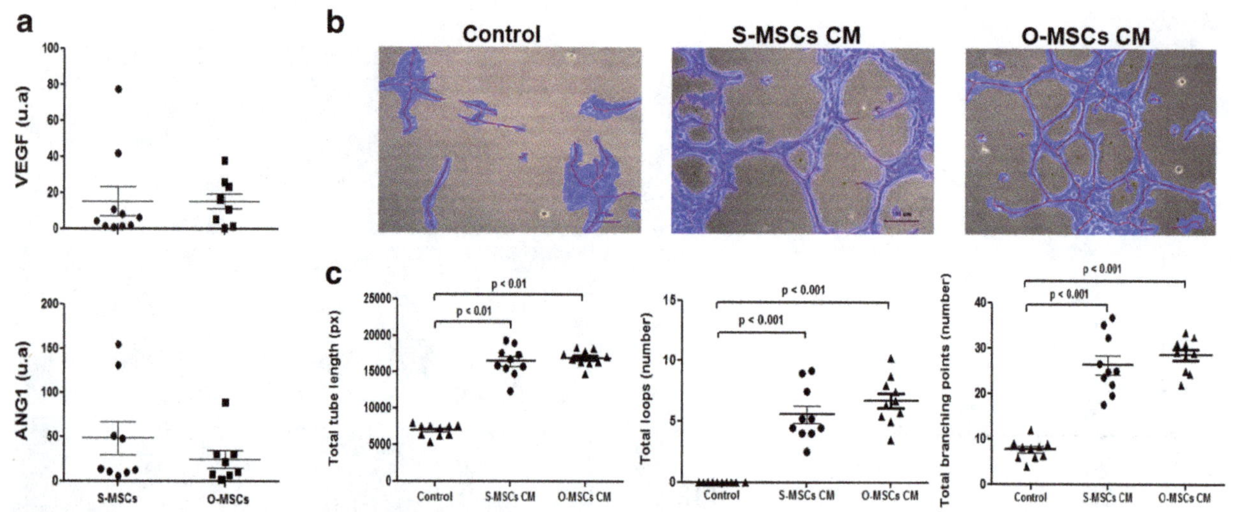

Fig. 4 MSCs derived from omental and subcutaneous adipose tissues have similar vasculogenic properties. **a** Quantitative analysis of mRNAs levels of vasculogenic factors. **b** Representative photomicrographs of tube assay performed with 3D collagen-embedded human umbilical endothelial cells cultivated 5 h with S-MSCs CM or O-MSCs CM and analyzed by Wimasis software. **c** Quantitative analysis of total tube length, total branching point and total loops of tube assay among the different conditions. Abbreviations: S-MSCs: mesenchymal stem cells derived from subcutaneous adipose tissue; O-MSCs: mesenchymal stem cells derived from omental adipose tissue; CM: conditioned medium; **VEGF**: vascular endothelial growth factor; **ANG1** angiopoietin 1

Vasculogenesis is a crucial step in the wound healing process [44, 45]. The formation of new blood vessels is necessary to sustain the newly formed granulation tissue and the survival of keratinocytes. In this study, we found that adipose tissue derived MSCs express VEGF and ANG1. Both stimulate endothelial cell proliferation, migration, and organization into tubules [46, 47]. Our functional study showed that MSCs either form omental or subcutaneous tissue secreted active factors that promote vasculogenesis.

Since in the functional assays we used human fibroblasts or human endothelial cells as target cells, our data

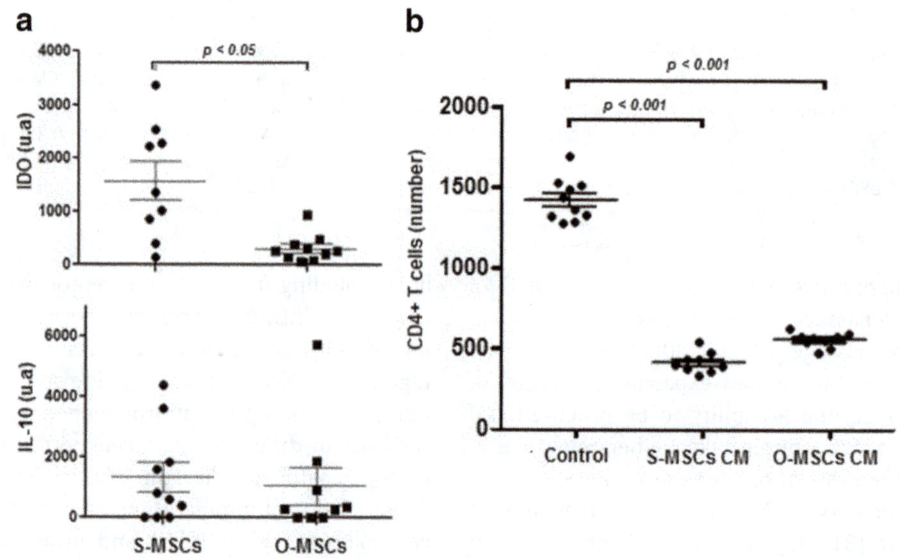

Fig. 5 MSCs derived from omental and subcutaneous adipose tissues have similar immunomodulatory properties. **a** Quantitative analysis of the mRNAs levels of immunomodulatory factors. Each value was normalized to 18S expression. **b** Quantitative analysis of total CD4+ T-cells stimulated and cultivated with S-MSC CM and O-MSC CM after 5 days. Abbreviations: S-MSCs: mesenchymal stem cells derived from subcutaneous adipose tissue; O-MSCs: mesenchymal stem cells derived from omental adipose tissue; CM: conditioned medium; **IDO** indoleamine-pyrrole 2,3-dioxygenase; **IL-10** interleukin 10

prove than trophic and vasculogenic factors secreted by MSCs isolated from dog omental or subcutaneous adipose tissue overcome species-specificity barrier. In order to further characterize the products secreted by canine MSCs it would be relevant to perform the functional experiments using target cells from dogs and other species.

Much attention has been paid to the immunomodulatory properties of MSCs. Several studies have shown a paracrine suppressive effect on T cells, B cells, monocytes and macrophages [48–50]. We showed similar gene expression levels of IL-10 in MSCs from both sources studied. Though, the expression of IDO in MSCs derived from subcutaneous adipose tissue was 11-fold higher than in MSCs derived from omentum. IDO catalyzes the conversion of tryptophan to kynurenine and inhibits T cell proliferation due to tryptophan depletion [51]. Nevertheless, this is not the unique mechanism supporting the immunosuppresive potential of MSCs [52–55]. That should explain why, despite of the differences observed in IDO mRNA levels, in the functional assay MSCs from both sources inhibit at the same magnitude CD4+ T cell proliferation. Our results appear consistent with previous findings for human and canine MSCs [4, 56, 57].

Data here presented not only shall be useful for evidence based-selection of MSC source but also to expand the frontiers of the use of canine MSCs as they prove to produce active trophic, vasculogenic and immunomodulator soluble factors.

Conclusion

Compared to subcutaneous adipose tissue, omental adipose tissue is a more suitable source of MSCs in dogs. Since it can be procured from donors with any body condition, its collection procedure is always feasible, its cell yield is high and the MSCs isolated from it have desirable differentiation and paracrine potentials.

Abbreviations

ANG1: Angiopoietin 1; bFGF: Basic fibroblast growth factor; CDPL: Cumulative population doubling level; CFU-F: Fibroblastic-like colony forming unit; CM: Conditioned medium; EDTA: Ethylenediaminetetraacetic acid; HGF: Hepatocyte growth factor; HUVEC: Human umbilical vein endothelial cells; IDO: Indoleamine-pyrrole 2,3-dioxygenase; IL-10: Interleukin 10; MSCs: Mesenchymal stem cells; OM: Omental adipose tissue; O-MSCs: Omental mesenchymal stem cells; PBS: Phosphate-buffered saline; PDGF: Platelet-derived growth factor; SC: Subcutaneous adipose tissue; S-MSCs: Subcutaneous mesenchymal stem cells; VEGF: Vascular endothelial growth factor

Acknowledgements

We thank the dog owners for their disposition to participate in this study. Also, we are grateful with the people that work at the Center of Regenerative Medicine, Facultad de Medicina Clinica Alemana - Universidad del Desarrollo for their technical assistance.
This study was presented in part as an abstract at the International Society for Stem Cell Research Annual Meeting, Stockholm, june 2015.

Funding

This study was supported by CONICYT Grant No. 21110863 and by CONICYT Doctoral Scholarship to FB.

Authors' contributions

FB designed the study, performed the experiments, analyzed data and wrote the manuscript. EF and GC participated in animal management and adipose tissue sampling. FBr performed RT-qPCR. PC designed the study, supervised all procedures, analyzed data and revised the manuscript versions. All authors read and approved the final manuscript.

Competing interests

The authors declare that they have no competing interests.

Consent for publication

Not applicable.

References

1. Dominici M, Le Blanc K, Mueller I, Slaper-Cortenbach I, Marini F, Krause D, Deans R, Keating A, Prockop DJ, Horwitz E. Minimal criteria for defining multipotent mesenchymal stromal cells. The International Society for Cellular Therapy position statement. Cytotherapy. 2006;8:315–7.
2. Le Blanc K, Tammik L, Sundberg B, Haynesworth SE, Ringdén O. Mesenchymal stem cells inhibit and stimulate mixed lymphocyte cultures and mitogenic responses independently of the major histocompatibility complex. Scand J Immunol. 2003;57:11–20.
3. Caplan AI, Dennis JE. Mesenchymal stem cells as trophic mediators. J Cell Biochem. 2006;98:1076–84.
4. Kang JW, Kang KS, Koo HC, Park JR, Choi EW, Park YH. Soluble factors-mediated immunomodulatory effects of canine adipose tissue-derived mesenchymal stem cells. Stem Cells Dev. 2008;17:681–93.
5. Sutton MT, Bonfield TL. Stem cells: innovations in clinical applications. Stem Cells Int. 2014; doi:10.1155/2014/516278.
6. Zuk PA, Zhu M, Ashjian P, De Ugarte DA, Huang JI, Mizuno H, Alfonso ZC, Fraser JK, Benhaim P, Hedrick MH. Human adipose tissue is a source of multipotent stem cells. Mol Biol Cell. 2002;13:4279–95.
7. Strem BM, Hicok KC, Zhu M, Wulur I, Alfonso Z, Schreiber RE, Fraser JK, Hedrick MH. Multipotential differentiation of adipose tissue-derived stem cells. Keio J Med. 2005;54:132–41.
8. Baer PC, Geiger H. Adipose-derived mesenchymal stromal/stem cells: tissue localization, characterization, and heterogeneity. Stem Cells Int. 2012;812693
9. Reich CM, Raabe O, Wenisch S, Bridger PS, Kramer M, Arnhold S. Isolation, culture and chondrogenic differentiation of canine adipose tissue- and bone marrow-derived mesenchymal stem cells–a comparative study. Vet Sci Commun. 2012;36:139–48.
10. Neupane M, Chang C-C, Kiupel M, Yuzbasiyan-Gurkan V. Isolation and characterization of canine adipose-derived mesenchymal stem cells. Tissue Eng. 2008;14:1007–15.
11. Vieira N, Brandalise V, Zucconi E, Secco M, Strauss B, Zatz M. Isolation, characterization, and differentiation potential of canine adipose-derived stem cells. Cell Transplant. 2010;9:279–89.
12. Astor D, Hoelzler M, Harman R, Bastian R. Patient factors influencing the concentration of stromal vascular fraction (SVF) for adipose-derived stromal cell (ASC) therapy in dogs. Canine J Vet Res. 2013;77:177–82.
13. Trzil JE, Masseau I, Webb TL, Chang CH, Dodam JR, Liu H, Quimby JM, Dow SW, Reinero CR. Intravenous adipose-derived mesenchymal stem cell therapy for the treatment of feline asthma: a pilot study. J Feline Med Surg. 2015; doi:10.1177/1098612X15604351.

14. Russo V, Yu C, Belliveau P, Hamilton A, Flynn LE. Comparison of human adipose-derived stem cells isolated from subcutaneous, omental, and intrathoracic adipose tissue depots for regenerative applications. Stem Cells Transl Med. 2014;2:206–17.
15. Guercio A, Di Bella S, Casella S, Di Marco P, Russo C, Piccione G. Canine mesenchymal stem cells (MSCs): characterization in relation to donor age and adipose tissue-harvesting site. Cell Biol Int. 2013;37:789–98.
16. Thengchaisri N, Wutthiwong T, Kaewmokul S, Sastravaha A. Abdominal obesity is associated with heart disease in dogs. BMC Vet Res. 2014;10:131.
17. Kobatashi T, Koie H, Kusumi A, Kitagawa M, Kanayama K, Otsuji K. Comparative investigation of body composition in male dogs using CT and body fat analysis software. J Vet Med Sci. 2014;76:439–46.
18. Requicha JF, Viegas CA, Albuquerque CM, Azevedo JM, Reis RL, Gomes ME. Effect of anatomical origin and cell passage number on the stemness and osteogenic differentiation potential of canine adipose-derived stem cells. Stem Cell Rev. 2012;8:1211–22.
19. García-Gómez I, Goldsmith H, Angulo J, Prados A, López-Hervás P, Cuevas B, Dujovny M, Cuevas P. Angiogenic capacity of human omental stem cells. Neurogical Res. 2005;27:807–11.
20. Jung S, Kleineidam B, Kleinheinz J. Regenerative potential of human adipose-derived stromal cells of various origins. J Craniomaxillofac Surg. 2015;43:2144–51.
21. Contador D, Ezquer F, Espinosa M, Arango-Rodriguez M, Puebla C, Sobrevia L, Conget P. Dexamethasone and rosiglitazone are sufficient and necessary for producing functional adipocytes from mesenchymal stem cells. Exp Biol Med (Maywood). 2015;240:1235–46.
22. Vellasamy S, Sandrasaigaran P, Vidyadaran S, George E, Ramasamy R. Isolation and characterisation of mesenchymal stem cells derived from human placenta tissue. World J Stem Cells. 2012;4(6):53–61.
23. Conget PA, Minguell JJ. Phenotypical and functional properties of human bone marrow mesenchymal progenitor cells. J Cell Physiol. 1999;181(1):67–73.
24. Ezquer FE, Ezquer ME, Simon V, Conget P. The antidiabetic effect of MSCs in not impaired by insulin prophylaxis and is not improved by second dose of cells. PLoS One. 2011; doi:10.1371/journal.pone.0016566.
25. Wagner W, Horn P, Castoldi M, Diehlmann A, Bork S, Saffrich R, Benes V, Blake J, Pfister S, Eckstein V, Ho AD. Replicative senescence of mesenchymal stem cells: a continuous and organized process. PLoS One. 2008; doi:10.1371/journal.pone.0002213.
26. Livak KJ, Schmittgen TD. Analysis of relative gene expression data using real-time quantitative PCR and the 2(–Delta Delta C(T)). Method. 2001;25:402–8.
27. Jing L, Rui W, Lei Y, Qi W, Qinwan W, Zhengchao N, Yongchun Y, Ji M, Qiuhui P. Knochdown of nestin inhibits proliferation and migration of colorectal cancer cells. Int J Clin Exp Pathol. 2015;8:6377–86.
28. Ponce ML. Tube formation: an in vitro matrigel angiogenesis assay. Methods Mol Biol. 2009;467:183–8.
29. Yoo KH, Jang IK, Lee MW, Kim HE, Yang MS, Eom Y, Lee JE, Kim YJ, Yang SK, Jung HL, Sung KW, Kim CW, Koo HH. Comparison of immunomodulatory properties of mesenchymal stem cells derived from adult human tissues. Cell Immunol. 2009;259:150–6.
30. Gruber HE, Somayaji S, Riley F, Hoelscher GL, Norton HJ, Ingram J. Human adipose-derived mesenchymal stem cells: serial passaging, doubling time and cell senescence. Biotech Histochem. 2012;87:303–11.
31. Murphy MB, Moncivais K, Caplan AI. Mesenchymal stem cells: environmentally responsive therapeutics for regenerative medicine. Exp Mol Med. 2013; doi:10.1038/emm.2013.94.
32. Haynesworth SE, Baber MA, Caplan AI. Cytokine expression by human marrow-derived mesenchymal progenitor cells *in vitro*: effects of dexamethasone and IL-1 alpha. J Cell Physiol. 1996;166:585–92.
33. Nalldijk Y, Johnson AA, Ishak S, Meisel HJ, Hohaus C, Stolzing A. Migrational changes of mesenchymal stem cells in response to cytokine, growth factors, hypoxia and aging. Exp Cell Res. 2015;338:97–104.
34. Kilroy GE, Foster SJ, Wu X, Ruiz J, Shrwood S, Heifetz A, Ludlow JW, Stricker DM, Potiny S, Green P, Halvorsen YD, Cheatham B, Storms RW, Gimble JM. Cytokine profile of human adipose-derived stem cells: expression of angiogenic, hematopoietic, and pro-inflammatory factors. J Cell Physiol. 2007;212(3):702–9.
35. Antoniades H, Scher C, Stiles C. Purification of human platelet-derived growth factor. Proc Natl Acad Sci U S A. 1979;76:1809–13.
36. Claesson-Welsh L, Ronnstrand L, Heldin C. Biosynthesis and intracellular transport of the receptor for platelet-derived growth factor. Proc Natl Acad Sci U S A. 1987;84:8796–800.
37. Heldin C. Platelet-derived growth factor–an introduction. Cytokine Growth Factor Rev. 2004;15:195–6.
38. Lubinus M, Meier K, Smith E, Gause K, LeRoy E, Trojanowska M. Independent effects of platelet-derived growth factor isoforms on mitogen-activated protein kinase activation and mitogenesis in human dermal fibroblasts. J Biol Chem. 1994;269:9822–5.
39. Walker T, Moore S, Lawson M, Panettieri R, Chilvers E. Platelet-derived growth factor-BB and thrombin activate phosphoinositide 3-kinase and protein kinase B: role in mediating airway smooth muscle proliferation. Mol Pharmacol. 1998;54:1007–15.
40. Bottaro DP, Rubin JS, Faletto DL, et al. Identification of the hepatocyte growth factor receptor as the c-met proto-oncogene product. Science. 1991;251:802–4.
41. Schuldiner M, Yanuka O, Itskovitz-Eldor J, Melton DA, Benvenisty N. Effects of eight growth factors on the differentiation of cells derived from human embryonic stem cells. Proc Natl Acad Sci U S A. 2000;97:11307–12.
42. Neuss S, Becher E, Woltje M, Tietze L, Jahnen-Dechent W. Functional expression of HGF and HGF receptor/c-met in adult human mesenchymal stem cells suggests a role in cell mobilization, tissue repair and wound healing. Stem Cells. 2004;22:405–14.
43. Forte G, Minieri M, Cossa P, Antenucci D, Sala M, Gnocchi V, Fiaccavento R, Carotenuto F, De Vito P, Baldini PM, Prat M, Di Nardo P. Hepatocyte growth factor effects on Mesenchymal stem cells:proliferation, migration, and differentiation. Stem Cells. 2006;24:23–33.
44. Arnold F, West DC. Angiogenesis in wound healing. Pharmacol Ther. 1991; 52:407–22.
45. Fam NP, Verma S, Kutryk M, Stewart DJ. Clinician guide to angiogenesis. Circulation. 2003;108:2613–8.
46. Chen L, Tredget EE, Wu PYG, Wu Y. Paracrine factors of mesenchymal stem cells recruit macrophages and endothelial lineage cells and enhance wound healing. PLoS One. 2008; doi:10.1371/journal.pone.0001886.
47. Pikula M, Langa P, Kosikowska P, Trzonkowski P. Stem cells and growth factors in wound healing. Postepy Hig Med Dosw. 2015;69:874–85.
48. Keating A. How do mesenchymal stromal cells suppress T cells? Cell Stem Cell. 2008;2:106–8.
49. Le Blanc K, Mougiakakos D. Multipotent mesenchymal stromal cells and the innate immune system. Nat Rev Immunol. 2012;12:383–96.
50. English K, Mahon BP. Allogeneic mesenchymal stem cells: agents of immune modulation. J Cell Biochem. 2011;112:1963–8.
51. Munn DH, Zhou M, Attwood JT, Bondarev I, Conway SJ, Marshall B, Brown C, Mellor AL. Prevention of allogeneic fetal rejection by tryptophan catabolism. Science. 1998;281:1191–3.
52. Chinnadurai R, Copland IB, Patel SR, Galipeau J. IDO-independent suppression of T cell effector function by IFN-γ-licensed human mesenchymal stromal cells. J Immunol. 2014;192:1491–501.
53. Yan Z, Zhuansun Y, Chen R, Li J, Ran P. Immunomodulation of mesenchymal stromal cells on regulatory T cells and its possible mechanism. Exp Cell Res. 2014;15:65–74.
54. Bloom DD, Centanni JM, Bhatia N, Emler CA, Drier D, Leverson GE, McKenna DH Jr, Gee AP, Lindblad R, Hei DJ, Hematti P. Cytotherapy. 2015;17:140–51.
55. Selleri S, Dieng MM, Nicoletti S, Louis I, Beausejour C, Le Deist F, Haddad E. Cord-blood-derived mesenchymal stromal cells downmodulate CD4+ T-cell activation by inducing IL-10-producing Th1 cells. Stem Cells Dev. 2013;22:1063–75.
56. Ren G, Su J, Zhang L, Zhao X, Ling W, L'huillie A, Zhang J, Lu Y, Roberts AI, Ji W, Zhang H, Rabson AB, Shi Y. Species variation in the mechanisms of mesenchymal stem cell-mediated immunosuppression. Stem Cells. 2009;27:1954–62.
57. Keating A. Cell how do mesenchymal stromal cells suppress T cells? Stem Cell. 2008;2:106–8.

4

Efficacy and safety of oral robenacoxib (tablet) for the treatment of pain associated with soft tissue surgery in client-owned dogs

Gabriele Friton[1*], Caryn Marie Thompson[2], Daniela Karadzovska[3], Stephen King[2] and Jonathan N. King[1]

Abstract

Background: Non-steroidal anti-inflammatory drugs (NSAIDs) have been proven to be effective in controlling peri-operative pain in dogs. Robenacoxib is an NSAID with high selectivity for the cyclooxygenase (COX)-2 isoform. The objective of this study was to assess the efficacy and safety of an oral tablet formulation of robenacoxib in client-owned dogs undergoing soft tissue surgery. The study was a prospective, multi-center, randomized, masked, placebo-controlled, parallel-group clinical trial. A total of 239 dogs were included and randomly allocated in a 1:1 ratio to receive either robenacoxib or placebo. Each dog received an oral tablet administration of either robenacoxib, at a target dose of 2 mg/kg, or placebo once prior to surgery and for two additional days post-operatively. All dogs also received a pre-anesthetic dose of 0.2 mg/kg butorphanol (intravenous or intramuscular). Pain assessments were performed using the short form of the Glasgow Composite Measure Pain Scale. Robenacoxib was compared to the placebo group on a success/failure basis. Treatment failure was defined as the need for rescue therapy to control post-operative pain.

Results: Significantly ($P = 0.019$) more dogs administered robenacoxib were considered treatment successes (89 of 116, 76.72%) compared to dogs given placebo (74 of 115, 64.35%). The percentage of treatment failure was therefore 23.28% in the robenacoxib and 35.65% in the placebo group. The least squares mean total pain scores were significantly different between groups and in favor of robenacoxib at 3 and 5 hours ($P < 0.05$) and 8 hours post-extubation ($P < 0.01$). Pain at the surgery sites (response to touch) was also significantly improved at 3, 5 and 8 hours post-extubation in dogs receiving robenacoxib versus placebo ($P < 0.01$). In addition, a significant overall improvement in posture/activity was revealed with robenacoxib having lower scores versus placebo ($P < 0.01$). No significant differences between the robenacoxib and placebo groups in the frequency of reported adverse events were observed.

Conclusions: Robenacoxib by oral (tablet) administration was effective and well tolerated in the control of peri-operative pain and inflammation associated with soft tissue surgery in dogs.

Keywords: Analgesia, Dog, NSAID, Robenacoxib, Peri-operative, Soft tissue surgery

* Correspondence: gabriele.friton@elanco.com
[1]Elanco Animal Health Inc., Companion Animal Development, CH-4058 Basel, Switzerland
Full list of author information is available at the end of the article

Background

Non-steroidal anti-inflammatory drugs (NSAIDs) have been proven to be effective in controlling post-operative pain in dogs when used either alone or in combination with opioids [1–3]. Robenacoxib is an NSAID which produces highly selective inhibition of the cyclooxygenase (COX)-2 isoform of COX, and significantly inhibits COX-2 and spares COX-1 in vivo when administered orally at the recommended dosages [4–6]. Robenacoxib has a fast onset of action, achieves maximal blood concentrations within 0.25–0.5 h after both oral and subcutaneous dosing, and has a high bioavailability (84% oral; 88% subcutaneous) [7]. The dose and concentration-effect relationships for single oral doses of robenacoxib over the dose range 0.5–8.0 mg/kg were established in a urate crystal-induced acute synovitis model in dogs; robenacoxib increased the weight-bearing and decreased pain and swelling [6].

The safety of robenacoxib was investigated in the dog in two randomized, placebo-controlled, parallel-group studies. Robenacoxib was administered orally once daily to healthy young beagle dogs at 0 (placebo), 10, 20 and 40 mg/kg for 1 month (Study 1) and at 0 (placebo), 2, 4, 6 and 10 mg/kg for 6 months (Study 2) [8]. Relative to placebo, no significant adverse effects of robenacoxib were recorded in either study for clinical observations, clinical chemistry and hematological variables, and macroscopic or microscopic lesions at necropsy. In Study 2, additional examinations identified no adverse effects of robenacoxib on buccal bleeding time, electrocardiographic and ophthalmoscopic examinations, urinalysis or stifle joint tissues. The lack of adverse events (AEs) at doses as high as 40 mg/kg versus recommended doses ranging from 1 to 4 mg/kg indicates a high safety index of robenacoxib in dogs, attributed to a combination of its high COX-2 selectivity and short residence time in the central compartment [8–10].

In view of its pharmacological properties, robenacoxib has the potential to provide optimal peri-operative pain control in dogs. Previous studies investigated robenacoxib for the management of peri-operative pain and inflammation in dogs undergoing various surgeries [11, 12]. Robenacoxib has been approved for the control of pain and inflammation associated with soft tissue surgery in many countries (e.g. http://www.ema.europa.eu/ema/) [13]. The most recent registration was in the USA (https://www.fda.gov/) [14], which was supported by the results of the study described in this manuscript.

The objective of this study was to demonstrate the field effectiveness and safety of robenacoxib tablets, administered orally at a dose of 2 mg/kg (an inherent dose band of 2–4 mg/kg) once daily for three days, for the control of post-operative pain and inflammation associated with soft tissue surgery in dogs. We hypothesized that robenacoxib administered prior to surgery and for two additional days post-operatively would have superior analgesic effects when compared to a placebo. Efficacy was measured by success/failure criteria based on pain assessments and the need for rescue therapy.

Methods

Study design

The study was a prospective, multi-center, randomized, masked, placebo-controlled, parallel-group clinical trial at 11 companion animal veterinary clinics located at various geographic locations within the USA. The study was conducted in accordance with guidelines for Good Clinical Practice (VICH GL9), Adequate and Well-controlled Studies (21 CFR 514.117), and New Animal Drugs for Investigational Use (21 CFR 511.1).

The protocol was reviewed and approved by the Sponsor's Institutional Animal Care and Use Committee. All owners provided written consent at the pre-enrollment visit (Day −14 to −2) for their dog to enter the study. This manuscript was prepared after consideration of the CONSORT guidelines on randomized trials [15].

Selection criteria

The inclusion criteria comprised dogs aged ≥6 months, either sex, any breed, weighing at least 2.5 kg at the time of enrollment and scheduled to undergo soft tissue surgery (e.g. ovariohysterectomy, cryptorchidectomy, splenectomy, cystotomy, or major external surgeries, such as mastectomy or skin tumor removal (mass ≥ 8 cm in size)). Aside from needing soft tissue surgery, dogs were clinically healthy and had acceptable clinical pathology results as determined by the Investigator. Dogs meeting any of the following exclusion criteria were not enrolled in the study: those that had a known hypersensitivity to NSAIDs or sulfonamide drugs; were being used for breeding, or were pregnant or lactating; were receiving anticonvulsant, behavioral or cardiac medications; were dehydrated or were receiving concomitant diuretic therapy; had existing cardiovascular, gastrointestinal tract, hepatic and/or renal dysfunction; had uncontrolled endocrine or systemic disorders such as diabetes mellitus, hypothyroidism, or other systemic disorders (dogs requiring treatment for diabetes mellitus or hypothyroidism had to be stabilized for at least 28 days prior to enrollment; stable status was documented by clinical pathology); within 14 days prior to enrollment had undergone invasive surgical procedures or procedures that would interfere with an accurate assessment of pain; had a concurrent painful condition other than the presenting condition, which could have interfered with pain assessments; had been treated with topical or systemic anti-inflammatory products such as NSAIDs within 14 days prior to enrollment, short-acting (systemic or local) corticosteroids within 30 days prior to enrollment or long-acting corticosteroids within 60 days prior to enrollment; had been treated with anesthetics, sedatives, tramadol or tranquilizers within 2 days prior to enrollment; exhibited aggressive or frightened behavior that would cause difficulty in clinical examinations, collection of clinical specimens or administration of treatments; had a known intolerance to the anesthetics used in the study or had received alternative forms of pain relief (e.g. acupressure, acupuncture, chiropractic manipulation, clinical therapy) within 14 days prior to enrollment. Dogs belonging to an employee of the sponsoring company or other animal health drug manufacturer, an Investigator or the Food and Drug Administration were also not eligible for enrollment in the study.

Dogs meeting any of the following criteria after inclusion were withdrawn from the study: those that required pain intervention with a Glasgow Composite Measure Pain Scale - Short Form (CMPS-SF) score of ≥6 (considered a treatment failure); exhibited an AE that compromised their ongoing treatment or the integrity of the study; were fractious and unable to continue in the study; received forbidden concomitant treatment; were affected by protocol deviation(s) that compromised the integrity of the study or a disorder that could have interfered with the evaluation of their response to treatment, or for any other reason as determined by the Investigator in consultation with the Sponsor. Owners or Investigators could also decide to withdraw the dog for efficacy or safety reasons and the study could have been stopped by the Sponsor at any time point if required.

Anesthesia and analgesia protocol

All dogs were adequately hydrated prior to and during surgery. As an anesthetic pre-medication, all dogs received intravenous or intramuscular administration of butorphanol at a dose of 0.2 mg/kg body weight after dosing with robenacoxib or placebo approximately 45 min prior to surgery. Agents including propofol, thiopental, sevoflurane and isoflurane were allowed to facilitate induction, maintenance and recovery from anesthesia. Local anesthesia was not permitted for any dog.

Randomization and treatment

Dogs were formally included on Day 0 and allocated randomly to treatment groups in a 1:1 ratio in blocks of four in order of enrollment. Dogs were administered either the oral (tablet) formulation of robenacoxib (Onsior®, Elanco Animal Health, Greenfield, USA) or placebo tablet (Elanco France, Huningue, France) once daily for 3 days. Robenacoxib was administered orally, as whole tablets (10 mg, 20 mg and 40 mg), at a target dose of 2 mg/kg of body weight (an inherent dose band of 2 to 4 mg/kg) once daily for three consecutive days. For the first dose, food was withheld overnight. For the second and third doses, robenacoxib was administered without food or with a small amount of food. The dose administered to each dog was calculated from the pre-anesthetic body weight measured at Day −1 or Day 0. The first treatment was given approximately 45 min prior to surgery at the time of pre-anesthetic medication. Subsequent once daily treatments were given at approximately the same time each day. Re-dosing was performed if the dog vomited within 5 min of administration and the tablet was recognizable in the vomitus. If the dog vomited and the tablet was not recognizable, the dog was not re-dosed. The administration methods for the placebo tablet were the same as those described for robenacoxib tablets.

The randomization list was computer-generated by the statistician using SAS/STAT® software (Version 9, SAS Institute Inc., Cary, NC, USA). Blinding was accomplished by the identical appearance of the tablets (same formulation except that the placebo tablets had no active ingredient) and packaging in both groups, and in addition by separation of functions: a treatment administrator (i.e. dispenser) at each clinic was responsible for dispensation and administration of test items and reconciliation of used and unused products. All study site personnel were masked to treatment assignment except the dispenser.

Clinical examination and follow-up

Clinical examinations were performed at enrollment, at scheduled study completion, in cases of early withdrawal, and for any animal which experienced a serious AE. The examination included a routine assessment of general appearance, major systems and body weight. A description of scheduled study activities is depicted in Table 1.

Surgical procedures

Surgery start time was defined as the time of first (skin) incision. If surgery start time was delayed and was ≥60 min after the first dose of robenacoxib or placebo administration, the Investigator was instructed to stop study procedures, and observe at least a 2-day washout period prior to re-dosing and surgery.

Rescue therapy

Intervention treatment ("rescue therapy") was administered at any time the Investigator determined that a dog was excessively uncomfortable or in pain, and/or a score of ≥6 was determined for the CMPS-SF during pain assessment. Intervention treatment could include any product (except other NSAIDs or corticosteroids) used to control pain.

Table 1 Schedule of study activities

Study Days	Activity
Day −14 to −2	Pre-enrollment visit
	Blood and urine sample collection
Prior to enrollment	Review clinical pathology results for animal eligibility
Day −1 to 0	Physical examination
	Body weight determination
	Begin acclimatization at least 2 h before performing the baseline CMPS-SF assessment
Day 0	Baseline pain assessment using CMPS-SF
	First treatment
	Administration of butorphanol
	Induction of anesthesia, perform soft tissue surgery, extubation
	Pain assessment using CMPS-SF
	- 1.5, 3, 5 and 8 h (± 30 min) post-extubation
	- between scheduled assessments, if pain intervention required[a]
Day 1	Pain assessment using CMPS-SF 24 h (± 1 h) after initial treatment and prior to second treatment
	Second treatment
	Pain assessment using CMPS-SF
	- 2 h and 8 h (± 30 min) post-treatment
	- between scheduled assessments, if pain intervention required[a]
Day 2	Pain assessment using CMPS-SF 48 h (± 1 h) after initial treatment and prior to third treatment
	Third treatment
	Pain assessment using CMPS-SF
	- 2 h and 4 h (± 30 min) post treatment - between scheduled assessments, if pain intervention required[a]
	- if pain intervention not required within 4 h (± 30 min) post treatment: - Exit physical examination - Body weight determination - Blood and urine sample collection
Day 3 to 10 after study exit	Post-study follow up phone call

CMPS-SF Glasgow Composite Measure Pain Scale - Short Form, *h* hours, *min* minutes

[a]if pain intervention required: administer intervention treatment, exit physical examination, determine body weight, collect blood and urine sample, remove dog from the study and monitor in clinic for 24 h

Premature completion and follow-up

Dogs could be withdrawn from the study and/or receive rescue therapy at any time at the discretion of the veterinarian. Dogs receiving intervention treatment were observed in the clinic for a minimum of 24 h post-intervention and any potential AEs were documented. The owners of study dogs received a follow-up phone call approximately 3 to 10 days after normal or premature completion to assess the animal's general well-being.

Efficacy assessments

The primary outcome variable was treatment failure, which was defined as the need for rescue therapy to control post-operative pain or premature withdraw of the dog from the study due to an AE which was considered possibly or probably related to treatment. Need for rescue therapy was decided by the Investigator based on either a score of ≥6 on the CMPS-SF [16] (Appendix) or if the Investigator determined at any time that rescue (pain) therapy was needed. Robenacoxib was compared to the placebo group on a success/failure basis. Investigators were instructed that the same clinician should make all efficacy assessments for all cases at each site.

Secondary outcome variables included the total CMPS-SF score and the six components of the CMPS-SF (vocalization, attention to wound area, mobility, response to touch, demeanor and posture/activity). A categorical score was assigned within each behavior category based on the severity of the behavior or response by the dog.

A baseline evaluation was performed on Day 0 after the dog had acclimatized for at least 2 h in the clinic, and prior to administration of the test items and pre-anesthetic agents. Thereafter evaluations for the primary and secondary outcome variables were conducted: on Day 0 post-surgical extubation at 1.5, 3, 5 and 8 h (±30 min); on Day 1 at 24 h (±1 h) after initial administration and prior to second treatment, and thereafter at 2 and 8 h (±30 min); on Day 2 at 48 h (±1 h) after initial administration and prior to third treatment, and thereafter at 2 and 4 h (±30 min).

Safety assessments

Safety was analyzed in all dogs that had received at least one dose of robenacoxib or placebo, from reported AEs, post-study owner follow-up findings, clinical pathology variables (hematology, serum chemistry and urinalysis) and changes in body weight.

Statistical analysis

The study was planned to include a minimum of 220 dogs, with 110 dogs from each group receiving either robenacoxib or placebo. All analyses were performed using SAS/STAT® software (Version 9.2, SAS Institute Inc., Cary, NC, USA). Unless stated otherwise, data are presented as mean ± standard deviation (SD). Statistical significance was concluded with two-tailed *P* values less than 0.05. The experimental unit was each individual dog.

Primary outcome variable

The primary outcome variable was treatment failure, with superiority established by a statistically significant lower proportion of failures in the robenacoxib group compared to the placebo group. A random effects generalized linear mixed model was utilized (SAS PROC GLIMMIX) with 'treatment' as a fixed effect and 'site' and 'treatment by site' as random effects. The analysis involved a binary response; therefore a binomial distribution with a logit link was utilized. The covariance was modeled using the variance components structure. All sites had multiple evaluable subjects in each treatment group (at least 8 evaluable cases per site) and were therefore included in the primary efficacy analysis.

In addition, the 'time to rescue therapy' for each dog was assessed via a Kaplan-Meier time to event plot with comparison of groups using the log-rank, generalized Wilcoxon and likelihood ratio tests (SAS PROC LIFETEST).

Secondary outcome variables

A total pain score was calculated for each animal at each time point as the sum of the pain category scores at that time where total pain score = vocalization + attention to wound area (surgical site) + mobility + response to touch + demeanor + posture/activity scores.

The last observation carried forward (LOCF) method was applied to the data for the first 8 h after extubation for any animal that required rescue therapy on the day of surgery. Repeated measures analysis of covariance (RMANCOVA; SAS PROC MIXED) was utilized with 'treatment', 'time' and 'treatment x time' as fixed effects, and 'site' and 'treatment x site', 'site x time', and 'treatment x site x time' as random effects. The pre-treatment total pain score was included in the model as a fixed covariate. Models incorporating the covariance structures Compound Symmetry and Heterogeneous Compound Symmetry were explored, with the structure yielding the lower Akaike Information Criterion selected for the final analysis.

The individual component variables contributing to the total pain score were also analyzed using LOCF data from the day of surgery (extubation to hour 8) and the same statistical model described for the total pain score analysis.

The Shapiro Wilks test (SAS PROC UNIVARIATE) was used to assess normality of the residuals from the linear mixed models for total pain score and each of the contributing component variables. Where non-normality was observed, the non-parametric Wilcoxon Rank Sum test was used to compare the groups.

Body weight was evaluated statistically using analysis of covariance (ANCOVA; SAS PROC MIXED) with the pre-treatment body weight used as a covariate. The model included the fixed effect of 'treatment'. In addition, summary statistics for body weight at baseline and at study exit, and the difference between the study exit and baseline body weights, were calculated for each group.

Hematology, serum chemistry, and urinalysis variables were evaluated statistically using ANCOVA (SAS PROC MIXED) with the pre-treatment value as covariate. The model included the fixed effect of 'treatment', with 'site' and the interaction 'treatment x site' as random effects.

The incidence of AEs in the two groups was compared with Fisher's Exact test (SAS PROC FREQ).

Results

Study dogs and drugs administered

A total of 239 client-owned dogs were enrolled in the study (119 dogs received robenacoxib and 120 received placebo) and included in the demographic and safety analyses. Efficacy analyses were performed on 231 animals (116 in the robenacoxib group and 115 in the placebo group). The number of cases enrolled per investigational site for safety (efficacy) analyses was 1(0), 10 (9), 10 (10), 11 (11), 20 (19), 20 (20), 24 (22), 28 (28), 30 (28), 41 (41) and 44 (43). Eight cases were excluded from the efficacy analyses due to the use of forbidden concomitant treatments (n = 2), staff-owned pet (n = 2), surgery complications leading to death/euthanasia (n = 2), inaccurate dosing (n = 1) and insufficient number of enrolled cases at site (n = 1).

Demographic and baseline variables are shown in Table 2. Differences between groups were not significant, and it was concluded that the randomization had effectively created balanced groups.

The mean (range) ages of dogs were 6.2 years (6 months to 14 years) in the robenacoxib group and 5.5 years (6 months to 16 years) in the placebo group. The weight range at pre-treatment was 2.7–55.0 kg in the robenacoxib group and 3.2–63.7 kg in the placebo group. There were more female than male dogs in the study.

The most common breeds were Labrador Retriever, Golden Retriever, Mix-Labrador Retriever and Shih Tzu. The predominant soft tissue surgeries in both treatment groups were skin tumor removal of mass ≥ 8 cm in size (n = 70), ovariohysterectomy (n = 55), cystotomy (n = 35) and gastropexy (n = 28).

All cases received butorphanol as a pre-operative medication. Propofol was used as the anesthesia medication for induction; isoflurane and sevoflurane were used as the anesthesia mediations for maintenance. Antibiotics were administered to 55.7% of dogs at the time of surgery. The most frequently used concomitant treatments were analgesics, fluids and antibacterials.

Primary outcome variable

During the study, a total of 163 dogs were considered treatment success with 89 of 116 cases (76.72%) in the

Table 2 Demographic, breed and surgery variables; data are mean (± SD) or number of dogs (%)

Variable	Robenacoxib	Placebo	Total	*P* value*
Number of dogs	119 (49.8%)	120 (50.2%)	239 (100.0%)	
Age (years)	6.2 (±4.3)	5.5 (±3.8)	5.8 (±4.0)	0.23
Body weight (kg), pre-enrollment	20.0 (±12.2)	22.9 (±15.1)	21.5 (±13.8)	0.10
Sex and neutered status				0.068
Female intact	40 (33.6%)	33 (27.5%)	73 (30.5%)	
Female spayed	36 (30.3%)	34 (28.3%)	70 (29.3%)	
Male intact	7 (5.9%)	20 (16.7%)	27 (11.3%)	
Male castrated	36 (30.3%)	33 (27.5%)	69 (28.9%)	
Breed				0.65
Labrador Retriever	11 (9.2%)	14 (11.7%)	25 (10.5%)	
Golden Retriever	10 (8.4%)	5 (4.2%)	15 (6.3%)	
Mix-Labrador Retriever	5 (4.2%)	7 (5.8%)	12 (5.0%)	
Shih Tzu	6 (5.0%)	5 (4.2%)	11 (4.6%)	
Various other breeds	87 (73.1%)	89 (74.2%)	176 (73.6%)	
Type of surgery				0.62
Skin tumor removal (≥ 8 cm in size)	31 (26.1%)	39 (32.5%)	70 (29.3%)	
Ovariohysterectomy	29 (24.4%)	26 (21.7%)	55 (23.0%)	
Cystotomy	18 (15.1%)	17 (14.2%)	35 (14.6%)	
Gastropexy	12 (10.1%)	16 (13.3%)	28 (11.7%)	
Other soft tissue surgery	29 (24.4%)	22 (18.3%)	51 (21.3%)	

*Significance of differences between treatment groups (based on t-test for continuous variables and χ^2 test for categorical variables)

robenacoxib group compared to 74 of 115 cases (64.35%) in the placebo group. The percentage of treatment failure was therefore 23.28% with robenacoxib and 35.65% with placebo. There was a significant difference in the proportion of success/failures in the robenacoxib group compared to the placebo group (P = 0.019) (Table 3). All treatment failures were due to administration of rescue therapy with CMPS-SF scores ≥6; no dogs received rescue therapy with a CMPS-SF <6 and none were classified as a treatment failure due an AE.

Table 3 Primary outcome variable: the frequency of success and failure outcomes by group

Group	Outcome		Total	*P* value
	Success	Failure (Withdrawn from study)		
Robenacoxib	89 (76.72%)	27 (23.28%)	116	0.019
Placebo	74 (64.35%)	41 (35.65%)	115	
Total	163	68	231	

The Kaplan-Meier plot of 'time to rescue analgesia therapy' is presented in Fig. 1. All rescues occurred at or before 8 h post-extubation, with 51/68 (75.0%) at ≤1.5 h, 64/68 (94.1%) at ≤3 h and 65/68 (95.6%) at ≤5 h. The number of dogs receiving rescue therapy at the 1.5, 3, 5 and 8 h time points (or in the interval since the previous time point) was respectively 23, 3, 1 and 0 in the robenacoxib group (total 27) and 28, 10, 0 and 3 in the placebo group (total 41).

In the time to event analysis, the log-rank and likelihood ratio tests were both statistically significant (P = 0.046 and P = 0.016) in favor of the robenacoxib group, while the generalized Wilcoxon test also provided some evidence of a favorable effect of robenacoxib (P = 0.072). The robenacoxib group had a lower probability of failures (rescues) beginning at 1.5 h post-extubation and at all subsequent remaining time periods compared to the placebo group.

Secondary outcome variables

The least squares mean (LSMean) total pain scores showed statistically significant differences between groups and in favor of robenacoxib (experiencing less pain) at 3 and 5 h (P < 0.05) and 8 h post-extubation (P < 0.01) (Fig. 2, Table 4), including the mean total pain score (with LOCF) over time between both groups. Analyses for the six individual components contributing to the total pain score using analogous models were conducted, again utilizing LOCF through the first 8 h after extubation (Table 4). Pain at the surgery sites (response to touch) was significantly improved at 3, 5 and 8 h post-extubation in dogs receiving robenacoxib versus placebo (P < 0.01). Furthermore, a significant overall improvement in posture/activity was revealed with robenacoxib having lower scores versus placebo (P < 0.01).

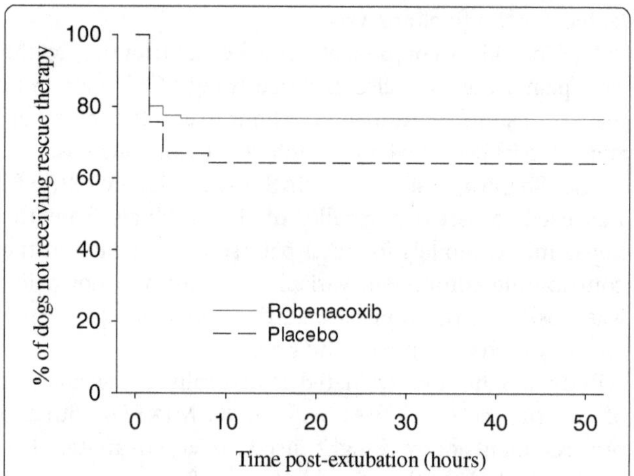

Fig. 1 Kaplan-Meier plot of time to rescue analgesia therapy

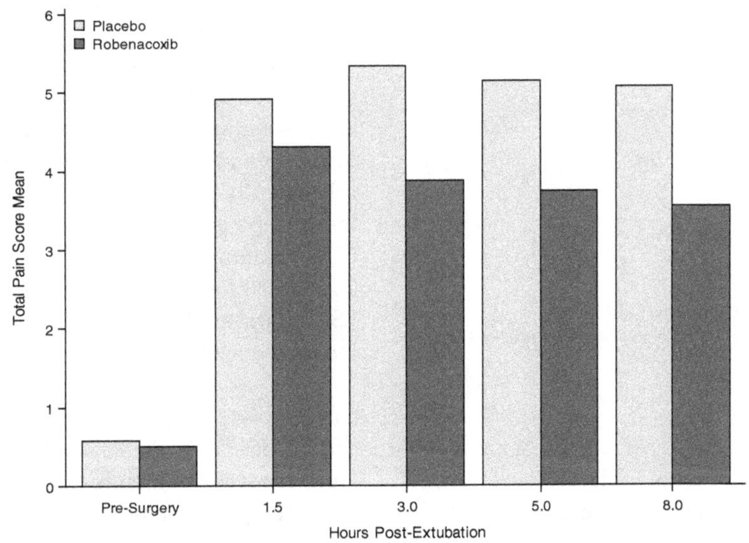

Fig. 2 Mean total pain score

Significant non-normality ($P < 0.01$) was detected in the residuals from the linear mixed models for total pain score and each of the component variables contributing to the total score. Re-analysis for each of these variables using the Wilcoxon Rank Sum test produced similar results to those obtained via the generalized linear model (Table 4).

Other observations

The percentage of dogs receiving rescue therapy by the predominant surgery types skin tumor removal, ovariohysterectomy, cystotomy and gastropexy was respectively 22.6%, 20.7%, 11.1% and 30.8% in the robenacoxib group and 21.1%, 39.1%, 37.5% and 44.4% in the placebo group.

Table 4 Secondary outcome variables

Variable	Time Point (Day: Time)	Robenacoxib LSMean	Placebo LSMean	LSMean Difference	*P* value (RMANCOVA)	*P* value (Wilcoxon Rank Sum)
Total Pain Score	0: 1.5 h	3.89	4.53	−0.648	0.27	0.558
	0: 3 h	3.44	4.95	−1.51	0.011*	0.003**
	0: 5 h	3.32	4.76	−1.44	0.015*	0.008**
	0: 8 h	3.12	4.69	−1.56	0.008**	0.014*
Vocalization	Overall[a]	0.252	0.309	−0.057	0.55	0.482
Attention to Wound/Surgical Site	Overall[a]	0.166	0.208	−0.042	0.47	0.435
Mobility	0: 1.5 h	0.960	0.867	0.093	0.57	0.276
	0: 3 h	0.745	0.945	−0.200	0.18	0.392
	0: 5 h	0.668	0.936	−0.268	0.072	0.170
	0: 8 h	0.607	0.884	−0.276	0.058	0.132
Response to Touch	0: 1.5 h	0.878	1.22	−0.342	0.098	0.128
	0: 3 h	0.846	1.46	−0.612	0.003**	0.001**
	0: 5 h	0.843	1.45	−0.612	0.003**	0.002**
	0: 8 h	0.796	1.48	−0.682	0.001**	0.001**
Demeanor	Overall[a]	0.995	1.13	−0.138	0.17	0.251
Posture/Activity	Overall[b]	0.463	0.816	−0.353	0.006**	0.028*

The Last Observation Carried Forward (LOCF) method was used (see Methods); *h* hour, *LSMean* Least Squares Mean

LSMean difference = *LSMean* of the robenacoxib group - *LSMean* of the placebo group, *RMANCOVA* Repeated Measures Analysis Of Covariance

[a]Treatment x time interaction was not statistically significant ($P > 0.05$). Therefore, results for the main effect of treatment are presented. The Wilcoxon rank sum test was performed on the median scores for each component obtained for each dog over the period 1.5 h to 8.0 h post-extubation

[b]Treatment x time interaction was not statistically significant ($P = 0.11$). However, a statistically significant overall effect of treatment was observed ($P = 0.006$ via RMANCOVA; $P = 0.028$ via the Wilcoxon rank sum test)

*Statistically significant at $P < 0.05$

**Statistically significant at $P < 0.01$

Table 5 Adverse events reported during the study

Adverse event[a]	Robenacoxib		Placebo		*P* value
	N	% of total (*n* = 119)	*N*	% of total (*n* = 120)	
Vomiting	6	5.0%	4	3.3%	0.544
Diarrhea	6	5.0%	3	2.5%	0.330
Decreased appetite	3	2.5%	0	0%	0.122
Weight loss	1	0.84%	0	0%	0.505
Hypotension	1	0.84%	0	0%	0.505

P values were calculated with the Fisher's Exact test

[a]Dogs may have experienced more than one type or occurrences of an event

Safety - adverse events

A summary of the number and percentage of cases with each reported AE is depicted in Table 5. The frequency of dogs with recorded AEs did not differ significantly between the two groups (P = 0.100). Gastrointestinal tract disorders (particularly diarrhea and vomiting) were the most commonly observed AEs in both groups. Three serious AEs were reported (one case in the robenacoxib group and two cases in the placebo group). One dog treated with robenacoxib died due to circulatory collapse after surgical resection of a chronic intestinal blockage with extensive tissue devitalization. One placebo-treated dog was euthanized due to diagnosis of advanced neoplasia during surgery. These two cases were considered unrelated to treatment. Finally, one dog in the placebo group had dramatically elevated liver enzymes at study exit; follow up blood work showed these returned to values within or close to normal ranges.

A total of 10 post-intervention AEs were experienced in 2 dogs in the robenacoxib group and in 6 dogs in the placebo group. In the robenacoxib group, one dog had diarrhea, while vomiting was reported in a second dog. In the placebo group, two dogs vomited, two dogs had elevated liver enzymes, one dog showed signs of redness and swelling at the surgical site, and for one dog hematoma at the dorsal aspect of the incision was reported with grade II lameness of the left hind limb and painful general appearance.

Based on results from follow-up phone calls, owners reported abnormal findings in 29 dogs (12 dogs that received robenacoxib and 17 dogs that received placebo). The majority of signs reported were consistent with those associated with surgery (e.g. local swelling at surgical site, skin and tissue infection or inflammation) or digestive tract disorders (e.g. vomiting and diarrhea).

Safety - clinical pathology

Summary data for selected hepatic, hematologic and renal variables are shown in Table 6. Mean values for all hepatic and hematology variables at pre-treatment and study exit were within the normal reference ranges in both groups. There were no significant differences between the robenacoxib and placebo groups.

In both groups, mean values for all serum chemistry and urine variables were within normal reference ranges at pre-treatment and study exit, with the exception of blood urea nitrogen (BUN)/creatinine ratio (higher in the robenacoxib group, P = 0.035) and urine pH (higher in the placebo group, P = 0.018). The LSMean difference in BUN/creatinine ratio for both groups at study exit was 2.23 (19.70 for robenacoxib versus 17.47 for placebo). The LSM difference for urine pH at study exit was −0.24 (6.52 for robenacoxib versus 6.76 for placebo).

Safety - body weight change

The change in body weight was similar between groups (i.e. body weight at study exit minus body weight at baseline). There were no significant (P = 0.512) differences in mean study exit body weight between the robenacoxib and placebo groups after adjusting for pre-enrollment body weight.

Discussion

Robenacoxib tablets, administered orally at a dose of 2 mg/kg (an inherent dose band of 2–4 mg/kg) prior to soft tissue surgery and again once daily for up to two days after surgery, provided superior analgesic effects when compared to a placebo as measured by the need for rescue therapy. There was a statistically significant reduction in the proportion of dogs requiring rescue therapy (P = 0.019) in favor of robenacoxib (23.28%) compared to placebo (35.65%). Furthermore, oral robenacoxib administration was well tolerated.

The study was designed as a prospective, multi-center, randomized, masked, placebo-controlled, parallel-group clinical trial. The study was adequately powered as superiority of robenacoxib versus placebo was statistically proven for the primary outcome variable with a balanced 1:1 ratio of cases between the two treatment groups.

All surgical procedures were performed by experienced surgeons from 11 clinics at different locations in the USA. Dogs enrolled were of various breeds and the types of soft tissue surgery performed are representative of cases in general practice. More female dogs were enrolled than male dogs due to the inclusion and exclusion criteria, i.e., including ovariohysterectomy but not castration (the later surgery type considered to be less painful) [1]. Efforts were taken to minimize the pain potentially suffered by dogs receiving placebo. All dogs were hospitalized and received butorphanol as pre-anesthetic medication pre-operatively, there were relatively frequent obligatory observation time points and rescue (pain) therapy could be given any time at the veterinarians' discretion.

It is generally accepted that surgery-associated pain is most severe in the early post-operative period [2, 3],

Table 6 Selected hepatic, hematologic and renal variables at pre-treatment and study exit (mean ± SD)

Variable (Laboratory reference range)	Time	Robenacoxib (*n* = 118)			Placebo (*n* = 119)			*P* value
		Mean (±SD)	Cases[a]		Mean (±SD)	Cases[a]		
			High	Low		High	Low	
Serum								
Urea nitrogen, mg/dL (6–31 mg/dL)	Pre-Treatment	18.1 (±7.3)	5	0	18.3 (±6.5)	5	0	0.078
	Study Exit	14.9 (±4.8)	1	0	13.6 (±4.1)	0	0	
Creatinine, mg/dL (0.5–1.6 mg/dL)	Pre-Treatment	0.91 (±0.25)	2	1	0.96 (±0.28)	2	2	0.763
	Study Exit	0.79 (±0.21)	0	5	0.81 (±0.20)	0	1	
Alkaline phosphatase, U/L (5–131 U/L)	Pre-Treatment	141.8 (±239.7)	26	0	112.0 (±214.7)	23	0	0.233
	Study Exit	162.1 (±281.5)	30	0	116.4 (±176.3)	21	0	
Alanine aminotransferase, U/L (12–118 U/L)	Pre-Treatment	55.3 (±41.6)	6	0	54.0 (±50.0)	7	1	0.613
	Study Exit	53.7 (±49.4)	5	0	59.1 (±101.2)	5	1	
Aspartate aminotransferase, U/L (15–66 U/L)	Pre-Treatment	29.6 (±10.5)	1	1	28.8 (±7.8)	0	1	0.449
	Study Exit	37.5 (±46.6)	6	1	41.7 (±41.3)	11	0	
Total bilirubin, mg/dL (0.1–0.3 mg/dL)	Pre-Treatment	0.14 (±0.06)	1	0	0.15 (±0.05)	0	0	0.431
	Study Exit	0.15 (±0.07)	3	0	0.15 (±0.07)	2	0	
Total protein, g/dL (5.0–7.4 g/dL)	Pre-Treatment	6.6 (±0.54)	7	0	6.5 (±0.57)	7	0	0.806
	Study Exit	6.4 (±0.53)	4	0	6.4 (±0.57)	6	0	
Albumin, g/dL (2.7–4.4 g/dL)	Pre-Treatment	3.6 (±0.34)	0	1	3.6 (±0.34)	0	1	0.501
	Study Exit	3.5 (±0.32)	0	1	3.4 (±0.36)	0	2	
Hematology								
Hemoglobin, g/dL (12.1–20.3 g/dL)	Pre-Treatment	16.2 (±2.1)	2	3	16.4 (±1.8)	0	1	0.380
	Study Exit	15.1 (±1.8)	0	8	15.0 (±1.8)	0	8	
Hematocrit, % (36–60%)	Pre-Treatment	49.8 (±6.4)	5	1	50.2 (±5.5)	2	0	0.302
	Study Exit	46.5 (±5.2)	0	5	46.2 (±4.9)	1	1	
Red blood cell count, 10^{12}/L (4.8–9.3 10^{12}/L)	Pre-Treatment	6.8 (±0.89)	0	0	6.9 (±0.76)	0	0	0.406
	Study Exit	6.3 (±0.78)	0	2	6.4 (±0.70)	0	0	
White blood cell count, 10^9/L (4.0–15.5 10^9/L)	Pre-Treatment	10.9 (±3.7)	13	0	10.4 (±3.0)	6	1	0.454
	Study Exit	13.5 (±4.0)	32	0	13.6 (±4.4)	37	0	
Urine								
Urine specific gravity (1.015–1.050)	Pre-Treatment	1.03 (±0.02)	23	8	1.03 (±0.01)	13	15	0.839
	Study Exit	1.04 (±0.02)	27	5	1.04 (±0.02)	25	5	

P values were obtained from an analysis of covariance of the study exit values for each variable, with the pre-treatment value for each variable used as a covariate. Only cases for which both pre-treatment and study exit results were available were included in the analysis

[a]Number of cases with values higher and lower than the reference range pre-treatment and at study exit

and then decreases with time as inflammation subsides and healing occurs. In several studies the duration of post-operative assessments did not proceed beyond 24 h after surgery [17–21] or was considerably shorter, lasting only a few hours after tracheal extubation [22]. Furthermore, it is recommended to start analgesic therapy before the potentially painful event rather than attempt to regain control of pain after it occurs [23–27]. Depending on the surgery type, the perception of pain can be different [1]. Interestingly, in our study the percentage of dogs requiring rescue therapy was highest after gastropexy in both groups indicating that pain was perceived to be more severe for this surgery type.

Behavioral assessments were performed as accurately as manageable under practical field conditions, and pain assessments were made using the CMPS-SF. Dogs were hospitalized throughout the study and kept in a quiet location. The assessments for the primary outcome variable were based on the opinion of the clinician and not of the owner. To ensure interpretative consistency for pain assessments, the person selected to evaluate the efficacy variables was trained and was the same individual for each assessment from the Day 0 clinical baseline to study exit for a given animal. The CMPS-SF was selected as it is a validated composite scale for assessing acute pain in dogs in a hospital setting based on observations and behaviors [2, 16, 21, 28]. In addition, the CMPS-SF provides guidance with regard to need for analgesia i.e. rescue therapy is required if the total score is 6 or greater. In this study, no case was judged by the Investigators to require rescue therapy with a CMPS-SF < 6, although it was permitted at any time at the discretion of the Investigators.

A limitation of the study was that analyses of the secondary outcome variables were challenging due to the unequal frequency of withdrawal of cases after administration of rescue therapy between the two groups, with the placebo group having more rescues within the first 8 h than those dogs treated with robenacoxib. The data were therefore analyzed using the LOCF method. The LOCF method [29] has limitations, but was justified in this study since it was used for cases proactively withdrawn due to lack of efficacy and for a limited period (up to 8 h post-extubation).

Robenacoxib, like other NSAIDs, decreases inflammation, but direct measurement of inflammation is generally not possible in clinical studies as the principle site of inflammation is frequently not visible. Inflammation was evaluated indirectly in our study as part of the CMPS-SF. Robenacoxib has been shown to have anti-inflammatory properties, evidenced from inhibition of swelling in model studies in rodents [10] and dogs [5, 6].

The efficacy of various NSAIDs in peri-operative pain management has been investigated previously in clinical studies in dogs [11, 12, 25, 26]. Comparison of results between studies is difficult due to different study designs, anesthetic procedures, concomitant drugs, NSAID treatment durations, types of surgeries as well as pain assessment methods. In a previous study, the efficacy of robenacoxib and meloxicam was investigated in dogs undergoing soft tissue surgery [12]. The efficacy of robenacoxib was at least as good (i.e. statistically non-inferior) to the positive control, meloxicam. In that study, pain and inflammation were assessed subjectively by clinicians using the Glasgow Composite Pain Scale (GCPS) [30]; unweighted results were reported since weighting factors for the indices had not been published at the time the study was initiated [21, 28]. There were no specific criteria defined when rescue therapy should be used and no dog received such therapy. The effect of two other NSAIDs, administered as a single oral dose pre-surgery followed by 2 days post-surgery, for the control of pain and inflammation in soft tissue surgery in dogs was investigated in the following two studies. For firocoxib, superior efficacy versus a negative control was reported with a comparable design to our study and pain assessment using the CMPS-SF [26]. The frequency of rescue therapy was 16.4% for the active and 50.0% for the negative control. For deracoxib, superior efficacy versus a placebo control was reported. The frequency of rescue therapy was 12.5% (2/16) compared to placebo 56.3% (9/16) [25]. However in that study, pain was assessed using a different method (GCPS). The incidence of rescue therapy (range 12.5 to 23.28%) in clinical trials testing NSAIDs in dogs undergoing soft tissue surgery indicates that pain is a complex phenomenon which may differ between individuals [3] and, although NSAIDs provide an important contribution to pain management, it is not surprising that NSAIDs alone may not produce optimal results. It is well established that optimal peri-operative pain management regimens should incorporate drugs from several classes i.e. multi-modal therapy [1, 3].

Reported AEs, clinical pathology variables and results of clinical examinations by the Investigators indicated that oral administration of robenacoxib was well tolerated. The most frequently reported AEs were gastrointestinal tract disorders such as vomiting and diarrhea.

Robenacoxib has a good safety index in healthy dogs, producing no biologically relevant toxicity at oral doses as high as 40 mg/kg daily for 1 month and up to 10 mg/kg daily for 6 months [8]. There was no evidence from this study of any toxicity of robenacoxib to target organs that are most sensitive to NSAID toxicity (gastrointestinal tract, kidney and liver). Although some statistically significant differences in clinical chemistry (BUN/creatinine ratio was higher in the robenacoxib group) and urinalysis (pH was higher in the placebo group) were found between groups, the means of all these variables remained within normal clinical ranges at the end of the study and findings were not considered to be clinically relevant.

Conclusions

Robenacoxib by oral (tablet) administration at a target dose of 2 mg/kg (an inherent dose band of 2–4 mg/kg) prior to soft tissue surgery and again once daily for up to two days after surgery was effective and well tolerated in the control of peri-operative pain and inflammation in dogs undergoing soft tissue surgeries.

Appendix

The short form of the Glasgow Composite Measure Pain Scale (CMPS-SF) [16] used by the clinicians to assess the dogs

Circumstance	Assessment and Scale
Look at the dog in kennel	Vocalization: Is the dog: [0] quiet [1] crying or whimpering [2] groaning [3] screaming Attention to wound area: Is the dog: [0] ignoring any wound or painful area [1] looking at wound or painful area [2] licking wound or painful area [3] rubbing wound or painful area [4] chewing wound or painful area
Dog out of kennel on lead	Mobility: When the dog rises/walks is it: [0] normal [1] lame [2] slow or reluctant [3] stiff [4] it refuses to move
Response to touch	Response to touch: Does the dog: [0] do nothing [1] look around [2] flinch [3] growl or guard area [4] snap [5] cry
Overall assessment	Demeanor: Is the dog: [0] happy and content or happy and bouncy [1] quiet [2] indifferent or non-responsive to surroundings [3] nervous or anxious or fearful [4] depressed or non-responsive to stimulation Posture: Is the dog: [0] comfortable [1] unsettled [2] restless [3] hunched or tense [4] rigid

Abbreviations

AE: Adverse Event; ANCOVA: Analysis Of Covariance; BUN: Blood Urea Nitrogen; CMPS-SF: Glasgow Composite Measure Pain Scale - Short Form; COX: Cyclooxygenase; GCPS: Glasgow Composite Pain Scale; LOCF: Last Observation Carried Forward; LSMean: Least Squares Mean; NSAID: Non-Steroidal Anti-Inflammatory Drug; RMANCOVA: Repeated Measures Analysis Of Covariance; SD: Standard Deviation

Acknowledgements

The authors thank Drs Butan, Buzhardt, Daigle, Dinges, Fly, Geller, Lively, Lukof, Phillips, Sifferman and Trevor for undertaking the clinical work; the staff at Midwest Veterinary Services Inc. for monitoring the study; Dr. Stephen Bienhoff for work on the protocol; Shane Coble for data management; Dr. Elizabeth Roberts for compiling the safety assessment; Dr. Theresa Real for support on the study protocol and preliminary analysis.

Funding

Not applicable. The role of the sponsor was to lead all activities associated with the conduct of the study (design the study protocol, manage the study with the contract research organization, conduct the statistical analysis and compile the study report).

Authors' contributions

The study was designed by DK, SK and JNK. DK managed the study with the contract research organization and compiled the study report. CT conducted the statistical analysis. All authors interpreted the results. GF drafted the manuscript. All authors contributed to later versions and agreed with the manuscript.

Competing interests

All authors are employees of Elanco Animal Health, a division of Eli-Lilly and company, which manufactures and markets robenacoxib (Onsior®).

Consent for publication

Not applicable.

Author details

[1]Elanco Animal Health Inc., Companion Animal Development, CH-4058 Basel, Switzerland. [2]Elanco Animal Health Inc., Companion Animal Development, Greenfield, IN 46140, USA. [3]Elanco Australasia Pty Limited, Food Animal Development, Kemps Creek, NSW 2178, Australia.

References

1. Mathews K, Kronen PW, Lascelles D, Nolan A, Robertson S, Steagall PV, et al. Guidelines for recognition, assessment and treatment of pain. J Small Anim Pract. 2014;55:E10–68.
2. Berry SH. Analgesia in the perioperative period. Vet Clin Small Anim. 2015;45:1013–27.
3. Epstein M, Rodan I, Griffenhagen G, Kadrlik J, Petty M, Robertson S, et al. AAHA/AAFP pain management guidelines for dogs and cats. J Am Anim Hosp Assoc. 2015;51:67–84.
4. King JN, Rudaz C, Borer L, Jung M, Seewald W, Lees P. In vitro and ex vivo inhibition of canine cyclooxygenase isoforms by robenacoxib: a comparative study. Res Vet Sci. 2010;88:497–506.
5. Schmid VB, Spreng DE, Seewald W, Jung M, Lees P, King JN. Analgesic and anti-inflammatory actions of robenacoxib in acute joint inflammation in the dog. J Vet Pharmacol Therap. 2010;33:118–31.
6. Borer LR, Seewald W, Peel JE, King JN. Evaluation of the dose-response relationship of oral robenacoxib in urate crystal-induced acute stifle synovitis in dogs. J Vet Pharmacol Therap. doi:10.1111/jvp.12348.
7. Jung M, Lees P, Seewald W, King JN. Analytical determination and pharmacokinetics of robenacoxib in the dog. J Vet Pharmacol Therap. 2009;32:41–8.
8. King JN, Arnaud JP, Goldenthal EI, Gruet P, Jung M, Seewald W, et al. Robenacoxib in the dog: target species safety in relation to extent and duration of inhibition of COX-1 and COX-2. J Vet Pharmacol Therap. 2011;34:298–311.
9. Brune K, Furst DE. Combining enzyme specificity and tissue selectivity of cyclooxygenase inhibitors: towards better tolerability? Rheumatol. 2007;46:911–9.
10. King JN, Dawson J, Esser RE, Fujimoto R, Kimble EF, Maniara W, et al. Preclinical pharmacology of robenacoxib: a novel selective inhibitor of cyclooxygenase-2. J Vet Pharmacol Therap. 2009;32:1–17.
11. Gruet P, Seewald W, King JN. Evaluation of subcutaneous and oral administration of robenacoxib and meloxicam for the treatment of acute pain and inflammation associated with orthopedic surgery in dogs. Am J Vet Res. 2011;72:184–93.
12. Gruet P, Seewald W, King JN. Robenacoxib versus meloxicam for the management of pain and inflammation associated with soft tissue surgery in dogs: a randomized, non-inferiority clinical trial. BMC Vet Res. 2013;9:92.
13. Onsior Summary of Product Characteristics. European Public Assessment Report (EPAR). The European Medicines Agency. EMEA/V/C/127, 2008. Accessed Aug 2014.

14. Onsior Freedom of Information Summary. U.S. Food and Drug Administration (FOI). NADA 141–463, May 2016.
15. CONSORT 2010 Checklist of information to include when reporting a randomised trial. www.consort-statement.org. Accessed 10 Feb 2015.
16. Reid J, Nolan AM, Hughes JML, Lascelles D, Dawson P, Scott EM. Development of the short-form Glasgow composite measure pain scale (CMPS-SF) and derivation of an analgesic intervention score. Anim Welf. 2007;16(S):97–104.
17. Conzemius MG, Hill CM, Sammarco JL, Perkowski SZ. Correlation between subjective and objective measures used to determine severity of postoperative pain in dogs. Am Vet Med Assoc. 1997;210:1619–22.
18. Hardie EM, Hansen BD, Carroll GS. Behaviour after ovariohysterectomy in the dog: what's normal? Appl Anim Behav Sci. 1997;51:111–28.
19. Lascelles BD, Cripps PJ, Jones A, Waterman AE. Post-operative central hypersensitivity and pain: the pre-emptive value of pethidine for ovariohysterectomy. Pain. 1997;73:461–71.
20. Kyles AE, Hardie EM, Hansen BD, Papich MG. Comparison of transdermal fentanyl and intramuscular oxymorphone on post-operative behaviour after ovariohysterectomy in dogs. Res Vet Sci. 1998;65:245–51.
21. Morton CM, Reid J, Scott EM, Holton LL, Nolan AM. Application of a scaling model to establish and validate an interval pain scale for assessment of acute pain in dogs. Am J Vet Res. 2005;66:2154–66.
22. Fox SM, Mellor JD, Stafford KJ, Lowoko CR, Hodge H. The effects of ovariohysterectomy plus different combination of halothane anaesthesia and butorphanol analgesia on behaviour in the bitch. Res Vet Sci. 2000;68:265–74.
23. Welsh EM, Nolan AM, Reid J. Beneficial effects of administering carprofen before surgery in dogs. Vet Rec. 1997;141:251–3.
24. Lascelles BDX, Cripps PJ, Jones A, Waterman-Pearson AE. Efficacy and kinetics of carprofen, administered preoperatively or postoperatively, for the prevention of pain in dogs undergoing ovariohysterectomy. Vet Surg. 1998;27:568–82.
25. Bienhoff SE, Smith ES, Roycroft LM, Roberts ES. Efficacy and safety of deracoxib for control of postoperative pain and inflammation associated with soft tissue surgery in dogs. Vet Surg. 2012;41:336–44.
26. Kondo Y, Takashima K, Matsumoto S, Shiba M, Otsuki T, Kinoshita G, et al. Efficacy and safety of firocoxib for the treatment of pain associated with soft tissue surgery in dogs under field conditions in Japan. J Vet Med Sci. 2012;74:1283–9.
27. Delgado C, Bentley E, Hetzel S, Smith LJ. Carprofen provides better post-operative analgesia than tramadol in dogs after enucleation: a randomized, masked clinical trial. J Am Vet Med Assoc. 2014;245:1375–81.
28. Murrell JC, Psatha EP, Scott EM, Reid J, Hellebrekers LJ. Application of a modified form of the Glasgow pain scale in a veterinary teaching centre in the Netherlands. Vet Rec. 2008;162:403–8.
29. Kim Y. Missing data handling in chronic pain trials. J Biopharm Stat. 2011;21:311–25.
30. Holton L, Reid J, Scott EM, Pawson P, Nolan A. Development of a behaviour-based scale to measure acute pain in dogs. Vet Rec. 2001;148:525–31.

Antimicrobial resistance patterns of *Staphylococcus* species isolated from cats presented at a veterinary academic hospital in South Africa

Daniel Nenene Qekwana[1], Dikeledi Sebola[1], James Wabwire Oguttu[2] and Agricola Odoi[1,3*]

Abstract

Background: Antimicrobial resistance is becoming increasingly important in both human and veterinary medicine. This study investigated the proportion of antimicrobial resistant samples and resistance patterns of *Staphylococcus* isolates from cats presented at a veterinary teaching hospital in South Africa. Records of 216 samples from cats that were submitted to the bacteriology laboratory of the University of Pretoria academic veterinary hospital between 2007 and 2012 were evaluated. Isolates were subjected to antimicrobial susceptibility testing against a panel of 15 drugs using the disc diffusion method. Chi square and Fisher's exact tests were used to assess simple associations between antimicrobial resistance and age group, sex, breed and specimen type. Additionally, associations between *Staphylococcus* infection and age group, breed, sex and specimen type were assessed using logistic regression.

Results: *Staphylococcus* spp. isolates were identified in 17.6% (38/216) of the samples submitted and 4.6% (10/216) of these were unspeciated. The majority (61.1%,11/18) of the isolates were from skin samples, followed by otitis media (34.5%, 10/29). Coagulase Positive *Staphylococcus* (CoPS) comprised 11.1% (24/216) of the samples of which 7.9% (17/216) were *S. intermedius* group and 3.2% (7/216) were *S. aureus*. Among the Coagulase Negative *Staphylococcus* (CoNS) (1.9%, 4/216), *S. felis* and *S. simulans* each constituted 0.9% (2/216). There was a significant association between *Staphylococcus* spp. infection and specimen type with odds of infection being higher for ear canal and skin compared to urine specimens. There were higher proportions of samples resistant to clindamycin 34.2% (13/25), ampicillin 32.4% (2/26), lincospectin 31.6% (12/26) and penicillin-G 29.0% (11/27). Sixty three percent (24/38) of *Staphylococcus* spp. were resistant to one antimicrobial agent and 15.8% were multidrug resistant (MDR). MDR was more common among *S. aureus* 28.6% (2/7) than *S. intermedius* group isolates 11.8% (2/17). One *S. intermedius* group isolate was resistant to all β-lactam antimicrobial agents tested.

Conclusion: *S. intermedius* group was the most common cause of skin infections and antimicrobial resistance was not wide spread among cats presented at the veterinary academic hospital in South Africa. However, the presence of MDR-*Staphylococcus* spp. and isolates resistant to all β-lactams is of both public health and animal health concern.

Keywords: *Staphylococcus* spp., Antimicrobial resistance, Veterinary hospital, Cats, South Africa

* Correspondence: aodoi@utk.edu
[1]University of Pretoria, Faculty of Veterinary Science, Department of Paraclinical Sciences, SectionVeterinary Public Health, Pretoria, Gauteng, South Africa
[3]University of Tennessee, College of Veterinary Medicine, Department of Biomedical and Diagnostic Sciences, Knoxville, TN, USA
Full list of author information is available at the end of the article

Background

Although *Staphylococcus* are commensals of the skin, mucous membranes, alimentary and urogenital tracts of a diverse group of mammals and birds, they have been implicated in clinical infections of humans and animals [1–3]. Transmission of *Staphylococcus* between animals and humans are known to occur [1, 4]. Cats have been reported as carriers of both Coagulase positive (CoPS) and coagulase negative *Staphylococc*us species (CoNS) [2, 3, 5–7]. However, coagulase positive *Staphylococcus* species infections seem to be more prominent in feline medicine than CoNS infections [1]. Among the CoPS species in cats, *S. pseudintermedius* are the most common followed by *S. aureus* [5, 8]. These infections have been associated with pyoderma, postoperative wound infections and otitis [9]. In addition, *S. felis*, is a cause of urinary tract infections [10].

Although resistance to β-lactam antimicrobials among *Staphylococcus* isolates from cats has been reported [6, 8], other antimicrobial agents such as gentamycin, enrofloxacin and doxycycline have been reported to be effective against *Staphylococcus* infections in cats [5, 11, 12]. However, information on the proportion of antimicrobial resistant isolates and resistance patterns of *Staphylococcus* species in clinical cases of cats in developing economies in general and South Africa in particular is very limited. Therefore, the objective of this study was to investigate the proportion of antimicrobial resistant isolates and resistance patterns among *Staphylococcus* species isolates from cat samples submitted to a veterinary academic hospital in South Africa between 2007 and 2012.

Methods

Data collection

Data containing records of cat samples submitted to the University of Pretoria Bacteriology Laboratory at the Veterinary Teaching Hospital in South Africa between January 2007 and December 2012 for routine diagnostic tests were evaluated. The following variables were captured: breed, age, sex, specimen type, staphylococcus species isolated, antimicrobial included in the antimicrobial susceptibility test panel and the susceptibility profile of the isolates.

Staphylococcus identification and antimicrobial susceptibility testing

Culture of samples was done using sheep blood agar incubated at 37 °C for at least 24 h. All media used were quality controlled using *S. aureus* ATCC 25923. Suspected *Staphylococcus* colonies were identified based on phenotypic characteristics including colony characteristics, catalase, D-mannitol, maltose, deoxyribonuclease (DNase) tests, polymyxin-B and Gram-staining as described by Quinn [13]. *S. intermedius* and *S. delphini* were classified as *S. intermedius* group (SIG) as described by Sasaki et al. [14].

Isolates were subjected to antimicrobial susceptibility testing against a panel of 15 drugs using the disc diffusion method (discs supplied by Oxoid) [15]. Included in the panel were the following drugs: 30 μg amikacin (AK), 30 μg doxycycline (DOX30), 5 μg enrofloxacin (ENR), 10 μg gentamicin (CN), 10 μg penicillin G (P), 25 μg sulpha-trimethroprim (SXT), 30 μg chloramphenicol (C), 30 μg cephalothin/lexin (KF), 30 μg kanamycin (K), 2 μg clindamycin/lincomycin (MY), 100 μg lincospectin (Espectinomycine-lincomycine) (LS100), 5 μg orbifloxacin (OBX5), 20/10 μg synulox (Amoxicillin-Clavulanic acid) (AMC20/10) and 15 μg tylosin (TY). The results, based on the diameter of the inhibition zones, were classified as sensitive, intermediate or resistant in accordance with the Clinical and Laboratory Standards Institute [15]. For the purposes of the study, intermediate susceptibility was considered as susceptible. Multidrug resistance (MDR) was defined as resistance to at least one antimicrobial agent in three or more antimicrobial categories [16].

Data analysis

All the statistical analyses were performed using SAS 9.4 (SAS Institute Inc., Cary, NC, USA) statistical package. The dataset was assessed for missing data and inconsistencies such as improbable values. Shapiro-Wilk test of normality was used for evaluation of distributions of age that was found to be non-normally distributed and hence median and interquartile ranges were reported. Age was also categorised into two categories: <2 years and ≥2 years. The frequencies and proportions of all categorical variables were calculated and presented in a table. Associations between antimicrobial resistance of *Staphylococcus* spp. isolates and a number of host factors (breed, age, sex, specimen type) and other categorical variables were assessed using the Chi-square and Fisher's Exact tests. Statistical significant was assessed using a critical *p*-value of 0.05. The variables specimen type and breed had too many categories to include in the model in their original form and hence they were re-coded (Table 1).

Univariable and multivariable models

Investigation of the predictors of *Staphylococcus* spp. infections was done in two steps. In the first step, univariable logistic regression model was fit to assess the relationships between sex, age, specimen type and breed, and the outcome variable, *Staphylococcus* status. The potential predictors of *Staphylococcus* spp. infection at this stage were identified using a relaxed $\alpha \leq 0.20$. Thus variables with $p \leq 0.20$ in the univariable model were considered for inclusion in the multivariable model in the 2nd step. Therefore, the 2nd step involved fitting a multivariable logistic regression

Table 1 Distribution of *Staphylococcus* isolates among cat specimens tested at an academic veterinary hospital laboratory, 2007–2012

		Number of cats tested		*Staphylococcus* positive	
Variable	Category	Frequency	Percent	Frequency	Percent
Breed (n = 212)					
	Domestic Short Hair	132	62.3	24	18.2
	Persian	21	9.9	4	19.1
	Siamese	15	7.1	1	6.7
	Domestic Long Hair	12	5.7	3	25.0
	All others	32	15.1	6	18.8
Sex (n = 205)					
	Male	122	59.5	17	13.9
	Female	83	40.5	20	24.1
Specimen type (n = 215)					
	Urine	95	44.2	3	3.2
	Ear canal swab	29	13.5	10	34.5
	Skin	18	8.4	11	61.1
	All others	73	34.0	14	19.2
Age (n = 216)					
	≥2 years	123	56.9	21	17.1
	<2 years	93	43.1	17	18.3

model using manual backwards selection method with the significance set at $\alpha \leq 0.05$.

Confounding was assessed by comparing the change in model coefficients with and without the suspected confounders. If the removal of a suspected confounding variable resulted in a 20% or greater change in another model coefficient, the removed variable was considered a confounder and retained in the model regardless of its statistical significance. In addition, two-way interaction terms between variable in the final main effects model were assessed.

Odds ratios (ORs) and their 95% confidence intervals were computed for variables included in the final model. The differences between categories of statistically significant predictors for *Staphylococcus* spp. were also assessed by changing the reference categories of the predictors. Hosmer-Lemeshow goodness-of-fit test was used to assess model fit.

Results

A total of 216 samples were submitted to the bacteriology lab during the study period, of which, 17.6% (38/216) tested positive for *Staphylococcus* spp. each of which had single isolates (i.e. no mixed infections were identified).The majority of samples tested were urine (44.2%, 95/215), followed by ear canal swab (13.5%, 29/215) and skin samples (8.4%, 18/215). Significantly (p = 0.0065) more samples originated from males (59.5%, 122/205) than female cats (40.5, 83/205). Similarly, a significantly (p = 0.0412) higher proportion of samples came from cats ≥2 years (56.9%, 123/216) compared to cats <2 years (43.1%, 93/216). The majority of samples were obtained from the domestic short hair breed (DSH) (62.3%, 132/212), followed by Persian breed (9.9%, 21/212) (Table 1).

Staphylococcus species were isolated from several cat breeds including domestic long hair (25.0% 3/12), domestic short hair (18.2%, 24/132) and persian breed (19.1%, 4/21). Skin samples yielded the highest (61.1%,11/18) percentage of *staphylococcus* isolates followed by ear swabs (34.5%,10/29).

Significantly (p = 0.02) more CoPS (11.1%, 24/216) were isolated compared to CoNS (1.9%, 4/216). Among the CoPS, *S. intermedius* group was most predominant (7.9%, 17/216) followed by *S. aureus* (3,2%, 7/216). Equal percentage of *S. felis* (0.9%, 2/216) and *S. simulans* (0.9%; 2/216) were observed among the CoNS. Five percent (4.6%, 10/216) of the *Staphylococcus* isolates identified were not characterized (Table 2).

Staphylococcus isolates exhibited relatively high levels of resistance towards ampicillin (32.4%, 12/26), penicillin-G (29.0%, 11/27), clindamycin (34.2%,13/25) and lincospectin (31.6%, 12/26) (Table 3). Overall, 63.2% (24/38) of *Staphylococcus* spp. were resistant to at least one antimicrobial agent and 21.1% (8/38) were multidrug resistant (MDR). *S. aureus* (85.7%, 6/7) had the highest level of resistance to at least one antimicrobial agent followed by *S. intermedius* group (52.9%, 9/17). Similarly, *S. aureus* (42.9%, 3/7) had a higher level of MDR than *S. intermedius* group (12.5%, 2/16). One *S.*

Table 2 Distribution of *Staphylococcus* species isolated from clinical specimens from cats presented at an academic veterinary hospital between 2007 and 2012 (n = 216)

	Isolate	Frequency	Percent (%)
CoPS n = 24 (11.1%)	*S. intermedius* group (SIG)	17	7.9
	S. aureus	7	3.2
CoNS n = 4 (1.9%)	*S. felis*	2	0.9
	S. simulans	2	0.9
Unspeciated	*S.* spp.	10	4.6
	Negative	172	82.4
	Total	216	100

intermedius group isolate was resistant to all β-lactam antimicrobial agents tested. This isolate was also resistant to 9 out of the 15 antimicrobial agents tested. Three *S. intermedius* group isolates were resistant to both clindamycin and lincosamides. Among the *S. aureus* isolates, one was resistant to five antimicrobial agents and two to four antimicrobial agents (Table 4).

Predictors of staphylococcus infections

Based on the univariable logistic model, only sex and specimen type stood out as potential predictors of *Staphylococcus* spp. infection based on a liberal $\alpha \leq 0.20$ (Table 5). Thus, only these two variables were assessed in the multivariable model. In the final model only specimen type was significantly associated with staphylococcus species infection based on $\alpha \leq 0.05$. The odds of testing positive for *Staphylococcus* spp. infections were significantly higher among ear canal (p = 0.0002) and skin samples ($p < 0.0001$) than urine samples (Table 6). However, there was no significant differences in the odds of *Staphylococcus* spp. infection between skin and ear canal samples (Table 7).

Discussion

The aim of this study was to investigate the proportion of antimicrobial resistant isolates and resistance patterns of *Staphylococcus* spp. isolates from clinical samples obtained from cats admitted to a veterinary academic

Table 3 Antimicrobial resistance profile of *Staphylococcus* isolates to antimicrobial agents from samples tested at an academic veterinary laboratory, 2007–2012

Group	Drug	Frequency	Percent (n/N) [b]
β-lactam		26	28.9 (26/90)
Penicillin	PenicillinG	11	29.0 (11/27)
	Ampicillin	12	32.4 (12/26)
Cephalosporin	Cephalothin	1	2.7 (1/37)
	Ceftiofur	1	2.7 (1/37)
Combination	Amoxicillin/Clavulanic acid	1	2.7 (1/37)
Tetracycline	Doxycycline	1	2.7 (1/37)
Fluoroquinolone		6	8.6 (6/70)
	Enrofloxacin	3	7.9 (3/35)
	Orbifloxacin	3	7.9 (3/35)
Aminoglycoside		4	3.6 (4/110)
	Gentamicin	1	2.7 (1/37)
	Amikacin	1	2.7 (1/37)
	Kanamycin	2	5.3 (2/36)
Potentiated sulfonamide	Sulfamethoxazole/trimethoprim	4	10.5 (4/34)
Amphenicols	Chloramphenicol	2	5.2 (2/36)
Lincosamides	Clindamycin	13	34.2 (13/25)
Aminoglycoside-lincosamide	Lincospectin	12	31.6 (12/26)
Macrolide	Tylosin	2	5.3 (2/36)

[b] = n is the number resistant, N is number tested

Table 4 Antimicrobial resistance patterns identified in *Staphylococcus* isolates from cat specimens tested at an academic veterinary hospital laboratory, 2007–2012

Species	Antimicrobial Resistance Percent (n/N)	Multidrug Resistance Percent (n/N)	B-Lactam resistance Percent (n/N)	Resistance patterns
S. aureus	85.7 (6/7)	42.9 (3/7)	0	AMP (1), AMP PEN (1), AMP PEN LIN (1), AMP PEN CLI LIN (1), AMP PEN CHL LIN (1), AMP SP KAN CLI LIN (1)
S. felis	0 (0/2)	0	0	
S. intermedius group	52.9 (9/17)	11.8 (2/17)	5.9 (1/17)	PEN (1), KAN (1), CLI LIN (3), SP LIN (1), AMP PEN SP (1), ENR LIN OR TYL (1), AMP CEF GEN PEN SP CEF KAN OR SU (1)
S. simulans	0 (0/2)	0	0	
S. spp.	90.0 (9/10)	30.0 (3/10)	0	CLI (2), LIN (1), CHL CLI (1), AMP PEN (1), CLI LIN OR (1), AMP AMP DOX ENR PEN CLI (1), AMP PEN CLI (1), AMP ENR PEN CLI LIN TYL (1),

n number of resistant samples, *N* number of samples tested, *AMP* ampicillin, *CEF* Ceftiofur, *ENR* Enrofloxacin, *GEN* Gentamicin, *PEN* PenicillinG, *SP* Sulpha/Trimethroprim, *CHL* Chloramphenicol, *KAN* Kanamycin, *CLI* Clindamycin/Lincomycin, *AMI* Amikacin, *DOX* Doxycycline, *LIN* Lincospectin, *ORB* Orbifloxacin, *SU* Amoxicillin/Clavulanic acid, *TYL* Tylosin

hospital in South Africa. The proportion of *Staphylococcus* spp. isolated from cat samples in this study was relatively low (17.6%). This is not directly comparable to findings from other previous studies on cats due to differences in isolation methods (use of enrichment media in particular), and differences in study designs. In the current study, we investigated *Staphylococcus* infections in hospitalised clinical cases only. However, the majority of similar published studies of *Staphylococcus* in cats have largely focused on methicillin resistance rather than *Staphylococcus* infections in general. In addition, past studies have focused on carriage rather than infections [8, 17].

Similar to findings from other studies [8, 17], in this study we observed that skin and ear canal samples had significantly higher odds of testing positive for *Staphylococcus* spp. than other samples. These results seem to suggest that *Staphylococcus* spp. are a major cause of skin related infections in cats [18–20]. Although there tended to be a higher proportion of *Staphylococcus* spp. isolated from the domestic short hair breeds, the final model indicated no significant association between breed and odds of *Staphylococcus* spp. infection. However, the lack of significant association might be due to small sample size involved in this study. It is worth noting that, there is evidence that certain diseases are more common in certain breeds of cats and we suspect that this might be the case with *Staphylococcus* infections [17, 21].

Consistent with other studies [3, 5, 17, 19], we observed a higher percentage of CoPS than CoNS. This is mainly due to the observed higher percentage of *S. intermedius* group, which are CoPS, isolated in this study. On the contrary, Abraham et al. [7] reported nearly equal proportions of *S. aureus* and *S. pseudintermedius*

Table 5 Results of the univariable logistic model showing predictors of *Staphylococcus* spp. infection among cats tested at an academic veterinary hospital laboratory, 2007–2012

Variable	OR[a]	95% CI[b]		p-value
Breed				
Domestic Long Hair	1.4	0.3	7.0	0.368
Domestic Short Hair	0.9	0.4	2.6	0.707
Persian	1.0	0.3	4.2	0.723
Siamese	0.3	0.03	2.8	0.237
All others	Ref	.	.	.
Sex				
Female	1.9	0.9	4.0	0.066
Male	Ref	.	.	.
Specimen type				
Ear canal swab	16.1	4.1	64.2	<0.0001
Skin	48.2	10.9	213.7	<0.0001
All others	7.3	2.0	26.4	0.003
Urine	Ref	.	.	.
Age				
< 2 years	1.1	0.5	2.2	0.818
> = 2 years	Ref	.	.	.

[a]Odds ratio
[b]95% Confidence Interval

Table 6 Multivariable logistic model showing predictors of *Staphylococcus* spp. infection among cats tested at an academic veterinary hospital laboratory, 2007–2012

Variable	OR[1]	95% CI[2]		p-value
Sex				
Female	1.9	0.8	4.3	0.117
Male	Ref	.	.	.
Specimen type				
Ear canal swab	14.8	3.6	60.5	0.0002
Skin	52.1	11.3	240.3	<.0001
All others	8.4	2.3	30.7	0.001
Urine	Ref	.	.	.

Table 7 Final multivariable logistic model showing the results of changing reference categories of specimen type

Variable	OR[1]	95% CI[2]		p-value
Specimen type				
Skin	3.519	0.969	12.78	0.0559
Urine	0.068	0.017	0.276	0.0002
All others	0.564	0.208	1.531	0.2611
Ear canal swab	Ref	.	.	.
Ear canal swab	0.284	0.078	1.032	0.0559
Urine	0.019	0.004	0.089	<.0001
All others	0.16	0.05	0.517	0.0022
Skin	Ref	.	.	.
Ear canal swab	1.773	0.653	4.81	0.2611
Skin	6.237	1.933	20.131	0.0022
Urine	0.12	0.033	0.439	0.0014
All others	Ref	.	.	.

isolates from asymptomatic cats. Consistent with our study, a Brazilian study by Lilenbaum et al. [8] reported a higher percentage of *S. intermedius* group (*S. pseudintermedius*) in cats compared to other *Staphylococcus* species. This may be related to the fact that SIG especially *S. pseudintermedius* is well adapted to the skin surface of dogs and cats than *S. aureus* [22–25].

The observed higher percentage of resistance towards β-lactam and lincosamide antimicrobial agents among the *Staphylococcus* isolates in cats has previously been reported [6, 8, 23]. Of particular concern is one *S. intermedius* group isolate that was resistant to all β-lactam antimicrobial agents tested in this study. Moreover, MRSA have an intrinsic resistance to β-lactams by virtue of newly acquired low-affinity penicillin-binding protein 2A (PBP2A). Therefore, it is possible that this isolate was MRSA [26, 27]. Unforunately, we could not assess this since the lab that supplied the data used in this study did not test for methicillin resistance. Almost 16 % (15.8%) of *Staphylococcus* isolates in this study were MDR. This is close to the 14.8% reported by Gandolfi-Decristophoris et al. [23] in Switzerland.

Since this is a retrospective study, these findings should be interpreted with caution. The history of previous use of antimicrobial agents was not included in the analysis and this could have affected the recovery rates of *Staphylococcus* species. The study also suffers from low samples size which impacted the precision of some of the estimates. Nonetheless, the results provide a useful preliminary indication of the burden and antimicrobial resistance patterns of *Staphylococcus* spp. infections in cats presented to the academic veterinary hospital in South Africa.

Conclusions

As has been observed in other studies, this study suggests that *S. intermedius* group is the most common cause of skin infections in cats investigated in this study. It also suggests that antimicrobial resistance is not so wide spread among cats presented at the veterinary academic hospital in South Africa. Considering the risk of cross-transmission of resistant organisms between cats and humans, the levels of resistance to β-lactams is of great concern from both a public health and animal health point of view. However, given the limited scope of this study, there is need for larger and more detailed primary base studies to specifically assess the extent of antimicrobial resistant infections in cats in South Africa and their role in the spread of antimicrobial drug resistance to humans.

Abbreviations

AMR: Antimicrobial resistance; CoNS: Coagulase negative staphylococci species; CoPS: Coagulase Positive *Staphylococcus*; DSH: Domestic Short Hair breed; MDR: Multidrug resistant resistance; SAS: Statistical Analysis System

Acknowledgements

The authors would like to thank the Department of Tropical Diseases and Companion Animal Clinical Studies for providing access to the records used in this study. We are also grateful to Ms. S Nxumalo and Mr. W Mbethe for helping with data entry and validation.

Funding

Not applicable.

Authors' contributions

DNQ was involved in study design and data management and performed all statistical analyses and interpretation as well as preparation of the manuscript draft. AO was involved in study design, data analysis and interpretation as well as extensive editing of the manuscript. JWO was involved in study design and editing of the manuscript. DS was involved in data collection and interpretation of results of the manuscript. All authors read and approved the final manuscript.

Consent for publication

The study does not involve human subjects and therefore no consent was required. However, the lab that supplied the study data provided consent for study results to be published.

Competing interests

The authors declare that they have no competing interests.

Author details

[1]University of Pretoria, Faculty of Veterinary Science, Department of Paraclinical Sciences, SectionVeterinary Public Health, Pretoria, Gauteng, South Africa. [2]University of South Africa, College of Agriculture and

Environmental Sciences, Department of Agriculture and Animal Health, Johannesburg, South Africa. [3]University of Tennessee, College of Veterinary Medicine, Department of Biomedical and Diagnostic Sciences, Knoxville, TN, USA.

References

1. Morris DO, Mauldin EA, O'Shea K, Shofer FS, Rankin SC. Clinical, microbiological, and molecular characterization of methicillin-resistant Staphylococcus Aureus infections of cats. Am J Vet Res. 2006;67:1421–5.
2. Hanselman BA, Kruth SA, Rousseau J, Weese JS. Coagulase positive staphylococcal colonization of humans and their household pets. Can Vet J. 2009;50:954–8.
3. Rich M. Staphylococci in animals: prevalence, identification and antimicrobial susceptibility, with an emphasis on methicillin-resistant Staphylococcus Aureus. Br J Biomed Sci. 2005;62:98–105.
4. Duquette RA, Nuttall TJ. Methicillin-resistant Staphylococcus Aureus in dogs and cats: an emerging problem? J Small Anim Pract. Blackwell Publishing Ltd. 2004;45:591–7.
5. Beça N, Bessa LJ, Mendes Â, Santos J, Leite-Martins L, Matos AJF, et al. Coagulase-positive staphylococcus: prevalence and antimicrobial resistance. J Am Anim Hosp Assoc. 2015;51:365–71.
6. Bierowiec K, Płoneczka-Janeczko K, Rypuła K. Is the colonisation of Staphylococcus Aureus in pets associated with their close contact with owners? PLoS One. 2016;11:e0156052.
7. Abraham J, Morris D, Griffeth G, Shofer F, Rankin S. Surveillance of healthy cats and cats with inflammatory skin disease for colonization of the skin by methicillin-resistant coagulase-positive staphylococci and staphylococcus schleiferi ssp. schleiferi. Dermatology. 2007;18:252–9.
8. Lilenbaum W, Nunes EL, Azeredo MA. Prevalence and antimicrobial susceptibility of staphylococci isolated from the skin surface of clinically normal cats. Lett Appl Microbiol. 1998;27:224–8.
9. Bannoehr J, Guardabassi L. Staphylococcus pseudintermedius in the dog: taxonomy, diagnostics, ecology, epidemiology and pathogenicity. Vet Dermatol. 2012;23:253–66.
10. Litster A, Moss SSM, Honnery M, Rees B, Trott DJD. Prevalence of bacterial species in cats with clinical signs of lower urinary tract disease: recognition of Staphylococcus Felis as a possible feline urinary tract pathogen. Vet Microbiol. 2007;121:182–8.
11. Ganiere JP, Medaille C, Mangion C. Antimicrobial drug susceptibility of Staphylococcus Intermedius clinical isolates from canine pyoderma. J Vet Med B Infect Dis Vet Public Health. 2005;52:25–31.
12. Lilenbaum W, Esteves AL, Souza GN. Prevalence and antimicrobial susceptibility of staphylococci isolated from saliva of clinically normal cats. Lett Appl Microbiol. Blackwell Science Ltd. 1999;28:448–52.
13. Quinn PJ, Carter ME, Markey B, Carter GR. Clinical veterinary microbiology. Edinburgh: Mosby Wolfe; 1994.
14. Sasaki T, Kikuchi K, Tanaka Y, Takahashi N, Kamata S, Hiramatsu K. Reclassification of phenotypically identified Staphylococcus Intermedius strains. J Clin Microbiol. 2007;45:2770–8.
15. Clinical Institute Laboratory Standards. Performance standards for antimicrobial disk and dilution susceptibility tests for bacteria isolated from animals; approved standard – fourth edition. CLSI document VET01-A. 2013.
16. Magiorakos AP, Srinivasan A, Carey RB, Carmeli Y, Falagas ME, Giske CG, et al. Multidrug-resistant, extensively drug-resistant and pandrug-resistant bacteria: an international expert proposal for interim standard definitions for acquired resistance. Clin Microbiol Infect. 2012;18:268–81.
17. Loeffler A, Boag AK, Sung J, Lindsay JA, Guardabassi L, Dalsgaard A, et al. Prevalence of methicillin-resistant Staphylococcus Aureus among staff and pets in a small animal referral hospital in the UK. J Antimicrob Chemother. 2005;56:692–7.
18. Scott DW, Paradis M. A survey of canine and feline skin disorders seen in a university practice: small animal clinic, University of Montréal, Saint-Hyacinthe, Québec (1987-1988). Can Vet J. 1990;31:830–5.
19. Devriese LA, Nzuambe D, Godard C. Identification and characteristics of staphylococci isolated from lesions and normal skin of horses. Vet Microbiol. 1985;10:269–77.
20. Biberstein EL, Jang SS, Hirsh DC. Species distribution of coagulase-positive staphylococci in animals. J Clin Microbiol. 1984;19:610–5.
21. Lekcharoensuk C, Osborne CA, Lulich JP. Epidemiologic study of risk factors for lower urinary tract diseases in cats. J Am Vet Med Assoc. 2001;218:1429–35.
22. Kawakami T, Shibata S, Murayama N, Nagata M, Nishifuji K, Iwasaki T, et al. Antimicrobial susceptibility and methicillin resistance in staphylococcus pseudintermedius and staphylococcus schleiferi subsp. coagulans isolated from dogs with pyoderma in Japan. J Vet Med Sci. 2010;72:1615–9.
23. Gandolfi-Decristophoris P, Regula G, Petrini O, Zinsstag J, Schelling E. Prevalence and risk factors for carriage of multi-drug resistant staphylococci in healthy cats and dogs. J Vet Sci. 2013;14:449–56.
24. Schmidt VM, Williams NJ, Pinchbeck G, Corless CE, Shaw S, McEwan N, et al. Antimicrobial resistance and characterisation of staphylococci isolated from healthy Labrador retrievers in the United Kingdom. BMC Vet Res. 2014;10:17.
25. Paul NC, Bärgman SC, Moodley A, Nielsen SS, Guardabassi L. Staphylococcus pseudintermedius colonization patterns and strain diversity in healthy dogs: a cross-sectional and longitudinal study. Vet Microbiol. 2012;160:420–7.
26. Guignard B, Entenza JM, Moreillon P. β-Lactams against methicillin-resistant Staphylococcus Aureus. Curr Opin Pharmacol. 2005;5:479–89.
27. Lim D, Strynadka NCJ. Structural basis for the beta lactam resistance of PBP2a from methicillin-resistant Staphylococcus Aureus. Nat Struct Biol. 2002;9:870–6.

Residues of chlortetracycline, doxycycline and sulfadiazine-trimethoprim in intestinal content and feces of pigs due to cross-contamination of feed

Laura E. J. Peeters[1,2], Els Daeseleire[3†], Mathias Devreese[4†], Geertrui Rasschaert[3], Annemieke Smet[2], Jeroen Dewulf[5], Marc Heyndrickx[2,3], Hein Imberechts[1], Freddy Haesebrouck[2], Patrick Butaye[2,6] and Siska Croubels[4*]

Abstract

Background: Cross-contamination of feed with low concentrations of antimicrobials can occur at production, transport and/or farm level. Concerns are rising about possible effects of this contaminated feed on resistance selection in the intestinal microbiota. Therefore, an experiment with pigs was set up, in which intestinal and fecal concentrations of chlortetracycline (CTC), doxycycline (DOX) and sulfadiazine-trimethoprim (SDZ-TRIM) were determined after administration of feed containing a 3 % carry-over level of these antimicrobials.

Results: The poor oral bioavailability of tetracyclines resulted in rather high concentrations in cecal and colonic content and feces at steady-state conditions. A mean concentration of 10 mg/kg CTC and 4 mg/kg DOX in the feces was reached, which is higher than concentrations that were shown to cause resistance selection. On the other hand, lower mean levels of SDZ (0.7 mg/kg) and TRIM (< limit of detection of 0.016 mg/kg) were found in the feces, corresponding with the high oral bioavailability of SDZ and TRIM in pigs.

Conclusions: The relation between the oral bioavailability and intestinal concentrations of the tested antimicrobials, may be of help in assessing the risks of cross-contaminated feed. However, future research is needed to confirm our results and to evaluate the effects of these detected concentrations on resistance selection in the intestinal microbiota of pigs.

Keywords: Cross-contamination, Oral bioavailability, Chlortetracycline, Doxycycline, Sulfadiazine, Trimethoprim, Pigs, Intestinal content, Feces

Background

Group administration of veterinary drugs through feed and drinking water is frequently applied in the pig industry. Antimicrobials are often administered to pigs by mixing the feed with an oral powder or premix formulation [1–3]. The important role of group administration of antimicrobials in the selection of resistant bacteria is generally recognized [4]. Concerns about antimicrobial resistance selection have already led to the prohibition of use of antimicrobials as growth promoters in Europe since 2006 [5]. However, group medication is still used extensively in many countries for prophylactic, metaphylactic and therapeutic purposes [3]. Major disadvantages of group medication are the poor control over dosage due to differences in feed uptake between sick and healthy animals, inflexible therapy duration for medicated feed, the risk of carry-over and the inevitable contamination of the environment with antimicrobials [4]. Different types of antimicrobial formulations can be used to treat animals in group. Premixes (38.2 %), oral powders (33.7 %) and solutions (19.6 %) each accounted for a significant share of the total amount of sold antimicrobials in 26 European countries in 2013 [1]. However, the types of antimicrobial formulations used for group

* Correspondence: Siska.Croubels@ugent.be
†Equal contributors
4Department of Pharmacology, Toxicology and Biochemistry, Faculty of Veterinary Medicine, Ghent University, 9820 Merelbeke, Belgium
Full list of author information is available at the end of the article

treatment vary considerably between the individual countries. In some countries, such as Germany, Luxembourg, Estonia and Denmark, it seems that oral powders and solutions are preferred over premix formulations, whereas the opposite applies for countries like Spain, Portugal, Hungary, Cyprus and the UK [1]. In Belgium, both oral powders (70 %, for feed and drinking water) and premixes (20 %) are used frequently [1, 2]. In this study we focus on medicated feed produced in feed mills, and thus on premix formulations.

Carry-over of feed additives and veterinary drugs from a compound feed to a non-target feed is a problem inherent to the production of compound feed in feed mills and the transport, storage and delivery of these feeds [6, 7]. A batch of non-target feed that is produced directly after a compound feed, is generally called 'flushing feed'. So far, only coccidiostats and histomonostats are included in the European legislation regarding maximum allowed levels (3 %) in flushing feeds [8]. In Belgium, a covenant was established in 2013 between the Belgian Federal Agency for the Safety of the Food Chain (FASFC) and the Belgian Compound Feed Industry Association (BCFIA) [9], in which guidelines for maximum levels of carry-over were set for antimicrobials (1 % of the min. approved dose, except 2.5 % for some formulations in rabbit pellet feed), paracetamol (1 %) and anthelmintics (1–3 % of the max. approved dose, depending on the type of feed). Moreover, due to additional technical requirements for feed mills established in this covenant, namely adding the drugs or additives at the end of the production line instead of the middle, carry-over should be reduced significantly in Belgian feed mills. Unfortunately, carry-over between different feed batches occurs not only in feed mills, but also during transport and at farm level, which makes it a difficult issue to control [10]. A study by Putier et al. [11], investigating carry-over at transport level, indicated that this route should not be underestimated. In this study, two types of carry-over (inter-bin and intra-bin) of antimicrobials (oxytetracycline and chlortetracycline) were measured in ten different types of delivery trucks. Inter-bin carry-over of the two antimicrobials ranged from 0.04 to 1.41 % and intra-bin carry-over ranged from 0 to 0.44 %. Carry-over at farm level remains to be elucidated but could be of great importance, especially in countries with a focus on use of oral powders and solutions as these products are mixed with feed or water at the farm [1].

As a result of cross-contamination of feed, the intestinal microbiota of pigs can be exposed to unintended, low concentrations of antimicrobials [12]. It is known that low antimicrobial concentrations can evoke selection of resistant bacteria in vitro [13, 14] and in vivo [15]. Moreover, in vitro studies with tetracycline, trimethoprim, streptomycin, erythromycin and ciprofloxacin show that the fitness cost for resistance-conferring mutations or genes selected at sub-MIC (Minimum Inhibitory Concentration) concentrations is often lower than for those selected above the MIC [13, 14]. Therefore, these sub-MIC selected mutants would be more stable in bacterial populations and thus potentially more problematic than mutants selected above the MIC [16–18].

In order to assess the true effect of cross-contaminated feed on resistance selection in the intestinal microbiota, it is necessary to first determine the intestinal concentrations of antimicrobials after administration of such feed. Indeed, each type of antimicrobial has different pharmacokinetic (PK) properties that determine the fraction of the orally ingested antimicrobial that remains in the intestines or is excreted in the bile [19]. The oral bioavailability is a measure of the rate and extent of a drug reaching the systemic circulation in its unchanged form through intestinal absorption [20]. As such, this PK property has a significant impact on the fraction of drug that remains in the intestinal content. The oral bioavailability is strongly dependent on the active substance and may be influenced among others by the formulation type and prandial state of the animal. In this study, an in vivo experiment with pigs was set up to determine concentrations in the intestinal content and the feces of chlortetracycline (CTC), doxycycline (DOX) and sulfadiazine-trimethoprim (SDZ-TRIM) when administering feed that contains 3 % of the maximum recommended dose (MRD). This percentage was chosen considering the only legally applicable guideline in Belgium regarding maximum carry-over levels at the time of the experiment (2013) [8]. The choice of antimicrobials was based on two aspects. First, tetracyclines and sulfonamides are among the most used classes of antimicrobials in Belgium when considering oral administration [21]. Second, the oral bioavailability in pigs was taken into account. SDZ, typically used in a combined formulation with TRIM because of the synergistic mode of action, has a very high oral bioavailability in pigs, namely 85–100 % [22, 23]. The same applies to TRIM (73–92 %) [22, 23]. In contrast, tetracyclines have a low oral bioavailability in pigs, with CTC even lower (6 %) than DOX (21–50 %) [24–26].

In the past, studies have been performed to examine levels of antimicrobials and other drugs in tissues and eggs when poultry is fed with cross-contaminated feed [27–29]. Yet no data have been published regarding intestinal concentrations due to cross-contamination in pigs or other livestock. The aim of this study was therefore to determine intestinal concentrations in pigs of CTC, DOX and SDZ-TRIM, when they were fed a diet that contains a 3 % carry-over level of these antimicrobials.

Methods

Premixes, reagents and standards

The premixes used for the preparation of the experimental diets were Doxyprex® (active pharmaceutical ingredient, API: 100 mg DOX hyclate/g premix), provided by Kela Veterinaria (Sint-Niklaas, Belgium), Aurofac® (API: 250 mg CTC.HCl/g premix) and Tucoprim® (API: 125 mg SDZ/g premix and 25 mg TRIM/g premix), both provided by Zoetis (Brussels, Belgium). Analytical standards of DOX (doxycycline hyclate), CTC (chlortetracycline.HCl), SDZ and TRIM were obtained from Sigma-Aldrich (Bornem, Belgium). The internal standards (IS) were demethylchlortetracycline.HCl (DMCTC, Sigma-Aldrich) and $^{13}C_6$-sulfadimethoxine and d9-trimethoprim, both from Witega (Berlin, Germany). Methanol (CH_3OH) and acetonitrile (CH_3CN) were of LC-MS grade and obtained from Biosolve (Valkenswaard, The Netherlands). Water was of LC-MS grade and was obtained from Biosolve (Valkenswaard, The Netherlands) for tetracycline analysis, and was generated from a Milli Q gradient purification system (Millipore, Billerica, MA, U.S.) for SDZ and TRIM analysis. Acetic acid (CH_3COOH, >99.99 %) was from Sigma Aldrich, succinic acid ($C_4H_6O_4$) from VWR (Leuven, Belgium) and sodium sulphate (Na_2SO_4), formic acid (HCOOH), trichloroacetic acid (CCl_3COOH) and sodium hydroxide (NaOH) were from Merck (Darmstadt, Germany).

Preparation of standard solutions

Standard stock solutions of CTC, DOX and the IS DMCTC were prepared in CH_3OH at a concentration of 1 mg/ml and stored at ≤ −15 °C. Working solutions of DMCTC at a concentration of 100 μg/ml and 20 μg/ml, and of CTC and DOX at a concentration of 100 μg/ml were prepared by appropriate dilution with water. Standard stock solutions of SDZ and the IS $^{13}C_6$-sulfadimethoxine were prepared in CH_3CN/water (50/50, V/V) at a concentration of 1 mg/ml and stored at ≤ −15 °C. Standard stock solutions of TRIM and the IS d9-trimethoprim were prepared in CH_3OH and stored at ≤ −15 °C. For $^{13}C_6$-sulfadimethoxine and d9-trimethoprim, working solutions of 1 μg/ml were prepared in water making use of an intermediate working solution of 10 μg/ml in CH_3CN/water (50/50, V/V). SDZ and TRIM working solutions of 10 μg/ml, 1 μg/ml and 0.1 μg/ml were prepared in water and used for spiking the calibration samples. To prepare sodium succinate 0.1 M, 11.8 g of $C_4H_6O_4$ was dissolved in 600 ml of water, 10 M NaOH was added until pH 4.0 was reached, and water was added to obtain a final volume of 1000.0 ml. The solution was stored at 4.0 °C. Solutions of HCOOH (0.1 %), CCl_3COOH (20 %) and CH_3COOH (0.1 %) were prepared by appropriate dilutions with water.

Preparation of the experimental feed

Three different batches of experimental diets were prepared. Blank feed (meal n° 9231, AVEVE, Merksem, Belgium) was mixed with the DOX, CTC and SDZ-TRIM premixes, respectively. A custom made mixing device (Silobouw, Zulte, Belgium) was kindly provided by the Food Science and Technology Unit of Ghent University. The added amounts of antimicrobials were calculated to yield cross-contamination levels in the feed corresponding to 3 % of the MRD (CTC, 18.6 mg/kg BW (body weight)/day; DOX, 13.5 mg/kg BW/day; SDZ, 25.0 mg/kg BW/day; TRIM, 5.0 mg/kg BW/day). BW and daily feed intake were set at 25 and 1.5 kg respectively. Thus, a target concentration of 9.29 mg CTC/kg feed, 6.76 mg DOX/kg feed, 12.5 mg SDZ/kg feed and 2.50 mg TRIM/kg feed was aimed for. Each premix was first mixed manually with 10 kg of blank feed, which was then mixed with the remaining blank feed (120 kg) in the feed mixer for 25 min. The feed was collected from the mixer in 13 bags, each containing 10 kg. One sample of approximately 200 g was taken from bag n° 1, 2, 3, 5, 6, 8, 9, 11, 12 and 13 of each experimental feed to assess if the target concentration was achieved and to determine the homogeneity. In this way, samples were collected at the beginning, middle and at the end of the mixing stream, in order to monitor the whole mixing cycle. The samples were kept at room temperature (t_R, 15–25 °C) until analysis (within a time frame of 2 weeks).

Animal experiment

Twenty-four pigs with an average BW of 27.0 ± 4.0 kg were randomly divided into 4 equal groups (3 males and 3 females/group): one control group and three experimental groups. Each group was housed in a strictly separated 3 by 4 m pen with a concrete floor and natural light cycle. The temperature varied between 21 and 25 °C. The floor was cleaned with water every day just before sample collection. Ad libitum access to drinking water and feed was provided throughout the experiment. After a 1-week acclimatization period, each experimental group received during ten days experimental feed containing 3 % cross-contamination levels of either CTC, DOX or SDZ-TRIM. The control group received blank feed (no antimicrobials). Individual fecal samples were taken by rectal stimulation, just before the start of providing the experimental diets and at day 2, 4, 6, 8 and 10 of the experimental feeding period. In case no individual sample could be obtained (which was the case for in total 19 time points from 12 pigs), fresh fecal samples were collected from the cleaned floor. On day 11, all animals were euthanized through a combined IM injection of xylazine (4.4 mg/kg BW), zolazepam and tiletamine (both 2.2 mg/kg BW) followed by an intracardial injection of 0.3 ml/kg BW of T61® (MSD, Brussels, Belgium). Immediately after euthanasia, samples of cecal content and colonic content from different sampling segments [proximal colon ascendens (PCA), distal colon ascendens (DCA), colon descendens (CD)] were taken from each animal individually. The samples were directly stored at −80 °C without homogenization.

Quantitation of antimicrobials in feed and feces

In-house developed methods were applied for both analysis of tetracyclines [30, 31] and SDZ-TRIM [27, 28].

a) Tetracyclines analysis
Twenty-five ml of CH_3OH were added to 5.0 g of each feed sample. After 20 min of shaking on an in-house rotary shaker, samples were centrifuged (6261 *g*, 10 min, 4 °C). Two-hundred µl of supernatant were transferred into an Eppendorf tube and 800 µl of CH_3OH were added. After adding 50 µl of IS (20 µg/ml), samples were vortex mixed. Next, the samples were filtered (PVDF 0.22 µm Millex-GV, Millipore, Overijse, Belgium) and transferred to an autosampler vial and 5 µl was injected onto the LC-MS/MS instrument.
To 2.0 g of intestinal content or feces, 50 µl of IS (100 µg/ml) were added. After vortex mixing (15 s), 10.0 ml of sodium succinate solution (0.1 M) were added and the samples were again vortex mixed (15 s). Samples were then shaken (20 min, in-house rotary shaker) and centrifuged (6261 *g*, 10 min, 4 °C). The supernatant was transferred to a new plastic tube and vortex mixed (15 s) after adding 1.0 ml of 20 % CCl_3COOH. These tubes were centrifuged again (6261 *g*, 10 min, 4 °C) and the samples were filtered through a Whatman filter (Whatman n°541, VWR, Leuven). This filtrate was used for further solid-phase clean-up. After preconditioning an OASIS® HLB 60 mg/3 ml solid phase extraction column (Waters, Milford, MA, U.S.) with consecutively 3 ml of CH_3OH, 3 ml of HCl (1 M) and 3 ml of HPLC water, the filtrate was poured onto the HLB column. The column was then washed with 1 ml of water and dried. The analytes were eluted with 3 ml of CH_3OH. The eluate was passed through a PVDF filter, transferred to an autosampler vial and 5 µl was injected onto the LC-MS/MS instrument.
The LC system consisted of an Acquity autosampler and an Acquity binary solvent manager from Waters (Milford, U.S.). Chromatographic separation was achieved on an Acquity UPLC BEH C18 column (50 mm × 2.1 mm i.d., 1.7 µm) from Waters. The temperatures of the autosampler tray and column oven were set at 10 °C and 30 °C, respectively. Mobile phase A consisted of CH_3CN whereas mobile phase B was 0.1 % HCOOH in water. Flow rate was set at 0.3 ml/min and the following elution program was run: 0–4.0 min (10 % A), 4.0–5.0 min (linear gradient to 90 % A), 5.0–7.1 (90 % A), 7.1–7.2 (linear gradient to 10 % A), 7.2–9.0 min (10 % A). The detection was performed with a Quattro Premier XE triple quadrupole mass spectrometer, equipped with an electrospray ionization (ESI) probe operating in the positive ionization mode (Waters). Masslynx software v 4.1 was used to quantitate, based on the following MS-MS transitions: m/z 479.04 > 461.84 (CTC) and m/z 445.10 > 427.96 (DOX).

b) Sulfadiazine-trimethoprim analysis
After homogenization of the feed sample, 5.0 g of feed was weighed and 50 µl of each IS (1 mg/ml) and 25 ml of CH_3OH were added. The sample was vortex mixed, shaken on a horizontal shaker (Edmund Bühler, Hechingen, Germany) during 30 min, and centrifuged (4000 *g*, 15 min, t_R). Five ml of the supernatant were evaporated to dryness at 45 ± 5 °C under nitrogen. The sample was redissolved in 10 ml of CH_3CN/water (50/50 V/V), vortex mixed (30 s), diluted to 1/15 in CH_3CN/water (50/50, V/V), vortex mixed (30 s) and transferred to an autosampler vial.
For intestinal content or feces analysis, 2.0 g of sample was weighed after homogenization and 40 µl of each IS (1 µg/ml) were added. The sample was carefully mixed with 8 g of Na_2SO_4 with a spatula to obtain a dry mixture. If necessary, extra Na_2SO_4 was added until the sample was dry. After adding 10 ml of CH_3CN, the sample was vortex mixed, shaken during 30 min (horizontal shaker, Edmund Bühler) and centrifuged (15 min, 4000 *g*, t_R). Five ml of the supernatant were then transferred into a glass tube and evaporated to dryness under nitrogen in a water bath of 45 °C. Next, the sample was redissolved in 1 ml of an CH_3CN/water mixture (50/50, V/V) containing 0.1 % CH_3COOH in water, vortex mixed (30 s), sonicated (5 min), and filtered through a PVDF filter into an autosampler vial.
Chromatographic separation was performed on a Waters Acquity UPLC system. An Acquity UPLC BEH C18 column (100 mm × 2.1 mm i.d., 1.7 µm) was used and the analysis was performed with a gradient of water/CH_3CN (95/5, V/V) + 0.3 % CH_3COOH (mobile phase A) and water/CH_3CN (5/95, V/V) + 0.3 % CH_3COOH (mobile phase B). The following elution program was run: 0–8 min (100 % A), 8–12 min (70 % A), 12–13 min (0 % A), 13–13.01 min (linear gradient to 100 % A), 13.01–14.6 min (100 % A). Flow rate was set at 0.4 ml/min. A Xevo TQ-MS triple quadrupole mass spectrometer with an ESI probe operating in the positive ionization mode was used. Quantitation

was done with Masslynx software v 4.1. MS-MS transitions for SDZ were: *m/z* 250.89 > 155.94/107.96 and for TRIM: *m/z* 290.98 > 122.99/230.01. The detected ion ratio's for the different samples were within the permitted tolerances specified in Commission Decision 2002/657/EC [32].

Method validation

The methods were validated for feed and feces according to a set of parameters that were in compliance with the recommendations and guidelines defined by the European Community [32] and international standards for validation of analytical methods in residue depletion studies [33]. The following set of parameters was determined: limit of detection (LOD, $n = 6$), limit of quantification (LOQ, $n = 6$), linearity (R^2 and goodness-of-fit coefficient (g)), precision (repeatability, RSD_r ($n = 6$), and reproducibility, RSD_R ($n = 6$)) and trueness ($n = 6$). Validation samples were prepared with blank feed from the same batch as the feed that was administered during the experiment and blank feces were obtained from pigs that were not treated with antimicrobial drugs.

Statistical analysis

After determination of normality and homogeneity of variances, one-way analysis of variance (ANOVA) (SPSS 22, IBM, Chicago, IL, U.S.) was performed for each antimicrobial on the concentrations from the four different intestinal segments. A Scheffé test was performed as post-hoc test. The significance level was set at 0.05.

Results

Method validation

The results of the method validation are given in Additional file 1: Table S1. All values, except for the trueness in case of SDZ in feed, were within the acceptance ranges according to Commission Decision 2002/657/EC [32].

Concentrations in experimental feed

Ten samples of each batch of experimental feed were analyzed to assess if the target concentrations (3 % of the MRD) were achieved. Mean concentrations ± standard deviation (SD) in the feed were 7.33 ± 6.87 mg/kg (=3.26 % of MRD) for DOX, 9.98 ± 5.35 mg/kg (=3.23 % of MRD) for CTC, 12.99 ± 4.15 mg/kg (=3.12 % of MRD) for SDZ and 2.31 ± 0.90 mg/kg (=2.77 % of MRD) for TRIM. In all experimental diets, there was a high variation between sample concentrations.

Concentrations in feces

The mean (+ SD) concentrations of CTC, DOX and SDZ in the feces are shown in Fig. 1. A steady-state was reached around day 4 for CTC (±10 mg/kg), DOX (±4 mg/kg) and SDZ (±0.7 mg/kg). Concentrations of TRIM were very low; all results except two were lower than the LOD of 0.016 mg/kg. No traces of antimicrobials were found in the fecal samples taken on day 0, just before the start of the experimental period.

Transfer ratio's (TR), i.e. the mean concentration in feces taken over day 4 – day 10 of the experimental period, and divided by the mean concentration in feed, were 102.5, 55.4 and 4.7 % for CTC, DOX and SDZ, respectively (Table 1).

Concentrations in cecal and colonic content

CTC, DOX and SDZ concentrations in cecal content and contents of different segments of the colon after 10 days of feeding are presented in Fig. 2. Min/max/mean concentrations for CTC in the different intestinal segments were 4.06/9.15/6.95 mg/kg (caecum, CM), 5.20/13.89/8.41 mg/kg (PCA), 5.14/11.22/7.12 mg/kg (DCA) and 8.99/11.63/10.08 mg/kg (CD). For DOX, these concentrations were 1.01/3.07/1.78 mg/kg (CM), 1.47/5.86/3.31 mg/kg (PCA), 1.40/3.51/2.68 mg/kg (DCA) and 2.80/4.62/3.81 mg/kg (CD). SDZ concentrations were 0.23/0.83/0.47 mg/kg (CM), 0.21/0.67/0.45 mg/kg (PCA), 0.51/1.00/0.67 mg/kg (DCA) and 0.47/0.65/0.54 mg/kg (CD). All results for TRIM were again lower than the LOD of 0.016 mg/kg. Concentrations in the CD approached the average feces concentration found for CTC, DOX and SDZ. CTC concentrations found in the CD proved to be significantly higher compared to concentrations in the DCA and the CM, but not compared to the PCA. DOX levels in the CM were significantly lower than in the PCA and CD. SDZ levels in the DCA were significantly higher than in the PCA. The TR's, i.e. the mean concentration in CM, PCA, DCA or CD divided by the mean concentration in the feed, are given in Table 1.

Discussion

The aim of this study was to determine which concentrations of CTC, DOX, SDZ and TRIM could be found in intestinal content and feces of pigs when feed containing a 3 % carry-over concentration was administered.

In each experimental diet the target concentration of 3 % of the MRD was approached (2.77–3.26 %). Although the best possible sampling procedure [7] was applied, a large variation between the samples was found. Adequate mixing of the premixes depends on multiple factors, including physico-chemical properties such as particle size and electrostatic properties of the premix. Other factors that influence homogeneity are the composition of the final feed, type of mixing machinery, mixing in stages or trituration and precision and size of the samples taken for analysis [34]. Since very small volumes

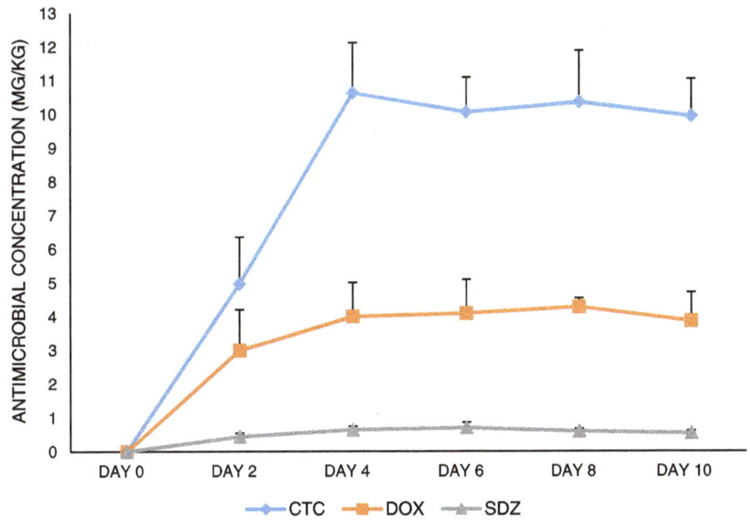

Fig. 1 Mean concentrations (mean of six pigs + standard deviation) of chlortetracycline (CTC), doxycycline (DOX) and sulfadiazine (SDZ) in pig feces during 10 days of ad libitum feeding with feed containing 3 % cross-contamination levels of these antimicrobials. For CTC, concentrations rose from 4.97 mg/kg to a steady-state of approximately 10 mg/kg. Mean concentrations of DOX rose from 2.99 mg/kg to a steady-state of approximately 4 mg/kg. Mean concentrations of SDZ rose from 0.44 mg/kg to a steady-state of approximately 0.70 mg/kg

of premix had to be mixed with large amounts of blank feed, it is not surprising that a large variability among samples was found. Moreover, studies on cross-contamination in feed mills show that antimicrobials are not homogenously divided in flushing feed either [6]. In contrast, concentrations found in intestinal content and feces showed a much lower variation.

In case of SDZ-TRIM, concentrations found in feces and intestinal content were very low (SDZ max. 0.995 mg/kg, TRIM < LOD). Except for two values, all results for TRIM were lower than the LOD. Since the administered dose was very low (2.31 mg/kg feed), the reported oral bioavailability for TRIM is high (73–92 % [22, 23]) and elimination occurs through renal excretion, very low intestinal concentrations were indeed expected. On the other hand, quantitative results for SDZ were obtained, although the oral bioavailability of SDZ in pigs is even higher than for TRIM. This can be explained by the higher absolute dosage of SDZ (12.99 mg/kg feed) compared to TRIM, as both compounds are present in a 5/1 ratio (SDZ/TRIM) in the used formulation. Interestingly, the calculated TR's from feed to gut of SDZ (3.5–5.2 %) correspond well to the high oral bioavailability reported in pigs (85–100 % [22, 23]), i.e. the higher the oral bioavailability the lower residual concentrations in the gut can be expected unless extensive biliary excretion or secretion in the gut takes place.

The concentrations of tetracyclines in feces and cecal and colonic content were found to be relatively high. In general, higher concentrations were seen in the distal part of the colon compared to the proximal part and the caecum. The main explanation for these observations is probably the progressive absorption of water throughout the intestinal tract. As in the case of SDZ, the calculated TR's from feed to gut (CTC 69.6–102.5 %, DOX 24.3–55.4 %) correspond well to the reported oral bioavailability in pigs (CTC 6 %, DOX 21–50 % [24–26]). It has to be taken into account though, that the bioavailability of tetracyclines is highly variable, most likely due to presence of feed in the gastrointestinal tract. It is known that oral absorption of tetracyclines may be reduced in the presence of bivalent ions [24, 35]. Also, the study design to calculate oral bioavailabilities may vary between different studies, e.g. the prandial state of the animals.

Table 1 Oral bioavailability (F) compared to transfer ratio's (TR) of chlortetracycline (CTC), doxycycline (DOX) and sulfadiazine (SDZ)

Antimicrobial	F	TR				
		CM	PCA	DCA	CD	Feces
CTC	6 % [25]	69.6 %	84.2 %	71.4 %	101.0 %	102.5 %
DOX	21–50 % [24, 26]	24.3 %	45.1 %	36.6 %	51.9 %	55.4 %
SDZ	85–100 % [22, 23]	3.7 %	3.5 %	5.2 %	4.2 %	4.7 %

TR's are calculated by dividing the mean concentration (6 pigs) in the content of an intestinal segment (*CM* caecum, *PCA* proximal colon ascendens, *DCA* distal colon ascendens, *CD* colon descendens) after 10 days of feeding by the mean concentration in the feed. The mean concentration in the feces was taken over day 4 - day 10 (steady-state)

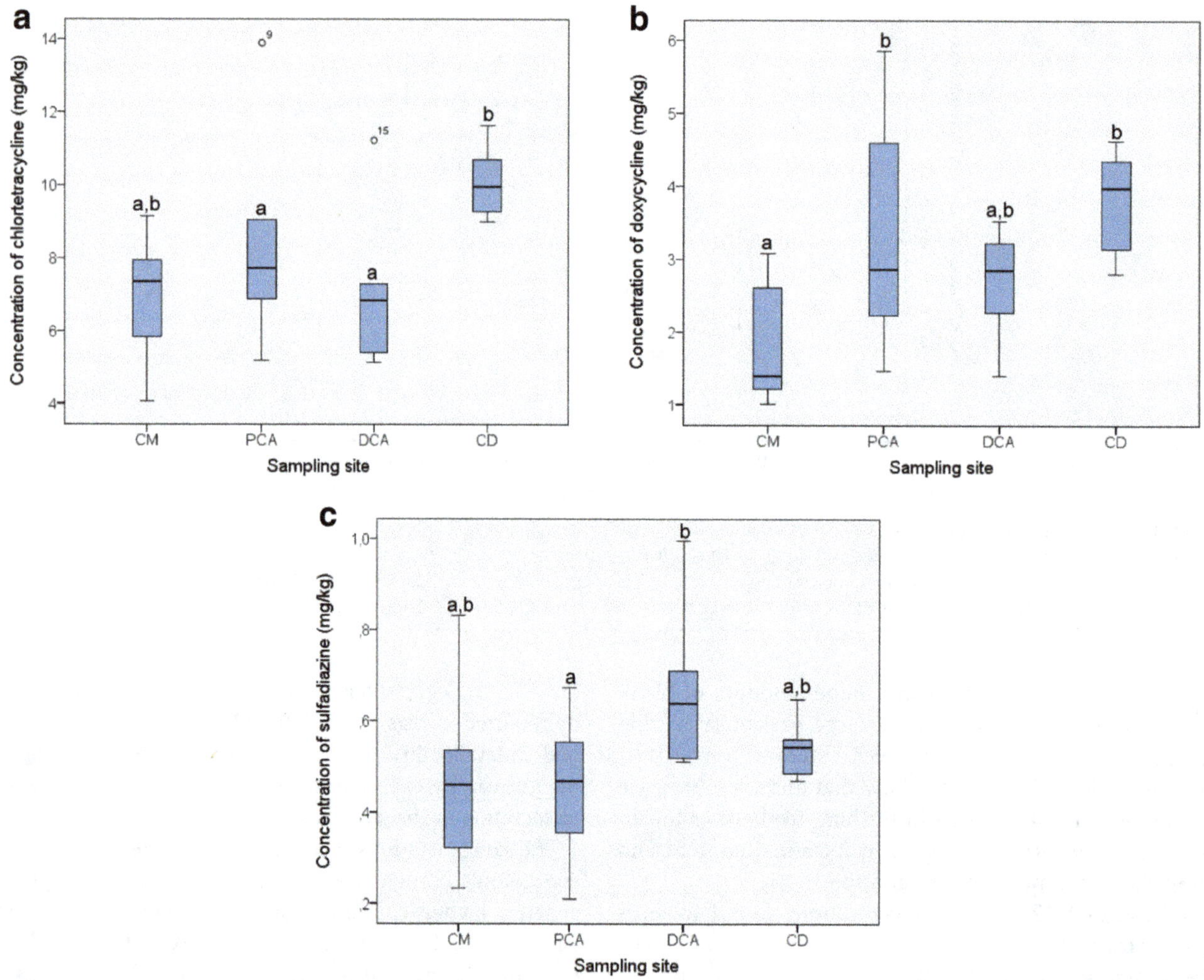

Fig. 2 Concentrations of A) chlortetracycline (CTC), B) doxycycline (DOX) and C) sulfadiazine (SDZ) in cecal content and colonic content from three different sampling segments (6 indepentent observations per sampling segment). Samples were taken from 6 pigs per group after 10 days of ad libitum feeding with feed containing 3 % cross-contamination levels of CTC, DOX and SDZ. Mean concentrations in caecum (CM), proximal colon ascendens (PCA), distal colon ascendens (DCA) and colon descendens (CD) were 6.95, 8.41, 7.12 and 10.08 mg/kg (CTC), 1.78, 3.31, 2.68 and 3.81 mg/kg (DOX) and 0.47, 0.45, 0.67 and 0.54 mg/kg (SDZ), respectively. The two outlying values for CTC (observation 9 and 15) belong to one animal. A different letter (a or b) denotes a significant difference in concentration between sampling segments ($p < 0.05$)

Taking into account that our experiment involves feed administration, references regarding oral bioavailability in non-fasted pigs in particular were consulted. Especially for DOX, the oral bioavailability seems to vary, even within the same study between individual animals (8.0–32.4 % [24], 40–50 % [26]). The intestinal concentrations of DOX in the present study correspond best to the oral bioavailability reported in a previous study that also used a premix formulation (40–50 %) [26] when compared to administration of an oral powder (8–32.4 %) [23]. Besides oral bioavailability, also the excretion route can influence the intestinal concentrations of a drug. SDZ-TRIM and CTC are renally excreted whereas up to 75 % of DOX is excreted unchanged in the intestinal tract [36]. It would therefore be expected that the TR ratio of DOX is higher than based solely on oral bioavailability. The large variability in reported oral bioavailabilities for DOX might explain the relatively low TR indicating that this TR only serves as a guidance value and depends on several factors.

The oral bioavailability of a drug is usually determined for its therapeutic dose. Given the inverse relation found between the oral bioavailability and intestinal concentrations of SDZ, CTC and DOX, it is rather likely that there is a linear relation between the administered dose and intestinal concentrations. This information can be used in the risk assessment of different cross-contamination levels of pig feed regarding potential resistance selection in the intestinal microbiota. However, this conclusion can only be drawn for the tested antimicrobials and animal species. Furthermore, additional experiments should be performed to confirm our results - ideally testing a range of antimicrobial concentrations - as there is no previous research available to compare. A non-peer reviewed report [37] though, estimated intestinal concentrations of CTC to be 1.68 mg/kg in case of administration of 12 mg CTC/kg feed. This is clearly lower compared to our results (min 5.1–max 13.9 mg/kg CTC in colonic content with 9.98 mg CTC/kg feed).

In a recent study [12], manure samples obtained from different pig, poultry and veal calve farms in the Netherlands were examined for the presence of antimicrobial residues. In 16 out of 20 of the sampled pig farms, residues were detected although no recent use of antimicrobials was reported. Tetracyclines were found in 14 of these farms, with DOX concentrations ranging from 2 to 95,000 μg/kg. Sulfonamides were detected in 6 out of 20 farms, with SDZ concentrations ranging from 1 to 216 μg/kg. In light of these data, it is clear that one should not focus on the absolute results based on 3 % carry-over levels obtained in this study, but rather on the relation found between the oral bioavailability of CTC, DOX and SDZ and intestinal concentrations.

In recent years, more attention has been paid to the possible effects of low antimicrobial concentrations on selection of resistant bacteria. Pioneer studies revealed important effects of very low concentrations on resistance selection in vitro. Gullberg et al. performed competition experiments between strains resistant and susceptible to tetracycline and found minimal selective concentrations of 15 ng/ml (competition between isogenic - except for the resistance determinant - *Salmonella* Typhimurium strains) [13] and 45 ng/ml tetracycline (competition between isogenic *E. coli* strains, with or without resistance plasmid pUUH239.2) [14]. The minimal selective concentration was in this case defined as the concentration where the fitness cost of the resistance is balanced by the antimicrobial-conferred selection for the resistant mutant. This would mean that even concentrations of tetracyclines 100× lower than those found in this study can cause resistance selection. Brewer et al. [15] investigated the effect of 1 μg/ml of different antimicrobials on transfer of resistance genes in vivo in pigs and found that 1 μg/ml of tetracycline and sulfamethazine increased transfer frequency, whereas 1 μg/ml of sulfathiazole did not. It is likely that intestinal concentrations of 1 μg/ml of tetracyclines can be found in pigs, considering our results and the maximum allowed carry-over level (1 %) established in the Belgian covenant [9].

Conclusions

This study showed an inverse relation between intestinal concentrations and the oral bioavailability for SDZ-TRIM as well as for CTC and DOX, which have a high, respectively low oral bioavailability in pigs. As different studies [6, 12] indicate there is a large variation in cross-contamination levels of feed, this result can be an important tool to evaluate possible risks of different contamination levels. Further research is needed to determine the effect on resistance selection in the intestinal microbiota. Furthermore, it would be interesting to perform additional experiments, confirming our results and analyzing other antimicrobials that are frequently used as premix formulation, such as penicillins, macrolides and polymyxins [2].

Abbreviations

API: Active pharmaceutical ingredient; BW: Body weight; $C_4H_6O_4$: Succinic acid; CCl_3COOH: Trichloroacetic acid; CD: Colon descendens; CH_3CN: Acetonitrile; CH_3COOH: Acetic acid; CH_3OH: Methanol; CM: Caecum; DCA: Distal colon ascendens; DMCTC: Demethylchlortetracycline.HCl; DOX: Doxycycline; HCOOH: Formic acid; IS: Internal standard; LOD: Limit of detection; LOQ: Limit of quantitation; MIC: Minimum inhibitory concentration; MRD: Maximum recommended dose; Na_2SO_4: Sodium sulphate; PCA: Proximal colon ascendens; PK: Pharmacokinetic; SD: Standard deviation; SDZ: Sulfadiazine; t_R: Room temperature; TR: Transfer ratio; TRIM: Trimethoprim

Acknowledgements

We gratefully acknowledge the technical assistance of An Maes (UGent) for the tetracyclines analyses and Marijke Hunninck and Petra De Neve (ILVO) for the SDZ-TRIM analyses, and the help of Nathan Broekaert, Thomas De Mil, Sophie Fraeyman and Heidi Wyns for the animal experiment.

Funding

This study is funded by the Belgian Federal Public Service of Health, Food Chain Safety and Environment through the contract RT 12/03 CROSSCONTAM.

Authors' contributions

Design of the study: SC, ED, JD, MH, FH, AS, GR, HI, PB. Executing the animal experiment: LP, MD. Development of the LC-MS/MS method: SC, ED. Analysis of the data: LP, MD, SC, ED. Preparation of the manuscript: LP, SC, MD, ED, GR, AS, JD, MH, HI, FH, PB. All authors read and approved the final manuscript.

Competing interests

The authors declare that they have no competing interests.

Consent for publication

Not applicable.

Author details

[1]Operational Directorate Bacterial Diseases, CODA-CERVA (Veterinary and Agrochemical Research Centre), 1180 Brussels, Belgium. [2]Department of Pathology, Bacteriology and Avian Diseases, Faculty of Veterinary Medicine, Ghent University, 9820 Merelbeke, Belgium. [3]Technology and Food Science Unit, Institute for Agricultural and Fisheries Research, 9090 Melle, Belgium. [4]Department of Pharmacology, Toxicology and Biochemistry, Faculty of Veterinary Medicine, Ghent University, 9820 Merelbeke, Belgium. [5]Veterinary Epidemiology Unit, Department of Reproduction, Obstetrics and Herd health, Faculty of Veterinary Medicine, Ghent University, 9820 Merelbeke, Belgium.

[6]Department of Biosciences, School of Veterinary Medicine, Ross University, Basseterre, Saint Kitts and Nevis.

References

1. Fifth ESVAC report: Sales of veterinary antimicrobial agents in 26 EU/EEA countries in 2013. http://www.ema.europa.eu/docs/en_GB/document_library/Report/2015/10/WC500195687.pdf. Accessed 3 May 2016.
2. Belgian Veterinary Surveillance of Antibacterial Consumption. National consumption report 2014. http://www.belvetsac.ugent.be/pages/home/BelvetSAC_report_2014%20finaal.pdf. Accessed 13 Oct 2015.
3. Callens B, Persoons D, Maes D, Laanen M, Postma M, Boyen F, Haesebrouck F, Butaye P, Catry B, Dewulf J. Prophylactic and metaphylactic antimicrobial use in Belgian fattening pig herds. Prev Vet Med. 2012;106(1):53–62.
4. Advice 19-2013 of the Scientific Committee of the FASFC on responsible use of antibacterial substances via group treatment of livestock and the effect on the selection of resistance. http://www.favv-afsca.fgov.be/scientificcommittee/opinions/2013/_documents/Advice19-2013.pdf. Accessed 13 Oct 2015.
5. Regulation (EC) No 1831/2003 of the European Parliament and of the Council of 22 September 2003 on additives for use in animal nutrition. Off J European Union. 2003;L268:29–43.
6. Stolker AAM, Manti V, Zuidema T, van Egmond H, Deckers ER, Herbes R, Hooglugt J, Heuvel EO, de Jong J. Carry-over of veterinary drugs from medicated to non-medicated feeds in commercial feed manufacturing plants. Food Addit Contam A. 2013;30(6):1100–7.
7. Borras S, Companyo R, Granados M, Guiteras J, Perez-Vendrell AM, Brufau J, Medina M, Bosch J. Analysis of antimicrobial agents in animal feed. Trac-Trend Anal Chem. 2011;30(7):1042–64.
8. Commission Directive 2009/8/EC amending Annex I to Directive 2002/32/EC of the European Parliament and of the Council as regards maximum levels of unavoidable carry-over of coccidiostats or histomonostats in non-target feed. Off J European Union 2002; L40:19–25
9. Convenant betreffende gemedicineerde voeders. BEMEFA. Belgian Compound Feed Industry Association; 2013. http://www.favv-afsca.fgov.be/dierlijkeproductie/dierenvoeding/gemedicineerdevoeders/_documents/2013-01-30_CONVENANT-FAVV-BEMEFA-gemedicineerde-voeders_finaal_jan-2013_NL.pdf. Accessed 13 Oct 2015.
10. McEvoy JDG. Contamination of animal feedingstuffs as a cause of residues in food: a review of regulatory aspects, incidence and control. Anal Chim Acta. 2002;473(1–2):3–26.
11. Putier F. Evaluation of cross-contamination in livestock feed delivery trucks. Technics. Feed magazine/Kraftfutter 2010:9–10.
12. Zuidema T, Stolker AAM, Van Ginkel LA. Kruiscontaminatie van antibiotica. Onderzoek naar de aanwezigheid van antibioticaresiduen in mest van vleesvarkens en vleeskalveren en op pluimveebedrijven, RIKILT-rapport 2014. 015. Wageningen: RIKILT; 2014. p. 48.
13. Gullberg E, Cao S, Berg OG, Ilback C, Sandegren L, Hughes D, Andersson DI. Selection of Resistant Bacteria at Very Low Antibiotic Concentrations. Plos Pathog. 2011;7(7), e1002158. doi:10.1371/journal.ppat.1002158.
14. Gullberg E, Albrecht LM, Karlsson C, Sandegren L, Andersson DI. Selection of a Multidrug Resistance Plasmid by Sublethal Levels of Antibiotics and Heavy Metals. Mbio. 2014;5(5), e01918-14. doi:10.1128/mBio.01918-14.
15. Brewer MT, Xiong N, Anderson KL, Carlson SA. Effects of subtherapeutic concentrations of antimicrobials on gene acquisition events in Yersinia, Proteus, Shigella, and Salmonella recipient organisms in isolated ligated intestinal loops of swine. Am J Vet Res. 2013;74(8):1078–83.
16. Sandegren L. Selection of antibiotic resistance at very low antibiotic concentrations. Upsala J Med Sci. 2014;119:103–7.
17. Liu A, Fong A, Becket E, Yuan J, Tamae C, Medrano L, Maiz M, Wahba C, Lee C, Lee K, et al. Selective Advantage of Resistant Strains at Trace Levels of Antibiotics: a Simple and Ultrasensitive Color Test for Detection of Antibiotics and Genotoxic Agents. Antimicrob Agents Chemother. 2011;55(3):1204–10.
18. Andersson DI, Hughes D. Antibiotic resistance and its cost: is it possible to reverse resistance? Nat Rev Microbiol. 2010;8(4):260–71.
19. Olofsson SK, Cars O. Optimizing drug exposure to minimize selection of antibiotic resistance. Clin Infect Dis. 2007;45:S129–36.
20. Hu M, Li X. Barriers to Oral Bioavailability-An Overview. In: Oral Bioavailability: Basic Principles, Advanced Concepts, and Applications. 1st ed. Hoboken: Wiley; 2011. p. 1–7.
21. Belgian Veterinary Surveillance of Antimicrobial Consumption. National consumption report 2012. http://www.belvetsac.ugent.be/pages/home/BelvetSAC_report_2012%20finaal.pdf. Accessed 13 Oct 2015.
22. Nielsen P, Gyrd-Hansen N. Oral bioavailability of sulphadiazine and trimethoprim in fed and fasted pigs. Res Vet Sci. 1994;56(1):48–52.
23. Baert K, De Baere S, Croubels S, Gasthuys F, De Backer P. Pharmacokinetics and bioavailability of sulfadiazine and trimethoprim (trimazin 30 %) after oral administration in non-fasted young pigs. J Vet Pharmacol Ther. 2001; 24(4):295–8.
24. Baert K, Croubels S, Gasthuys F, De Busser J, De Backer P. Pharmacokinetics and oral bioavailability of a doxycycline formulation (DOXYCYCLINE 75 %) in nonfasted young pigs. J Vet Pharmacol Ther. 2000;23(1):45–8.
25. Nielsen P, GyrdHansen N. Bioavailability of oxytetracycline, tetracycline and chlortetracycline after oral administration to fed and fasted pigs. J Vet Pharmacol Ther. 1996;19(4):305–11.
26. Sanders P, Gicquel M, Hurtaud D, Chapel AM, Gaudiche C, Bousquet E. Absolute bioavailability of doxycycline after oral administration in medicated feed to pigs. Bologna: Proceedings of the 14th IPVS Congress; 1996. p. 663.
27. Vandenberge V, Delezie E, Huyghebaert G, Delahaut P, Daeseleire E, Croubels S. Residues of sulfadiazine and doxycycline in broiler liver and muscle tissue due to cross-contamination of feed. Food Addit Contam Part A Chem Anal Control Expo Risk Assess. 2012;29(2):180–8.
28. Vandenberge V, Delezie E, Huyghebaert G, Delahaut P, De Backer P, Daeseleire E, Croubels S. Residues of sulfadiazine and doxycycline in egg matrices due to cross-contamination in the feed of laying hens and the possible correlation with physicochemical, pharmacokinetic and physiological parameters. Food Addit Contam A. 2012;29(6):908–17.
29. Segato G, Benetti C, Angeletti R, Montesissa C, Biancotto G. Doxycycline and sulfadimethoxine transfer from cross-contaminated feed to chicken tissues. Food Addit Contam A. 2011;28(7):860–8.
30. Cherlet M, De Backer P, Croubels S. Control of the keto-enol tautomerism of chlortetracycline for its straightforward quantitation in pig tissues by liquid chromatography-electrospray ionization tandem mass spectrometry. J Chromatogr A. 2006;1133(1–2):135–41.
31. Cherlet M, Schelkens M, Croubels S, De Backer P. Quantitative multi-residue analysis of tetracyclines and their 4-epimers in pig tissues by high-performance liquid chromatography combined with positive-ion electrospray ionization mass spectrometry. Anal Chim Acta. 2003;492(1–2):199–213.
32. European Commission. Commission Decision 2002/675/EC implementing Council Directive 96/23/EC concerning the performances of analytical methods and the interpretation of results. Off J European Union. 2002;L221:8–36.
33. VICH_GL_49: Studies to evaluate the metabolism and residue kinetics of veterinary drugs in food producing animals: validation of analytical methods used in residue depletion studies. http://www.fda.gov/downloads/AnimalVeterinary/GuidanceComplianceEnforcement/GuidanceforIndustry/UCM207942.pdf. Accessed 13 Oct 2015.
34. Note for guidance: Additional quality requirements for products intended for incorporation into animal feedingstuffs (medicated premixes). http://www.ema.europa.eu/docs/en_GB/document_library/Scientific_guideline/2009/10/WC500004466.pdf. Accessed 13 Oct 2015.
35. Santos MDF, Vermeersch H, Remon JP, Schelkens M, DeBacker HJJ, VanBree HJJ, Ducatelle R, Haesebrouck F. Pharmacokinetics and bioavailability of doxycycline in turkeys. J Vet Pharmacol Ther. 1996;19(4):274–80.
36. Ahrens FA, Martin RJ. Antimicrobial drugs. In: Hsu WH, editor. Handbook of Veterinary Pharmacology. 1st ed. Ames: Wiley-Blackwell; 2008. p. 357.
37. Potential effects of carryover of antimicrobials in pig feed. http://www.octagon-services.co.uk/articles/carryover.pdf. Accessed 13 Oct 2015.

Safety evaluation of the interchangeable use of robenacoxib (Onsior™) tablets and solution for injection in dogs

Céline E. Toutain[1*], Mark C. Heit[2], Stephen B. King[2] and Rainer Helbig[1]

Abstract

Background: Robenacoxib (Onsior™) is a non-steroidal anti-inflammatory drug developed for canine and feline use for the control of pain and inflammation. It is available as both tablets and solution for injection. The objective of this safety study was to investigate the interchangeable use of two robenacoxib formulations in dogs using a novel study design alternating between oral tablets and subcutaneous injections. Thirty-two naïve healthy 4-month dogs were enrolled in this 88-day study and were randomized among four groups to be untreated or to receive robenacoxib at the highest recommended or elevated dose rates. The dogs were administered three 20-day treatment cycles each separated by a 14-day washout period. Each 20-day cycle was comprised of 10 days of once daily oral administration, 3 days of subcutaneous administration, followed by further 7 days of oral administration (Groups 2 to 4). The control group (Group 1) received oral empty gelatin capsules or subcutaneous saline injections. Assessment of safety was based on general health observations, clinical observations, physical and neurological examinations including ophthalmological examinations, electrocardiographic examinations and clinical pathology evaluations, food and water consumption, body weight, and macroscopic and microscopic examinations. Blood samples were collected for pharmacokinetic evaluation.

Results: Blood concentrations of robenacoxib confirmed systemic exposure of all treated dogs. All dogs were in good health through study termination and there were no serious adverse events during the course of the study. No changes in body weight, food consumption, ophthalmic, neurological examinations, electrocardiograms, buccal mucosal blood times, clinical pathology or organ weight were attributable to robenacoxib formulation administration. Primary treatment-related abnormalities were of low incidence at all doses. They were confined to macroscopic and microscopic changes observed locally at the subcutaneous injection sites and microscopic findings within the gastrointestinal tract. These findings were as expected based on previous studies with robenacoxib solution for injection alone and the known properties of this class of compound and mode of administration. There were no adverse effects which could be attributed specifically to the interchangeable use of oral and injectable robenacoxib.

Conclusions: Alternating regimens of robenacoxib tablets and solution for injection were well tolerated in healthy young dogs.

Keywords: Robenacoxib, Onsior™, Tablet, Injection, NSAID, Dog, Safety, Interchangeable

Background

Robenacoxib is a non-steroidal anti-inflammatory drug (NSAID) of the cyclooxygenase (COX)-2 inhibitor (coxib) subclass with a fast onset of action in dogs and cats [1, 2]. It is a registered veterinary medicinal product available for dogs as an injectable (Onsior™ 20 mg/mL solution for injection, Elanco Animal Health, Greenfield, IN) and oral (Onsior™ 10 mg, 20 mg and 40 mg tablets, Elanco Animal Health, Greenfield, IN) formulation. Onsior™ is licensed in the US for use in dogs for the control of postoperative pain and inflammation associated with soft tissue surgery at a dose of 2 mg/kg subcutaneously or 2 mg/kg orally (2–4 mg/kg range) for a maximum of 3 days [3, 4]. Onsior™ tablet is registered in Europe for the treatment of pain and inflammation associated with chronic osteoarthritis in dogs at a dose of 1 mg/kg (1–2 mg/kg range) for up to 10 days. Onsior™ is also available in Europe as a solution for injection for the treatment of pain and inflammation

* Correspondence: celine.toutain@elanco.com
[1]Elanco Animal Health, a Division of Eli Lilly and Company, Mattenstrasse 24A, CH-4058 Basel, Switzerland
Full list of author information is available at the end of the article

associated with orthopedic or soft tissue surgery at a dose of 2 mg/kg [5]. The systemic bioavailability of robenacoxib solution is 88% and it is 62% with food or 84% without food, for the tablet [5].

Thanks to its pharmacodynamic and pharmacokinetic properties, robenacoxib displays a favorable safety profile in healthy dogs [6]. Indeed, robenacoxib targets COX-2 activity and is able to spare COX-1 activity [1, 6–8]. In addition, robenacoxib is characterized by a rapid elimination from the central compartment with a prolonged persistence at sites of inflammation [9, 10].

The safety of robenacoxib has been investigated in both cats [11, 12] and dogs [6, 13]. The safety of oral administration was demonstrated in individual studies in healthy young dogs (approximately 6 months of age) up to 40 mg/kg for 1 month and up to 10 mg/kg for 6 months [6]. In addition, the safety of subcutaneous administration in adult dogs was established up to 10 mg/kg once a day for 3 days [4].

This target animal safety study was a component of the safety data package presented to the Food and Drug Administration's Center for Veterinary Medicine (FDA-CVM) for the interchangeable use approval. Its objective was to apply a novel study design to establish the safety of the interchangeable use of Onsior™ tablets and Onsior™ solution for injection in dogs. By alternating between oral tablet and subcutaneous (SC) injection dosing, it was possible to demonstrate that tablets and injections can be used sequentially in either order. This is relevant for situations, in which for example a dog receives robenacoxib for surgery via injection and then continues for two additional days of postoperative pain therapy with tablets or when a dog treated with oral robenacoxib for osteoarthritis receives a single injection of robenacoxib for surgery and then continues with its oral osteoarthritis therapy. Because Onsior™ is a globally marketed product and dosages and indications vary in different geographies, the dose levels used in this study were selected to equal or exceed all potential scenarios of use and addressed both indications (postoperative pain and osteoarthritis). Group 1 was the negative control group. Groups 2 to 4 received three cycles of oral and subcutaneous treatments (separated by a washout period). During each cycle, Group 2 was administered ≥2 mg/kg orally for 7 days, ≥4 mg/kg orally for 3 days, 4 mg/kg subcutaneously for 3 days and ≥2 mg/kg orally for 7 days. Groups 3 and 4 received multiples thereof (2X and 3X). In addition, to investigate the minimum proposed label age for safe use of Onsior™, dogs were 4 months of age at start of treatment compared to 6 months of age in previous safety studies.

Methods

Objective and standards

The objective of the study was to establish the safety of the interchangeable use of robenacoxib (Onsior™) tablets and solution for injection in dogs starting at 4 months of age.

This study was conducted in compliance with Good Laboratory Practice [14, 15] and site procedures. It was designed in consultation with regulatory authorities (FDA-CVM) and according to the VICH guideline for evaluating the target animal safety of new pharmaceuticals (VICH Guideline 43 [16]). All animal procedures were in compliance with the U.S. Department of Agriculture's Animal Welfare Act [17], the Guide for the Care and Use of Laboratory Animals [18] and the Office of Laboratory Animal Welfare [19]. The study was reviewed and approved by the study site Institutional Animal Care and Use Committee.

Animal management

Young purpose-bred mongrel dogs (crossbred hounds) were used. Thirty-two naïve dogs (16 males and 16 females, weighing 13 kg to 19.3 kg and 11.9 kg to 13.8 kg, respectively at initiation of dosing) were selected and obtained commercially from a laboratory animal supplier (Marshall BioResources, North Rose, New York). Each animal was uniquely identified with a microchip and acclimatized to the study conditions for 4 weeks. Dogs were approximately 4 months old at initiation of dosing (Day 1). Suitability was evaluated by physical examination and clinical pathology and only healthy animals were included. Dogs were housed individually indoors in climate controlled facilities (20 to 26 °C, 30 to 70% humidity and 12-h light/12-h dark cycle) in accordance with accepted laboratory animal care and use guidelines. Dogs were fed ad libitum at least 8 h each day with an appropriate ration of a certified commercial canine feed and water was available ad libitum. Dogs were observed for general health, behavior and appetite at least once daily throughout the study. Environment enrichment included visual, auditory and olfactory contact with other animals and dogs were provided exercise opportunities in large kennel runs.

Experimental design

This was a randomized, controlled, blinded study with a parallel design (Fig. 1). The 32 dogs were randomized to the four dose groups and the four rooms used in the study within each sex, with an equal number of males and females within each room and an equal number of animals from each group within each room. Healthy mongrel dogs (4/sex/group) were administered three 20-day cycles (each separated by a 14-day washout period). Each 20-day cycle was comprised of 10 days of once daily oral robenacoxib administration, 3 days of subcutaneous robenacoxib treatment followed

Study days	1-7	8-10	11-13	14-20	21-34	35-41	42-44	45-47	48-54	55-68	69-75	76-78	79-81	82-88
Group	7-day oral	3-day oral	3-day SC	7-day oral	14-day	7-day oral	3-day oral	3-day SC	7-day oral	14-day	7-day oral	3-day oral	3-day SC	7-day oral
1	0 mg/kg	0 mg/kg		0 mg/kg	washout	0 mg/kg	0 mg/kg		0 mg/kg	washout	0 mg/kg	0 mg/kg		0 mg/kg
2	2 mg/kg	4 mg/kg		2 mg/kg		2 mg/kg	4 mg/kg		2 mg/kg		2 mg/kg	4 mg/kg		2 mg/kg
3	4 mg/kg	8 mg/kg		4 mg/kg		4 mg/kg	8 mg/kg		4 mg/kg		4 mg/kg	8 mg/kg		4 mg/kg
4	6 mg/kg	12 mg/kg		6 mg/kg		6 mg/kg	12 mg/kg		6 mg/kg		6 mg/kg	12 mg/kg		6 mg/kg

Fig. 1 Study design diagram

by 7 days of oral administration (Groups 2 to 4) to result in a total of 60 treatment days and 88 in-life days. The negative control group (Group 1) received empty gelatin capsules or saline injection consistent with the Group 4 animals.

Test articles and administration

Robenacoxib was orally administered as Onsior™ tablets (20 or 40 mg of robenacoxib) or by subcutaneous administration of Onsior™ solution for injection (20 mg/mL of robenacoxib) under fasted conditions. The excipients used in the Onsior™ formulations [5] are standard excipients and are widely used in veterinary and human pharmaceuticals. Appropriately sized whole tablets placed in one or two gelatin capsules (Torpac® no.12, Torpac Inc., Fairfield, NJ, USA) were used to provide the most accurate dosing based on the body weights of the study dogs. The number and strength of oral tablets were calculated to ensure that the minimum targeted dose level was achieved. For Group 2, this meant that dogs received a robenacoxib dose of at least 2 mg/kg during the first and last 7 days of each cycle and at least 4 mg/kg from the 8th to 13th day of each cycle (Fig. 1). The dose level for robenacoxib injections was in all cases delivered at the exact dosage (i.e. 4 mg/kg for Group 2). Dose levels within the study were determined as multiples (2X and 3X) of the dose levels received by Group 2. A different injection site was used on each dosing day (as recommended by the Joint Working Group on Refinement [20] and the product label [4]) in order to minimize the potential damage that could result from multiple injections at a single site. Injections were administered at nine distinct sites where three each were located at the left shoulder, the midline interscapular region and right shoulder.

Safety variables

Safety variables recorded and samples collected during the in-life phase are presented in Table 1. Clinical observations, body weight, food consumption, physical and neurological examinations, injection site scoring, ophthalmologic examinations, electrocardiographic examinations, buccal mucosal bleeding time (BMBT) and clinical pathology evaluations (hematology, clinical chemistry, coagulation and urinalysis) were performed prior to randomization, during and at the end of the dosing phase.

Animals were checked twice daily for mortality, abnormalities and signs of pain or distress. Cageside observations were made once daily throughout the study. Additionally, on each day of dosing, observations were performed 1 h (± 15 min) post-dose and on each day of subcutaneous dosing, animals were observed for an immediate response upon administration of the injection. Detailed observations included, but were not limited to: changes in skin, fur, eyes, and mucous membranes; occurrences of secretions and excretions; and autonomic activity (e.g., lacrimation, piloerection, pupil size and unusual respiratory pattern). For evaluation of gait, animals were allowed to walk freely.

Body weights were measured at least once a week during the study, at the same time in the morning (prior to dosing) on a calibrated balance. Food consumption was measured and recorded daily. Complete physical and neurological examinations were conducted five times during the study, by a veterinarian. Physical examinations included evaluation of general condition and behaviour, eyes without ophthalmoscope, integument, musculoskeletal and gastrointestinal systems, body temperature, cardiovascular and respiratory systems, including calculation of heart rate and assessment by auscultation and reproductive system. Neurological examinations included observation of nystagmus, pupillary response, extensor thrust (muscle tone), righting reflex, startle reflex and walking movement.

Injection sites were scored for erythema, edema, heat and pain on palpation and were measured (if necessary), on days of dosing and for 3 days following each injection. Electrocardiograms (ECGs) were performed to evaluate the cardiovascular system in accordance with VICH GL 43. They were digitally recorded from unanesthetized animals on Days 20 and 88 and the ECG traces from each animal were examined by a certified veterinary cardiologist for the following variables: PR interval, QRS duration, QT interval, RR interval, heart rate and heart rate-corrected QT (QTc) interval. A qualitative review for rhythm abnormalities and disturbances was performed.

Analyses of robenacoxib concentrations in blood

Whole blood (2 mL) was collected from fasted animals via a jugular or cephalic vein 1 and 5 h post dose on

Table 1 Safety variables recorded and samples collected during the in-life phase

Variables	Study days[a]
Clinical observations	General observations twice daily Cageside observations once daily Observations 1 h ± 15 min postdose Detailed observations (Days 7, 10, 13, 21, 28, 34, 41, 44, 47, 55, 62, 69, 75, 78, 81 and 89) 1 h ± 15 min postdose (on dosing days)
Body weight	Days 1, 8, 11, 14, 21, 28, 35, 42, 45, 48, 55, 62, 69, 76, 79, 82, 88 and 89
Food consumption	Daily
Physical and neurological examinations	Days 20, 34, 54, 68 and 88
Injection sites scoring	Days of injection (predose and 7 to 8 h postdose) and at 24, 48, and 72 h (±1 h) following each injection
Ophthalmologic examination	Day 88
Electrocardiographic examination	1 h ± 15 min postdose on Days 20 and 88
Buccal mucosal bleed times	Days 20 and 88
Clinical pathology	Days 21, 55 and 89
Bioanalytical collection	*Dose cycle 1:* On days 1 and 14, samples were collected predose and 1 and 5 h postdose On days 6, 8 and 11, samples were collected 1 and 5 h postdose *Dose cycle 3:* On days 69 and 82, samples were collected predose and 1 and 5 h postdose On days 74, 76 and 79, samples were collected 1 and 5 h postdose

[a]Dosing phase length was 88 days and necropsies were performed at study termination at Day 89

Days 1, 6, 8, 11, 14, 69, 74, 76, 79 and 82 (Table 1). Additionally, pre-dose samples were collected within 30 min prior to dose administration on Days 1, 14, 69 and 82. Samples were placed in tubes containing K_2 EDTA and were stored frozen (−10 to −30 °C) within 1 h after collection. Whole blood rather than plasma was chosen as smaller volumes of blood are needed which is an advantage not to interfere with primary safety endpoints and in terms of animal welfare. The blood: plasma concentration ratio is approximately 0.5: 1 in the dog, indicating lower concentration in blood than in plasma and that robenacoxib does not penetrate into cells [21] .

Robenacoxib was quantitatively analyzed in blood using a validated analytical method involving liquid chromatography with tandem mass spectrometry detection (LC-MS/MS). Each blood sample (50 μL) was prepared using protein precipitation and chromatographed by HPLC on an ACE 5 μm C18 column (50 × 2.1 mm). The samples were analyzed on an Applied Biosystems/ Sciex API 5000 triple quadrupole mass spectrometer system using the negative electrospray ionisation (TurboIonSpray®) mode and multiple reaction monitoring of the transition m/z 326 → 222 for robenacoxib. The method utilized an internal standard (i.e., deuterated robenacoxib) and quantification ranged from 2.00 ng/ mL (lower limit of quantitation; LLOQ) to 2000 ng/mL (upper limit of quantitation) based on peak area using linear regression with $1/x^2$ concentration weighting. Performance of the method was monitored by quality control samples at 6, 80 and 1600 ng/mL. Mean inter-day precision was 13.0% at LLOQ and ranged between 6.9 and 9.4% at the other levels and the mean inter-day accuracy ranged between 96.5 and 104.2%.

Pharmacokinetics and pharmacodynamics of robenacoxib

Only abbreviated pharmacokinetic sampling was performed so as not to interfere with the primary safety objective of the study. The limited sampling schedule did not allow calculation of half-life or extrapolation of AUC for the entire dose period (i.e., 0 to 24 h), therefore, exposure between 1 and 5 h was calculated ($AUC_{1\text{-}5h}$) using the loglinear trapezoidal rule. Concentrations below the limit of quantification were considered 0.

For levels of inhibition of COX-1 and COX-2, the standard sigmoid model:

$$\%\text{Inhibition} = (I_{max} \times C^n)/(C^n + IC50^n)$$

was used to predict inhibition of TxB_2 (as an index of COX-1 inhibition) and PGE_2 (as an index of COX-2 inhibition) at the robenacoxib concentrations observed during the study. In this model, I_{max} is the maximal inhibition (100%), IC50 is the concentration of robenacoxib providing 50% of Imax, C is the robenacoxib concentrations and n is the slope parameter. The parameters values were obtained from previously published work in dog [6, 8]. Mean values for n and IC50 were, respectively, 0.586 and 11,328 ng/mL for inhibition of TxB_2 and 1.273 and 280.3 ng/mL for inhibition of PGE_2. Inhibition level means and standard deviations at 1 and 5 h after treatment were calculated for each dose. The percent inhibition versus dose was analysed using analysis of variance and the statistical software GraphPad Prism 7.02 (GraphPad Software, La Jolla California USA).

Pathological examinations

At study termination on Day 89, complete necropsies were performed on all animals and macroscopic abnormalities for all tissues were recorded. Organs were weighed and tissues were processed for microscopic examination.

Statistical evaluations of safety variables

All data were analyzed with the statistical software package SAS (2002–2008) (Statistical analysis system. Version 9.2, Cary, North Carolina: SAS Institute Inc.). The following endpoints were analyzed: body weight, food consumption, injection site scoring, ECG variables, organ weights, clinical pathology and pharmacokinetic parameters. Except for the pharmacokinetic parameters, each treated group (Group 2 to 4) was analyzed compared to the control group (Group 1).

Endpoints measured once post-treatment (i.e., organ weight) were analyzed using analysis of variance (ANOVA) with treatment, sex and treatment by sex as fixed effects [22]. If a pre-treatment value was available (i.e., ECG), it was used as a covariate (analysis of covariance, ANCOVA). Endpoints measured multiple times postdose (i.e. injection site scoring) were analyzed using repeated measures analysis of variance (RMANOVA) with treatment, time and sex, the two-way interactions treatment x time, treatment x sex, and sex x time, and the three-way interaction treatment x time x sex all as fixed effects. If a pre-treatment measurement was available (i.e., bodyweights, food consumption, hematology, coagulation, urinalysis and clinical chemistry), it was used as a covariate (repeated measures analysis of covariance, RMANCOVA). The pre-treatment value closest to dosing was used as the covariate [23].

Depending on the significance of the interaction terms ($p \leq 0.10$ level for two-way interactions and $p \leq 0.05$ for the three-way interaction), treated groups were compared to the control either within each sex (treatment x sex significant), within each time point (treatment x time significant) or main effect only (neither treatment x sex nor treatment x time significant).

Results

Test article dosages

Ranges for individual robenacoxib dosages achieved using tablets are provided in Table 2 and were equal to or exceeded the minimum target oral dose levels in all treatment groups. Due to body weight gain of study dogs, the individual dose volumes of injected sterile saline (0.6 mL/kg) or robenacoxib solution (0.2, 0.4 and 0.6 mL/kg for Group 2 to 4) increased from the first dosing cycle through the last dosing cycle in all animals.

Table 2 Oral dosing table

Group	Target dosage (mg/kg/day)	Actual dosage range (mg/kg/day)
Group 2	≥2	2.0–3.4
	≥4	4.1–5.3
Group 3	≥4	4.0–5.3
	≥8	8.0–9.1
Group 4	≥6	6.0–7.3
	≥12	12.0–13.4

Ranges for individual injected dose volumes are provided in Table 3 where the maximum that any dog received was 17.0 mL. The maximum dose volume of 0.6 mL/kg administered in this study was below the administration volume considered good practice or maximal (1 and 2 mL/kg respectively) [24].

Physical, clinical and neurological observations

All mongrels were in good health through study termination. There were no serious adverse events during the course of the study and no treatment-related adverse findings in general health observations. No treatment-related abnormalities were noted during the physical examinations or neurological abnormalities other than injection site findings as described hereafter. Over the entire study, a total of 288 subcutaneous injections were administered and only occasional scratching (47 observations) or excessive licking of the dose site (27 observations) were noted. Additionally, there was a single observation each of twitching and vocalization, in a Group 4 female and Group 2 male, respectively during dosing.

Other clinical observations included liquid, mucoid, or non-formed feces, vomitus and various other findings on the skin and pelage. These observations appeared infrequently, were transient and lacked a dose relationship for incidence, or were reported at a comparable incidence in control animals and/or during the predose phase or

Table 3 Subcutaneous dosing volume table

Group	Study day	Dose volume (mL/day)
Group 1	11–13	7.9–10.9
	45–47	9.8–14.9
	79–81	10.9–16.7
Group 2	11–13	2.6–4.3
	45–47	3.3–5.6
	79–81	3.7–6.4
Group 3	11–13	5.5–7.7
	45–47	6.9–10.0
	79–81	7.6–11.7
Group 4	11–13	7.8–11.3
	45–47	10.4–14.4
	79–81	11.0–17.0

washout periods. They were therefore not considered test article-related.

Body weights and food consumption

All dogs gained weight during the study. Individual body weight gain in the treatment groups between dosing phase Day 1 and 88 ranged from 8.1 to 15.5 kg and 6.4 to 10.8 kg for males and females, respectively. No test article-related effects were noted in body weight for either sex as no statistically significant differences between control and treated animals were observed ($p = 0.2386$). A significant sex x time interaction was observed ($p = 0.0002$), which is expected in growing animals. No test article-related effects were noted in food consumption as no statistical significant differences between control and treated animals were observed ($p = 0.1233$).

Ophthalmology, electrocardiography and buccal mucosal bleeding time

No ophthalmic or ECG parameter abnormalities or changes in BMBT were noted during the study. During the two pre-test periods, BMBT ranged from 34 s to 2 min 44 s in all study animals. On Day 20 and 88, the times for all animals were within this range with two exceptions. On Day 20, the BMBT for a Group 2 female was 3 min and 16 s, but decreased to 1 min and 26 s on Day 88. This female had increased fibrinogen on Day 21 likely associated with the concurrent findings of a scab and swollen skin at the injection site on Days 19 and 21. On Day 88 the BMBT for a Group 3 female was 25 s which was considered not clinically relevant.

Injection sites

There was a greater number of injection sites with edema at 8 h post-injection and with erythema at 24, 48, and 72 h post-injection in Groups 3 and 4 compared to Groups 1 or 2. In some instances, the erythema continued as skin thickening and/or an ulcer/cyst developed followed by granulation. Ulcers or fluid-filled cysts occurred in one control dog, 2 dogs in Group 2, 4 dogs in Group 3 and in 4 dogs in Group 4. Ulcers tended to have a delayed occurrence, happening 6–8 days after injection out to 10–14 days after injection.

Microscopic findings at injection sites included subcutaneous necrosis, degeneration, and/or fibrosis with occasional involvement of the underlying panniculus muscle (Group 2–4). Minimal to moderate acanthosis/hyperkeratosis of the overlying skin was observed (Group 2–4). Minimal or slight acanthosis/hyperkeratosis in two Group 3 dogs and one Group 4 dog, and minimal to moderate ulceration of the skin (Groups 3 and 4) were also observed. Slight infiltrates of macrophages and an infiltrate of lipid within the axillary lymph nodes were noted in one control dog and all treated dogs. Axillary lymph node findings reflected drainage from the subcutaneous injection sites, therefore, they were considered secondary and not primary test article-related effects.

Clinical pathology and urinalysis

Summary data for selected haematology and clinical chemistry are presented in Tables 4 and 5. There were no notable differences present for haematology, clinical chemistry, coagulation profiles, or urinalysis parameters between control and treated groups. Any statistically significant differences (e.g. lower white blood cell count for Groups 2 and 4 when compared to the control ($p = 0.0154$ and 0.0467, respectively), and lower urea nitrogen for Groups 3 and 4 when compared to the control ($p = 0.0245$ and 0.0570, respectively) were considered incidental and were characterized by three or more of the following: small magnitude, absence of dose dependency, inconsistency between sexes, similarity to differences present before initiation of dosing and absence of correlative findings.

Several animals exhibited transient clinical pathology changes (i.e. increased fibrinogen concentration, increased white blood cell count, absolute neutrophil count, absolute monocyte count) consistent with inflammation at the injection sites.

Organ weights, gross and microscopic examinations

Summary data for organ weights are presented in Table 6. For prostate, a significant increase was only noted for Group 2 when compared to the control ($p = 0.0364$). In the absence of a dose relation and the lack of macroscopic or microscopic correlates, the observation was neither considered treatment related nor relevant.

Macroscopic observations consisted of red discoloration within multiple sections of the gastrointestinal tract in two dogs in Group 2 and two dogs in Group 3, with no corresponding histopathology findings. Microscopic findings included a jejunal ulcer with minimal inflammation in one Group 2 dog, minimal cecal hemorrhage with microscopic cecal inflammation in one Group 3 dog, slight duodenal congestion in one Group 3 dog and cecal inflammation in one Group 4 dog.

Treated male dogs exhibited an increased number and severity of lymphocyte depletion within the thymus compared to the controls. The lymphocyte depletion may have been a secondary, stress-related response to the injection site findings and not a direct effect of the test article.

Table 4 Summary of hematology data; mean (SD), $N = 8$

Variable (reference range and units) [a]	Day	Group 1		Group 2		Group 3		Group 4		*P* value	
										Treatment	Time
Red blood cell count (5.8–7.8 $10^6/\mu L$)	−17	6.23	(1.14)	5.85	(0.38)	5.75	(0.37)	5.84	(0.28)	0.3548	<0.0001
	−11	5.66	(0.34)	5.77	(0.19)	5.75	(0.27)	5.87	(0.23)		
	21	5.85	(0.49)	5.63	(0.46)	5.71	(0.48)	5.84	(0.46)		
	55	6.21	(0.59)	5.99	(0.36)	6.05	(0.42)	6.36	(0.38)		
	89	6.38	(0.51)	6.22	(0.47)	6.27	(0.26)	6.37	(0.48)		
Hemoglobin (14.1–18.7 g/dL)	−17	13.16	(2.23)	12.44	(0.72)	12.43	(0.77)	12.71	(0.56)	0.2896	<0.0001
	−11	12.05	(0.32)	12.31	(0.49)	12.55	(0.48)	12.79	(0.43)		
	21	12.49	(0.82)	12.18	(0.92)	12.50	(0.93)	12.88	(0.87)		
	55	13.68	(1.11)	13.33	(0.96)	13.70	(0.82)	14.51	(0.56)		
	89	13.88	(0.76)	13.50	(1.06)	14.13	(0.37)	14.16	(0.71)		
Hematocrit (41.0–55.3%)	−17	42.60	(7.67)	39.50	(2.38)	39.66	(2.68)	40.48	(1.89)	0.1645	<0.0001
	−11	38.48	(1.35)	38.93	(1.41)	39.68	(1.67)	40.64	(1.17)		
	21	39.18	(2.57)	37.68	(2.71)	38.98	(2.97)	40.18	(2.71)		
	55	42.58	(3.30)	41.06	(2.56)	42.58	(2.45)	44.84	(1.78)		
	89	43.29	(2.56)	41.90	(3.21)	43.86	(0.98)	44.24	(2.44)		
Platelet count (161.6–379.0 $10^3/\mu L$)	−17	297.13	(75.13)	268.00	(106.63)	384.75	(61.17)	318.63	(64.39)	0.9909	<0.0001
	−11	320.75	(63.09)	287.75	(54.84)	366.38	(50.36)	296.75	(71.34)		
	21	323.50	(57.94)	317.88	(63.30)	352.75	(42.68)	309.00	(93.97)		
	55	300.13	(43.28)	275.00	(47.67)	326.75	(34.01)	287.75	(56.39)		
	89	275.88	(36.74)	257.50	(31.27)	308.00	(31.60)	267.38	(66.42)		
White blood cell count (7.4–14.5 $10^3/\mu L$)	−17	9.64	(1.54)	8.27	(1.18)	9.93	(1.96)	9.34	(1.56)	0.0433	<0.0001
	−11	9.45	(1.67)	8.58	(2.08)	10.05	(2.91)	9.12	(1.53)		
	21	8.39	(1.40)	6.93	(0.70)	8.54	(2.15)	6.95	(0.91)		
	55	9.14	(2.13)	7.11	(0.98)	8.63	(2.10)	7.26	(0.51)		
	89	9.47	(1.01)	7.95	(1.20)	9.83	(2.20)	9.12	(1.62)		
Activated partial thromboplastin time (sec) [b]	−17	11.35	(0.67)	11.56	(0.83)	11.63	(0.71)	11.44	(0.75)	0.8555	0.0859
	−11	13.68	(1.36)	13.60	(1.71)	13.05	(1.20)	13.55	(0.95)		
	21	12.74	(0.78)	12.24	(1.01)	12.24	(0.35)	12.49	(1.22)		
	55	12.26	(1.05)	12.98	(2.25)	12.61	(2.20)	11.80	(1.30)		
	89	12.13	(0.91)	12.21	(1.85)	11.76	(0.57)	11.91	(0.67)		

[a] These reference ranges have been derived from healthy young mongrel dogs ($n = 124$) and have been provided by the animal supplier. They are to be used for information only and the two values collected before the dosing period (at Day −17 and −11) should be used for interpretation in the context of this study
[b] Not available in mongrel dogs

Pharmacokinetic and pharmacodynamic evaluation

Predose samples on Day 1 and 69 did not contain robenacoxib nor would they be expected to since Day 1 was the first dose and Day 69 followed a 14-day washout period. Predose samples on Day 14 and 82 followed subcutaneous dosing and had low but measureable concentrations of robenacoxib in 26 of the 48 samples obtained (< 40 ng/mL).

The robenacoxib concentrations observed throughout the study at 1 and 5 h are displayed in Table 7. Increased dose resulted in increased exposure as demonstrated by 1 h concentrations and $AUC_{1\text{-}5h}$. In view of the sparse data, there was no evidence for differences in dose-normalized exposure between the different tablet dose regimens or between tablet and subcutaneous administrations. Accumulation assessed by comparing concentrations achieved 5 h post oral administration (at Day 1 and 6 and Day 69 and 74), was not observed.

The predicted COX-1 and COX-2 inhibition levels corresponding to the robenacoxib concentrations observed at 1 and 5 h throughout the study were calculated (Table 8). At the dosages tested in this study and 1 h after the treatment, the mean inhibition was 23–29% for COX-1 and 79–87% for COX-2 but there

Table 5 Summary of clinical chemistry data; mean (SD), $N = 8$

Variable (reference range and units) [a]	Day	Group 1		Group 2		Group 3		Group 4		P value	
										Treatment	Time
Alanine aminotransferase (23.0–64.6 U/L)	−17	20.88	(7.12)	21.88	(4.91)	18.75	(4.65)	21.75	(5.01)	0.7693	<0.0001
	−11	21.75	(4.23)	22.00	(3.78)	21.00	(3.82)	24.38	(7.11)		
	21	25.50	(6.00)	26.50	(4.28)	24.13	(4.36)	26.88	(5.36)		
	55	28.50	(6.44)	29.25	(4.95)	27.63	(5.21)	29.50	(6.09)		
	89	32.00	(7.84)	31.13	(4.67)	29.50	(4.14)	31.13	(5.84)		
Aspartate aminotransferase (28.1–59.7 U/L)	−17	29.00	(5.04)	30.25	(4.06)	28.25	(4.27)	30.63	(2.97)	0.5585	0.0002
	−11	30.88	(3.68)	30.63	(3.46)	29.88	(2.85)	32.25	(4.46)		
	21	28.50	(3.74)	29.75	(2.60)	29.63	(3.74)	30.25	(4.62)		
	55	28.75	(3.24)	31.38	(4.50)	30.38	(6.23)	32.00	(5.50)		
	89	31.50	(5.86)	33.00	(4.07)	32.88	(3.44)	34.38	(5.04)		
Alkaline phosphatase (65.4–177.5 U/L)	−17	118.88	(22.90)	109.00	(30.81)	139.13	(32.89)	117.25	(23.92)	0.8396	<0.0001
	−11	126.88	(27.03)	114.88	(32.42)	146.63	(33.43)	120.00	(25.60)		
	21	92.88	(19.98)	86.00	(25.47)	104.50	(29.08)	88.50	(22.77)		
	55	80.13	(15.63)	75.13	(17.31)	89.13	(25.05)	76.25	(19.77)		
	89	62.75	(13.47)	56.38	(13.41)	73.63	(22.92)	59.13	(15.82)		
Urea nitrogen (10.0–22.0 mg/dL)	−17	10.25	(2.25)	10.75	(1.28)	9.75	(1.49)	10.38	(1.60)	0.0196	0.0823
	−11	12.00	(1.93)	11.50	(1.69)	11.00	(1.31)	12.38	(2.07)		
	21	16.00	(1.77)	15.50	(1.07)	13.13	(2.10)	14.50	(2.20)		
	55	16.00	(2.56)	17.13	(1.96)	14.75	(2.25)	14.88	(2.10)		
	89	16.63	(2.62)	16.38	(2.39)	14.25	(2.25)	14.63	(1.69)		
Creatinine (0.7–1.1 mg/dL)	−17	0.61	(0.06)	0.56	(0.05)	0.60	(0.08)	0.60	(0.05)	0.9290	<0.0001
	−11	0.60	(0.08)	0.59	(0.04)	0.59	(0.06)	0.59	(0.06)		
	21	0.79	(0.06)	0.78	(0.05)	0.78	(0.07)	0.81	(0.04)		
	55	0.95	(0.09)	0.94	(0.07)	0.90	(0.09)	0.93	(0.09)		
	89	1.00	(0.05)	1.00	(0.09)	0.99	(0.08)	0.98	(0.07)		
Total protein (5.3–6.4 g/dL)	−17	4.75	(0.15)	4.71	(0.14)	4.84	(0.32)	4.91	(0.20)	0.4983	<0.0001
	−11	4.71	(0.15)	4.74	(0.18)	4.85	(0.24)	4.80	(0.14)		
	21	4.98	(0.07)	4.99	(0.16)	5.09	(0.28)	5.11	(0.15)		
	55	5.23	(0.13)	5.24	(0.09)	5.35	(0.19)	5.36	(0.23)		
	89	5.10	(0.15)	5.25	(0.16)	5.36	(0.20)	5.24	(0.32)		
Albumin (2.9–3.9 g/dL)	−17	3.26	(0.15)	3.23	(0.10)	3.29	(0.19)	3.36	(0.18)	0.9691	0.1652
	−11	3.25	(0.14)	3.20	(0.09)	3.30	(0.19)	3.29	(0.12)		
	21	3.50	(0.09)	3.44	(0.13)	3.55	(0.12)	3.54	(0.15)		
	55	3.51	(0.15)	3.51	(0.19)	3.48	(0.16)	3.55	(0.15)		
	89	3.53	(0.10)	3.54	(0.13)	3.64	(0.14)	3.53	(0.20)		
Creatine kinase (127.5–869.4 U/L)	−17	365.38	(57.30)	359.38	(80.96)	342.75	(22.22)	417.88	(96.99)	0.6395	0.2253
	−11	318.38	(50.07)	322.88	(57.31)	324.75	(38.87)	403.50	(91.48)		
	21	240.88	(46.46)	289.75	(66.14)	277.88	(60.09)	336.25	(170.44)		
	55	223.25	(60.46)	248.13	(57.50)	254.00	(48.67)	302.38	(96.44)		
	89	270.00	(148.55)	255.50	(65.44)	314.38	(134.62)	285.88	(52.55)		

[a] These reference ranges have been derived from healthy young mongrel dogs (n = 124) and have been provided by the animal supplier. They are to be used for information only and the two values collected before the dosing period (at Day −17 and −11) should be used for interpretation in the context of this study

Table 6 Summary of organ (g) weights; mean (SD), $N = 8$ unless stated

Organ	Group 1		Group 2		Group 3		Group 4		*P* value Treatment
Heart	170.66	(20.62)	173.22	(25.40)	174.79	(17.99)	157.73	(24.55)	0.2398
Kidneys	77.27	(9.74)	90.93	(23.45)	85.75	(17.00)	79.50	(15.42)	0.1829
Liver/Gall bladder	527.00	(73.45)	534.15	(114.49)	549.49	(129.55)	532.26	(117.27)	0.9546
Lung	180.73	(21.52)	182.79	(23.98)	180.34	(20.64)	179.20	(26.20)	0.9707
Brain	84.18	(8.19)	81.16	(7.60)	83.58	(7.48)	83.25	(7.34)	0.6928
Thymus	27.45	(12.91)	25.51	(7.78)	26.01	(6.88)	28.21	(11.79)	0.9293
Spleen	85.57	(38.68)	85.69	(34.93)	69.05	(14.38)	84.36	(37.65)	0.7196
Thyroid/Parathyroid	1.72	(0.41)	1.83	(0.43)	1.67	(0.45)	2.15	(0.84)	0.3149
Adrenals ($N = 7$[a])	1.42	(0.24)	1.61	(0.19)	1.67	(0.27)	1.64	(0.17)	0.2064
Pituitary	0.11	(0.02)	0.10	(0.02)	0.11	(0.02)	0.09	(0.02)	0.3402
Ovary ($N = 4$)	1.39	(0.56)	1.26	(0.14)	1.17	(0.42)	1.30	(0.19)	0.8505
Uterus ($N = 4$)	6.35	(5.83)	3.04	(1.23)	3.19	(1.15)	2.88	(1.04)	0.3747
Testis ($N = 4$)	28.72	(6.37)	30.23	(4.96)	27.96	(0.90)	24.92	(6.97)	0.5779
Prostate ($N = 4$)	4.96	(2.03)	9.52	(4.75)	4.88	(1.30)	3.51	(0.87)	0.0462

[a] Adrenal was missing in one dog

were no significant differences among the dose groups for the inhibition levels ($p = 0.2694$ and 0.7723 for COX-1 and COX-2 inhibition, respectively). At 5 h after the treatment, inhibition decreased and the mean inhibition was 6–11% for COX-1 and 24–41% for COX-2 (Table 8). The difference between the groups was greater at 5 h and the level of inhibition for both COX-1 and COX-2 was statistically significantly higher with increasing doses ($p < 0.0001$).

Discussion

The primary objective of this study was to evaluate the safety of the interchangeable use of Onsior™ tablets and Onsior™ solution for injection containing robenacoxib in dogs. The dose levels and dose multiples (up to 3X) were chosen in accordance with Target Animal Safety Guidelines for Veterinary Pharmaceutical Products (VICH GL43 [16]) to identify a margin of safety. This modification from the traditional approach of using 1X, 3X and 5X dose levels in target animal safety studies was based on animal welfare concerns and preventing generation of data already available as well as assessing safety in young dogs.

Alternating regimens of robenacoxib tablets and injection (Onsior™) for three 20 day cycles (each separated by a 14-day washout) for 88 days to 4 month old dogs was well tolerated based on the overall good health of the dogs. Primary treatment-related abnormalities were confined to (i) microscopic findings in the gastrointestinal tract and (ii) macroscopic and microscopic findings at the subcutaneous injection sites.

The principal targets for toxicity of non-selective NSAIDs are the gastrointestinal tract, kidney, liver and inhibition of blood clotting [25, 26]. Robenacoxib-related gastrointestinal microscopic findings seen in this study were consistent with the known pharmacology of NSAID class of COX-2 inhibitors [27] and with previous studies evaluating the safety/toxicity of robenacoxib administered separately orally or via subcutaneous injection [4, 6]. They were mild and did not result in clinical signs, changes in body weight, or effects on haematology. Microscopic findings were generally higher in incidence and severity among dogs in Groups 3 and 4 compared to those in Group 2. In addition, there were no changes in serum total protein or albumin concentrations which could indicate protein-losing enteropathy.

There was no evidence from this study of toxicity of robenacoxib on the kidney. There were no post mortem gross changes and no relevant histological findings affecting the kidney. Plasma creatinine, urea concentrations and results of urinalysis were normal in the treated groups. There were no post mortem gross changes and no relevant histological findings affecting the liver. Analysis of alkaline phosphatase, alanine aminotransferase and aspartate aminotransferase did not indicate any effect on the liver function. Finally, there was no effect of robenacoxib on the coagulation parameters (i.e., activated partial thromboplastin time, BMBT) similar to what has been previously reported for robenacoxib in both cats and dogs [6, 11].

The clinical signs observed upon subcutaneous administration (twitching, scratching, licking or vocalization) were uncommon and, as they occasionally occur after subcutaneous injection in dogs, were not considered related to robenacoxib injectable or saline, but to the subcutaneous injection process itself.

Table 7 Summary of robenacoxib concentration (ng/mL); mean (SD), $N = 8$

Day	Time (h)	Group 2		Group 3		Group 4	
1	1	2514	(1339)	1760	(1401)	2761	(1728)
1	5	44	(32)	151	(223)	136	(87)
6	1	1447	(1473)	1608	(1164)	2610	(2083)
6	5	30	(15)	72	(74)	73	(37)
8	1	1039	(1026)	1677	(1477)	4991	(4129)
8	5	78	(80)	212	(149)	191	(154)
11	1	1564	(582)	2014	(573)	3015	(1336)
11	5	435	(202)	1126	(344)	1913	(1101)
14	1	2825	(3489)	1603	(1442)	1822	(1413)
14	5	38	(43)	110	(118)	103	(63)
69	1	2896	(1369)	2653	(2530)	3915	(2533)
69	5	53	(54)	128	(105)	154	(129)
74	1	1290	(955)	1232	(1632)	4759	(2889)
74	5	67	(52)	157	(180)	104	(61)
76	1	3467	(2004)	2791	(2447)	4492	(4924)
76	5	166	(178)	366	(276)	1047	(1421)
79	1	1269	(405)	1402	(386)	2245	(1137)
79	5	944	(299)	2050	(428)	3133	(999)
82	1	1130	(563)	2118	(1349)	2541	(2049)
82	5	45	(50)	110	(113)	114	(126)

The incidence of macroscopic findings at the subcutaneous dose sites was greater in Groups 3 or 4 than in Groups 1 or 2. Following injection, severity was generally dose-related and the findings at the subcutaneous injection sites were consistent with the observations in a previous target animal safety study using only Onsior™ solution for injection (unpublished report). In this study, 6-month old healthy beagles were administered subcutaneously Onsior™ solution for injection formulation at 0 (control), 2, 6 and 20 mg/kg of robenacoxib during three dosing cycles of one subcutaneous injection per day for three consecutive days separated by 11-day washout time. A dose-dependent increased frequency of thickening scabbing, scarring, discoloration foci, accentuated vasculature, and subcutaneous haemorrhage at the injection site, were observed at necropsy. Subcutaneous inflammation was dose-dependent and a progressive resolution of subcutaneous lesions over time was evident. Thus, it can be concluded that the interchangeable use with Onsior™ tablets does not result in additional effects compared to use of Onsior™ solution for injection only.

Table 8 Predicted inhibition percentage of COX-1 and COX-2 for the observed robenacoxib concentrations at 1 and 5 h; mean (SD) [max], $N = 80$

	Time	Group 2			Group 3			Group 4		
% inhibition COX-1	1	24	(9)	[50]	23	(10)	[44]	29	(11)	[53]
% inhibition COX-1	5	6	(5)	[22]	10	(8)	[30]	11	(10)	[36]
% inhibition COX-2	1	82	(23)	[99]	79	(27)	[98]	87	(20)	[99]
% inhibition COX-2	5	24	(27)	[88]	39	(32)	[95]	41	(32)	[97]

In the present study, none of these findings had a clinically significant effect on the health or well-being of the animals. Dogs were comfortable and healthy, bright, alert, and responsive, hydrated, and in good body condition, showing only some discomfort upon palpation of dose sites.

The findings of lipid infiltrates and infiltrates of vacuolated macrophages in axillary lymph nodes were considered secondary treatment-related effects because they represented drainage of the necrosis and degeneration that occurred at the subcutaneous injection sites (including a control dog). Likewise, depletion of lymphocytes in the thymus may have been a secondary response and not a direct effect of the treatment.

Toxicokinetic results confirmed consistent and appropriate exposure of the animals and thus allows conclusion to be made regarding the safety of interchangeable use. Further interpretation of the toxicokinetics in this study is made difficult by the limited sampling schedule. A maximum of three (one predose and two post dose) samples during a dosing interval is insufficient to accurately estimate C_{max}, half-life, or AUC. No accumulation was observed in this 88-day study. Previous studies have shown robenacoxib to be eliminated in the dog with a half-life of less than 1 h [21] therefore no accumulation would be expected with once daily dosing.

The predicted levels of COX-1 and COX-2 inhibition in this study were derived from the concentrations observed at 1 and 5 h. In general, the maximum inhibition of COX-1 and COX-2 was observed at 1 h where high average inhibition of COX-2 (i.e., ≥ 79%) and limited inhibition of COX-1 (≤ 41%) was predicted. The maximum predicted inhibition for COX-1 was 53%, in Group 4 (Table 8). Inhibition levels were higher when the blood concentrations were higher at 1 h after treatment, but without marked differences between the dose groups presumably because the concentrations achieved in all groups had saturated the enzyme and reflect maximum activity. Levels of COX-1 and COX-2 inhibition were decreased at 5 h compared to at 1 h corresponding to decreased blood concentrations. At these lower concentrations, the enzymes are not saturated and therefore at 5 h the level of inhibition was dose-dependent. The magnitude and duration of COX-1 inhibition needed to induce gastrointestinal toxicity is not known, however it was concluded in a previous study that approximately 50% inhibition of COX-1 for up to 3.5 h or 25% for up to 8 h was safe for robenacoxib and the canine gastrointestinal tract [6]. This is in alignment with the maximum inhibition of COX-1 predicted in the present study, in which gastrointestinal toxicity was not observed.

The results of this study indicate that injections of robenacoxib can be safely administered instead of a tablet to a dog receiving oral therapy or that robenacoxib injection(s) can be followed by oral robenacoxib therapy. The microscopic findings in the gastrointestinal tract and the clinical signs and microscopic findings at the injection site were as expected based on a previous study with robenacoxib solution for injection alone (unpublished report) and the known properties of this class of compound and mode of administration. There were no safety concerns caused by the interchangeable use of the oral and injectable robenacoxib formulations. To our knowledge, this is the first publication showing results of a study designed to establish the interchangeable use of two formulations in veterinary medicine.

Conclusions

This study supports the safe use of any combination of Onsior™ tablets or injectable once daily. There were no serious adverse events during the course of the study. No changes in body weight, food consumption, ophthalmic examinations, electrocardiograms, buccal mucosal blood times, clinical pathology or organ weight were attributable to robenacoxib administration. Primary treatment-related findings were confined to clinical signs upon subcutaneous administration, macroscopic and microscopic findings at the subcutaneous injection sites and microscopic findings in the gastrointestinal tract, typically seen with the individual use of oral or injectable robenacoxib or with this class of compound and mode of administration. It is concluded that alternating regimens of robenacoxib tablets and injection (Onsior™) were well tolerated in healthy young dogs when administered once a day.

Abbreviations

AUC: Area under the curve; BMBT: Buccal mucosal bleed times; C_{max}: Maximum blood drug concentration; COX: Cyclooxygenase; ECG: Electrocardiogram; FDA-CVM: Food and Drug Administration's Center for Veterinary Medicine; HPLC: high-performance liquid chromatography; K2-EDTA: Ethylenediaminetetraacetic acid dipotassium; LC-MS/MS: Liquid chromatography tandem mass spectrometry; LLOQ: Lower limit of quantification; NSAID: Non-steroidal anti-inflammatory drug; PGE_2: Prostaglandin E2; SC: Subcutaneous; T_{max}: Time to maximum blood concentration following drug administration; TxB_2: Thromboxane B2; VICH: Veterinary International Conference on Harmonization

Acknowledgements

The authors would like to thank the personnel of Covance Laboratories Inc., Madison, Wisconsin, US for conducting the study.

Funding

The study was funded by the Sponsor i.e. Novartis Animal Health which is now owned by Elanco Animal Health.

Authors' contributions

CET prepared the manuscript; MCH, SBK and RH revised it critically. SBK and RH were responsible for the conception and design of the study, MCH and CET conducted the pharmacokinetic and pharmacodynamic analysis, RH supervised the safety data analysis and interpretation. All the authors have read and approved the final version.

Consent for publication

Not applicable.

Competing interests

All authors are employees of Elanco Animal Health, a Division of Eli Lilly and Company.

Author details

[1]Elanco Animal Health, a Division of Eli Lilly and Company, Mattenstrasse 24A, CH-4058 Basel, Switzerland. [2]Elanco Animal Health, a Division of Eli Lilly and Company, 2500 Innovation Way, Greenfield, IN 64140, USA.

References

1. Schmid VB, Spreng DE, Seewald W, Jung M, Lees P, King JN. Analgesic and anti-inflammatory actions of robenacoxib in acute joint inflammation in dog. J Vet Pharmacol Ther. 2010;33(2):118–31.
2. Giraudel JM, King JN, Jeunesse EC, Lees P, Toutain PL. Use of a pharmacokinetic/pharmacodynamic approach in the cat to determine a dosage regimen for the COX-2 selective drug robenacoxib. J Vet Pharmacol Ther. 2009;32(1):18–30.
3. Food and Drug Administration Freedom of Information Summary: Original New Animal Drug Application NADA 141–463 (Onsior Robenacoxib Tablets Dogs) [https://www.fda.gov/downloads/AnimalVeterinary/Products/

ApprovedAnimalDrugProducts/FOIADrugSummaries/UCM504543.pdf]. Accessed 10 July 2017.

4. Food and Drug Administration Freedom of Information Summary: Supplemental New Animal Drug Application NADA 141–443 (Onsior Robenacoxib Injection Dogs) [https://www.fda.gov/downloads/AnimalVeterinary/Products/ApprovedAnimalDrugProducts/FOIADrugSummaries/UCM532540.pdf]. Accessed 10 July 2017.
5. European Medicines Agency: European Public Assessment Report, Onsior Summary of Product Characteristics [http://www.ema.europa.eu/docs/en_GB/document_library/EPAR_-_Product_Information/veterinary/000127/WC500067759.pdf]. Accessed 10 July 2017.
6. King JN, Arnaud JP, Goldenthal EI, Gruet P, Jung M, Seewald W, Lees P. Robenacoxib in the dog: target species safety in relation to extent and duration of inhibition of COX-1 and COX-2. J Vet Pharmacol Ther. 2011;34(3):298–311.
7. Borer LR, Seewald W, Peel JE, King JN. Evaluation of the dose-response relationship of oral robenacoxib in urate crystal-induced acute stifle synovitis in dogs. J Vet Pharmacol Ther. 2017;40(2):148–57.
8. King JN, Rudaz C, Borer L, Jung M, Seewald W, Lees P. In vitro and ex vivo inhibition of canine cyclooxygenase isoforms by robenacoxib: a comparative study. Res Vet Sci. 2010;88(3):497–506.
9. King JN, Dawson J, Esser RE, Fujimoto R, Kimble EF, Maniara W, Marshall PJ, O'Byrne L, Quadros E, Toutain PL, et al. Preclinical pharmacology of robenacoxib: a novel selective inhibitor of cyclooxygenase-2. J Vet Pharmacol Ther. 2009;32(1):1–17.
10. Brune K, Furst DE. Combining enzyme specificity and tissue selectivity of cyclooxygenase inhibitors: towards better tolerability? Rheumatology (Oxford). 2007;46(6):911–9.
11. King JN, Hotz R, Reagan EL, Roth DR, Seewald W, Lees P. Safety of oral robenacoxib in the cat. J Vet Pharmacol Ther. 2012;35(3):290–300.
12. King JN, King S, Budsberg SC, Lascelles BD, Bienhoff SE, Roycroft LM, Roberts ES. Clinical safety of robenacoxib in feline osteoarthritis: results of a randomized, blinded, placebo-controlled clinical trial. J Feline Med Surg. 2016;18(8):632–42.
13. Gruet P, Seewald W, King JN. Evaluation of subcutaneous and oral administration of robenacoxib and meloxicam for the treatment of acute pain and inflammation associated with orthopedic surgery in dogs. Am J Vet Res. 2011;72(2):184–93.
14. United States Food and Drug Administration, Code of Federal Regulations Title 21, Part 58, Good Laboratory Practice for nonclinical laboratory studies [https://www.accessdata.fda.gov/scripts/cdrh/cfdocs/cfcfr/CFRSearch.cfm?CFRPart=58]. Accessed 10 July 2017.
15. Organisation for Economic Cooperation and Development (OECD) Series on Principles of Good Laboratory Practice (GLP) and Compliance Monitoring [http://www.oecd.org/chemicalsafety/testing/oecdseriesonprinciplesofgoodlaboratorypracticeglpandcompliancemonitoring.htm]. Accessed 10 July 2017.
16. Veterinary International Conference on Harmonization (VICH) Guideline 43: Target Animal Safety for Veterinary Pharmaceutical Products [http://www.vichsec.org/guidelines/pharmaceuticals/pharma-safety/pharma-target-animal-safety.html]. Accessed 10 July 2017.
17. U.S. Department of Agriculture's Animal Welfare Act , 9 CFR Parts 1, 2 and 3 [https://www.federalregister.gov/topics/animal-welfare]. Accessed 10 July 2017.
18. Guide for the Care and Use of Laboratory Animals, Institute of Laboratory Animal Resources. Washington, D.C: National Academy Press; 1996.
19. Office of Laboratory Animal Welfare [https://grants.nih.gov/grants/olaw/olaw.htm]. Accessed 10 July 2017.
20. Morton DB, Jennings M, Buckwell A, Ewbank R, Godfrey C, Holgate B, Inglis I, James R, Page C, Sharman I, et al. Refining procedures for the administration of substances. Report of the BVAAWF/FRAME/RSPCA/UFAW joint working group on refinement. British veterinary association animal welfare foundation/Fund for the Replacement of animals in medical experiments/Royal Society for the Prevention of Cruelty to Animals/Universities Federation for Animal Welfare. Lab Anim. 2001;35(1):1–41.
21. Jung M, Lees P, Seewald W, King JN. Analytical determination and pharmacokinetics of robenacoxib in the dog. J Vet Pharmacol Ther. 2009; 32(1):41–8.
22. Snedecor GW, Cochran WG. Statistical methods, eighth edition. Ames (IA): Iowa State Press; 1989.
23. Milliken GA, Johnson DE. Analysis of messy data volume III: analysis of covariance. London: Chapman and Hall; 2002.
24. Diehl KH, Hull R, Morton D, Pfister R, Rabemampianina Y, Smith D, Vidal JM, van de Vorstenbosch C. A good practice guide to the administration of substances and removal of blood, including routes and volumes. J Appl Toxicol. 2001;21(1):15–23.
25. Flower RJ. The development of COX2 inhibitors. Nat Rev Drug Discov. 2003; 2(3):179–91.
26. Warner TD, Giuliano F, Vojnovic I, Bukasa A, Mitchell JA, Vane JR. Nonsteroid drug selectivities for cyclo-oxygenase-1 rather than cyclo-oxygenase-2 are associated with human gastrointestinal toxicity: a full in vitro analysis. Proc Natl Acad Sci U S A. 1999;96(13):7563–8.
27. Bergh MS, Budsberg SC. The coxib NSAIDs: potential clinical and pharmacologic importance in veterinary medicine. J Vet Intern Med. 2005; 19(5):633–43.

8

Optimisation of a double-centrifugation method for preparation of canine platelet-rich plasma

Hyeok-Soo Shin, Heung-Myong Woo and Byung-Jae Kang*

Abstract

Background: Platelet-rich plasma (PRP) has been expected for regenerative medicine because of its growth factors. However, there is considerable variability in the recovery and yield of platelets and the concentration of growth factors in PRP preparations. The aim of this study was to identify optimal relative centrifugal force and spin time for the preparation of PRP from canine blood using a double-centrifugation tube method.

Methods: Whole blood samples were collected in citrate blood collection tubes from 12 healthy beagles. For the first centrifugation step, 10 different run conditions were compared to determine which condition produced optimal recovery of platelets. Once the optimal condition was identified, platelet-containing plasma prepared using that condition was subjected to a second centrifugation to pellet platelets. For the second centrifugation, 12 different run conditions were compared to identify the centrifugal force and spin time to produce maximal pellet recovery and concentration increase. Growth factor levels were estimated by using ELISA to measure platelet-derived growth factor-BB (PDGF-BB) concentrations in optimised $CaCl_2$-activated platelet fractions.

Results: The highest platelet recovery rate and yield were obtained by first centrifuging whole blood at 1000 g for 5 min and then centrifuging the recovered platelet-enriched plasma at 1500 g for 15 min. This protocol recovered 80% of platelets from whole blood and increased platelet concentration six-fold and produced the highest concentration of PDGF-BB in activated fractions.

Conclusions: We have described an optimised double-centrifugation tube method for the preparation of PRP from canine blood. This optimised method does not require particularly expensive equipment or high technical ability and can readily be carried out in a veterinary clinical setting.

Keywords: Dog, Double centrifugation, Platelet-derived growth factor-BB, Platelet-rich plasma, Platelet recovery

Background

Investigations of the morphologic and biologic features of platelets have established their important role in wound healing through the release of various growth factors. These factors, which include platelet-derived growth factor (PDGF), transforming growth factor beta, vascular endothelial growth factor, epidermal growth factor and osteoconductive proteins (fibrin, fibronectin and vitronectin), are contained in platelet α granules and are released when platelets are activated or destroyed [1–3]. The release of these growth factors into damaged tissue facilitates tissue regeneration by stimulating cell proliferation, cell migration, angiogenesis and vascular ingrowth [4, 5]. Furthermore, platelets also release antimicrobial, anti-inflammatory and analgesic factors [6–8].

The use of platelet-rich plasma (PRP) to deliver growth factors has emerged as a convenient method for promoting wound healing and tissue regeneration. The autologous nature of PRP preparations makes them safer than other allogenic cell-based regenerative therapies and less expensive. As a result, PRP therapy is seeing widespread use in human medicine, with applications in dentistry, orthopaedic surgery, cardiac surgery, ophthalmology and plastic surgery [9–12]. PRP is also increasingly being used in veterinary medicine [13–15],

* Correspondence: bjkang@kangwon.ac.kr
College of Veterinary Medicine and Institute of Veterinary Science, Kangwon National University, Chuncheon 24341, Republic of Korea

prompting the need for development of simple and reproducible methods for preparation of high-quality PRP for use in veterinary patients.

Despite the popularity and advantages of PRP, there are conflicting reports in the literature regarding its efficacy [9–14, 16]. These differences may in part be attributable to variations in the composition of PRP preparations with respect to platelet yield, concentrations of beneficial growth factors and the presence of other blood components, particularly leukocytes [17–19]. Tube methods employing differential centrifugation to separate and concentrate platelets are most convenient clinical settings because they are low cost and do not require specific technical expertise. Considerable research effort has been focused optimising PRP protocols reproducible recovery, yield and cellular composition. Most of these studies have focused on PRP prepared from human blood [20–22]; relatively fewer studies have addressed optimisation of PRP for use in veterinary medicine [23, 24]. Several commercial products are available for producing PRP from human blood, but they have been found to produce variable results when used to prepare PRP from canine blood [25].

The purpose of this study was to identify optimal centrifugal force and spin times for the preparation of PRP from canine whole blood using a double-centrifugation tube method. The goal was to identify run conditions that will reproducibly recover large numbers of platelets capable of releasing large amounts of growth factor when activated and that are relatively free of other contaminating blood components. To determine which run conditions were optimal, preparations were assessed for platelet recovery and yield, concentrations of white blood cells (WBC) and red blood cells (RBC) and the amount of PDGF-BB released from activated platelets.

Methods

Experimental animals

Twelve, clinically healthy adult male beagles, bred for research purposes (Dreambio, Seoul, Republic of Korea), were included in this study. Dogs were evaluated at the Kangwon National University Veterinary Teaching Hospital by means of physical examination, thoracic and abdominal radiography, complete blood count (CBC), serum biochemistry profile and blood smear microscopic analysis by a veterinarian and were deemed healthy. All dogs in this experiment had normal blood count and morphological features. They ranged from 14.3–17.8 months of age. Body weights ranged were 9.3–10.1 kg. The dogs were individually housed in stainless steel cages at conventional housing facilities with controlled temperature (21 °C) and humidity of 55%. They received standard care and water and food. All dogs were under the care of a licensed veterinarian.

Blood collection

Whole blood was collected from the jugular vein of each dog using a 21-gauge multiple-use needle into blood collection tubes containing 1.5 mL anticoagulant acid citrate dextrose-A solution (BD Vacutainer system, Plymouth, UK). No more than 90 mL of blood was drawn from each dog per collection, with at least 4 weeks between collections.

Sampled whole blood was divided into 9-mL aliquots that were centrifuged in 15 mL conical centrifuge tubes. Centrifugation and analysis of samples was initiated within 1 h of blood collection.

Preparation of platelet concentrates

A double-spin preparation method was used for all samples. Samples were centrifuged at room temperature in a Hanil MF-550 centrifuge (HanilScience, Kimpo, Korea) and centrifugal brake was not applied. For the first spin, samples were centrifuged at one of 5 different RCFs (100, 200, 300, 500 or 1000 g) for 5 and 10 min at room temperature (RT), for a total of 10 RCF-time comparisons, with four replications for each comparison. Four replications were conducted on different days using blood drawn from different individuals, and CBC of both whole blood and PRP1 used in each experiment were performed.

After the first centrifugation, the whole plasma fraction above the buffy coat (PRP1) was transferred to an empty tube, its volume was measured, and after mixing this fraction well, a 1-mL aliquot was taken for CBC.

The second centrifugation step was performed with PRP1 prepared using the first-centrifugation RCF-time condition that recovered the highest percentage of platelets. The PRP1 fraction was divided into 1-mL aliquots, which were centrifuged at RT at either 500, 1000, 1500 or 3000 g for 10, 15 or 20 min, for a total of 12 RCF-time comparisons.

The second centrifugation produced a platelet-poor plasma (PPP) supernatant and a platelet-enriched pellet. A volume of 700 μL of PPP supernatant was removed, and the pellet was resuspended in 300 μL PPP; this concentrated platelet fraction was designated as PRP2.

Platelet activation and PDGF-BB quantification

There are so many activated PDGF such as EGF, PDGF and TGF-β. Because PDGF-BB is not included in the plasma, its concentration correlates well with the quantity of activated platelets. Therefore, PDGF-BB was chosen as an index of platelet activation. PDGF-BB levels were assessed in activated PRP1 and PRP2 samples as well as plasma that had been prepared by centrifuging whole blood at 1000 g for 5 min. To activate samples, they were activated using 20 mM $CaCl_2$ and incubated at 37 °C for 1 h followed by 4 °C for 16 h. Samples were then centrifuged at 3000 g for 20 min at 18 °C, and the supernatant collected for PDGF-BB measurement.

The supernatant for PDGF-BB measurement was diluted 20-fold with diluent buffer in kit and quantified by enzyme-linked immunosorbent assay (ELISA) using antibodies against canine PDGF-BB (Raybiotech, Norcross, GA, USA) according to the manufacturer's instructions. The detection limits ranged from 4 pg/mL to 1200 pg/mL, the interassay coefficient was <12%, and the intraassay coefficient was <10%.

Haematological analysis

A CBC of whole blood and PRP1 and PRP2 fractions was carried out using an automated laser flow cytometry haematology analyser (ProCyte Dx, IDEXX, ME, USA).

Statistical analysis

Statistical analysis was performed using Prism 5.00 software (Graphpad Software Inc. San Diego, CA, USA). Results are presented as mean ± standard deviation. Statistical significance was assessed using the Kruskal–Wallis test followed by the Mann–Whitney *post-hoc* test (to compare all pairs in group). $P < .05$ was considered significant for all tests.

Results

The 12 dogs from which blood was collected weighed between 9.3 and 10.1 kg. No significant weight changes and side effects occurred for any dog during the course of the study.

PRP1 after first centrifugation step

Table 1 shows the results for the 10 different RCF-time run conditions used for the first centrifugation. The percent of platelets recovered from whole blood progressively increased as the RCF increased when centrifugation time was held constant. Platelet recovery also increased when RCF was held constant but centrifugation time increased 5 min to 10 min for every RCF except the 1000 g condition. The greatest recovery was achieved with run condition 9 (1000 g, 5 min). Comparison of mean percent recoveries of run conditions 1–5 and 7 were all significantly lower than the recovery of condition 9. The mean percent platelet recoveries for conditions 6, 8, 9 and 10 were not significantly different. Furthermore, only 8.18 ± 0.98% of the whole blood WBCs remained in PRP1 obtained through condition 9, which was not significantly different from the WBC recovery rate of PRP1 obtained under conditions 1–8, and it was significantly lower than that of condition 10. Therefore, because the centrifugation time was shorter, condition 9 was chosen as optimal for the first centrifugation step. This condition was used to prepare PRP1 samples for use in optimising the second centrifugation step. (See Additional file 1)

Table 1 Platelet recovery after total blood centrifugation

Run	Parameters		Recovery (%)	*P* value
	RCF (× g)	Centrifugation time (minutes)		
1	100	5	16.33 ± 10.92	0.0286*
2	100	10	38.53 ± 15.46	0.0286*
3	200	5	31.05 ± 14.18	0.0286*
4	200	10	55.51 ± 12.14	0.0286*
5	300	5	42.62 ± 10.22	0.0286*
6	300	10	73.00 ± 12.10	0.1143
7	500	5	72.69 ± 6.90	0.0286*
8	500	10	76.62 ± 8.57	0.1143
9	1000	5	92.28 ± 4.88	-
10	1000	10	82.77 ± 8.35	0.3429

Values expressed as mean ± standard deviation; RCF, relative centrifugal force. Asterisk (*) indicates a recovery significantly different ($P < .05$) from condition 9, which produced the highest recovery

PRP2 after second centrifugation step

The purpose of second centrifugation step was to further concentrate platelets by reducing the volume of PPP. To identify the optimal RCF-time run conditions for the second centrifugation, PRP1 prepared by condition 9 (1000 g, 5 min) was used. The amount of PRP1 obtained by the first centrifugation varied depending on the packed cell volume of each individual, and mean volume of PRP1 was 4.2 ± 0.32 mL. The PRP1 fraction was divided into 1-mL aliquots and samples were subjected to 12 different centrifugation conditions to obtain PRP2 with four replications for each comparison.

Table 2 shows the percent recovery of platelets relative to PRP1 and yield (fold increase) relative to whole blood at each run condition. Lowest RCF resulted in less percent recovery. Recovery increased with increasing RCF and duration of centrifugation. Recovery was substantially reduced following centrifugation at 3000 g for 20 min due to platelet aggregation. Condition 8 (1500 g, 15 min) resulted in both highest recovery and increase in platelet concentration. Statistical analysis revealed that the recovery and yield for condition 8 was not significantly different from results obtained using condition 5 (1000 g, 15 min), condition 9 (1500 g, 20 min) or condition 10 (3000 g, 10 min). Based on these results, conditions 5, 8, 9 and 10 were chosen for additional assessment and each of these 4 run conditions were replicated 8 times.

Mean percent platelet recoveries relative to PRP1 and yields relative to whole blood under run conditions 5, 8, 9 and 10 are shown in Fig. 1a and b, respectively. Platelet recovery and yield were once again the highest when samples were centrifuged at 1500 g, 15 min (condition 8). The

Table 2 Platelet yield and recovery after the second centrifugation step

Run	Parameters		Yield (fold)	*P* value	Recovery (%)	*P* value
	RCF (x g)	Centrifugation time (min)				
1	500	10	4.42 ± 0.84	0.0286*	63.21 ± 4.66	0.0286*
2	500	15	4.65 ± 0.76	0.0286*	66.65 ± 3.64	0.0286*
3	500	20	5.60 ± 0.49	0.1143	74.50 ± 1.51	0.0286*
4	1000	10	5.41 ± 0.37	0.0286*	72.06 ± 2.68	0.0286*
5	1000	15	5.94 ± 0.36	0.3429	82.23 ± 6.51	0.4897
6	1000	20	5.65 ± 0.13	0.0286*	78.08 ± 2.85	0.0286*
7	1500	10	5.80 ± 0.48	0.1143	81.96 ± 2.58	0.0286*
8	1500	15	6.48 ± 0.46	-	91.70 ± 4.49	-
9	1500	20	5.93 ± 0.28	0.3429	86.73 ± 1.54	0.4897
10	3000	10	5.82 ± 0.39	0.3429	85.06 ± 3.28	0.1143
11	3000	15	5.75 ± 0.49	0.3429	85.87 ± 1.65	0.0286*
12	3000	20	4.34 ± 1.06	0.1143	64.79 ± 13.73	0.0286*

Values expressed as mean ± standard deviation; RCF, relative centrifugal force. Asterisk (*) indicates a recovery or yield significantly different ($P < .05$) from condition 8, which produced the highest recovery and yield

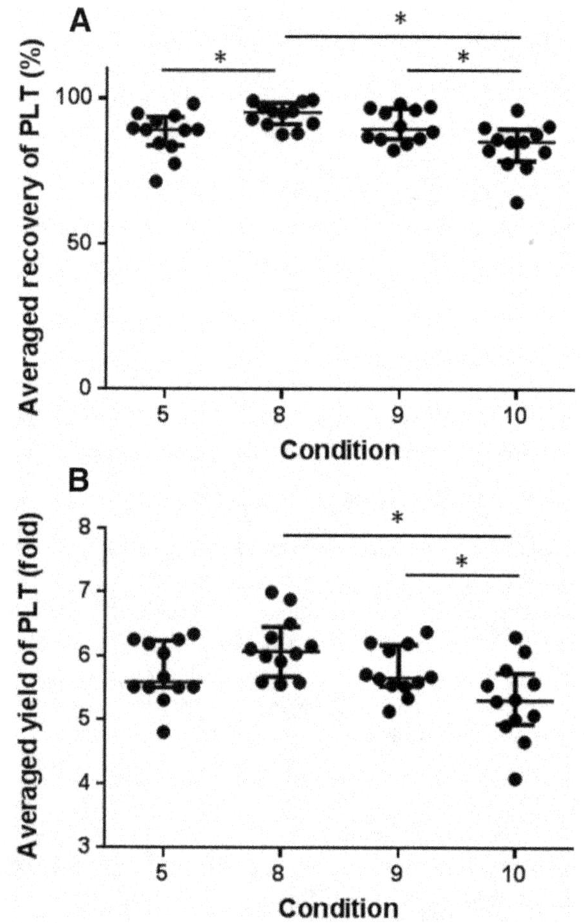

Fig. 1 Scatter plots for platelet recovery and yield of selected 4 conditions after the second centrifugation step. **a** Percent platelet recovery relative to PRP1 and (**b**) yield expressed as fold increase relative to whole blood. Data are presented by groups, the line represents the median of the group; error bars represent the interquartile range. Asterisk (*) indicates a recovery or yield significantly different ($P < .05$) between the two groups. Condition 5, 1000 g, 15 min; condition 8, 1500 g. 15 min; condition 9, 1500 g, 20 min; condition 10, 3000 g, 10 min

platelet recovery rate for condition 8 was significantly higher than those for conditions 5 and 10 but not higher than that for condition 9. The platelet yield for condition 8 was significantly greater than that for condition 10, but it was not significantly greater than the yield for conditions 5 and 9 (Fig. 1b). There was no statistically significant difference between conditions 8 and 9, but condition 8 could shorten centrifugation time by 5 min. Based on these results, condition 8 (1500 g, 15 min) was chosen as optimal for the second centrifugation step.

Table 3 shows the concentrations of platelets, RBC, total WBC and lymphocytes in whole blood and in PRP2 prepared using the centrifugation conditions identified as optimal for platelet recovery and yield (i.e. initial centrifugation of whole blood at 1000 g for 5 min to obtain PRP1, followed by centrifugation of PRP1 at 1500 g for 15 min). This centrifugation protocol recovered approximately 80% of the platelets from whole blood and increased platelet concentration approximately 6-fold. The concentration of platelets in the PRP preparation was 1748 ± 193 × 10^3 cells/μL, which was 6.1 ± 0.4 times higher than the concentration in the original whole blood sample. The PRP preparations contained negligible concentrations of RBCs, and WBC contents were 8.5 ± 1% neutrophils, 15.5 ± 4% monocytes and 73 ± 7% lymphocyte. (See Additional file 1)

PDGF-BB quantification

To determine the effects of the centrifugation protocol on the level of platelet-associated growth factors in activated fractions, concentrations of a representative growth factor, PDGF-BB, were measured in plasma, PRP1, and in the various PRP2 fractions prepared using conditions 5, 8, 9, 10 and 11. Figure 2 shows that condition 8 (1500 g, 15 min), which produced the highest recovery and yield of platelets, correspondingly also had the highest concentration of PDGF-BB. PRP2 prepared under condition 8 was the only PRP2 fraction that had a significantly higher PDGF-BB concentration than plasma or PRP1.

Discussion

In this study, we prepared PRP from canine blood using a double-centrifuge tube method. We found that the following protocol produced the greatest recovery and yield

Table 3 Descriptive results after double centrifugation

Variables	Whole blood	PRP1	PRP2
Red blood cells (cells × 10^6/μL)	5.8 ± 0.23	0.03 ± 0.05*	0.065 ± 0.02#
Lymphocytes (cells × 10^3/μL)	2.3 ± 0.54	1.05 ± 0.77	3.71 ± 2.4
Neutrophil (cells × 10^3/μL)	7.11 ± 1.67	0.15 ± 0.17*	0.44 ± 0.39#
Monocyte (cells × 10^3/μL)	0.7 ± 0.15	0.2 ± 0.13	0.79 ± 0.57
White blood cells (cells × 10^3/μL)	10.32 ± 2.4	1.45 ± 0.87*	5.09 ± 3.39#
Platelets (cells × 10^6/μL)	289 ± 35	523 ± 56*	1748 ± 193#

Values expressed as mean ± standard deviation (n = 12). Asterisk (*) indicates a significant difference (P < .05) between platelet-rich plasma-1 and whole blood. # indicates a significant difference (P < .05) between platelet-rich plasma-2 and whole blood

of platelets and highest concentrations of PDFG-BB in PRP preparations:

1. Collect blood samples in 10-mL tubes containing 3.2% sodium citrate to prevent coagulation. Retain a 0.5-mL small aliquot for initial CBC.
2. Centrifuge the blood sample at 1000 g for 5 min at RT.
3. Transfer the upper plasma and platelet fraction (PRP1) into a sterile tube and measure the volume. Retain an aliquot for determination of PRP1 platelet concentration.
4. Centrifuge the PRP1 fraction at 1500 g for 15 min at RT.
5. Draw off two-thirds of the PPP supernatant and resuspend the platelet-containing pellet PRP2 in the remaining PPP. Measure the PRP2 volume and take an aliquot for determination of PRP2 platelet concentration

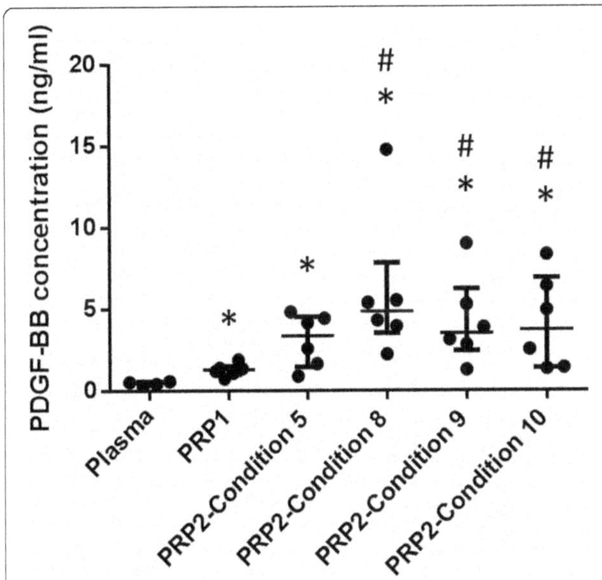

Fig. 2 Scatter plots for PDGF-BB concentrations in plasma, PRP1 and PRP2 * Indicates a statistically significant difference (P < 0.05) compared with plasma. # Indicates a statistically significant difference (P < 0.05) compared with PRP1. Data are presented by groups, the line represents the median of the group; error bars represent the interquartile range. Condition 5, 1000 g, 15 min; condition 8, 1500 g. 15 min; condition 9, 1500 g, 20 min; condition 10, 3000 g, 10 min

The purpose of the first spin is to separate as many platelets as possible from the whole blood. Centrifugation separates blood components on the basis of their density gradients. Platelets are the lightest components, followed by WBCs, and RBCs are heaviest [26]. Therefore, RCF and time must be appropriate to obtain optimal separation of blood components. In this study, a low RCF and short duration of centrifugation was insufficient to obtain good separation of platelets from other blood cells, resulting in low recovery. The highest platelet recovery in conditions 9 and 10, which were the highest RCF conditions, indicated that the 1000-g condition was the most suitable condition to sink RBCs and WBCs and separated platelets at the upper layer. However, in condition 10, the WBC recovery rate was also high because the high RCF and long centrifugation time caused the platelet to overlap with the WBC layer.

The purpose of the second spin is to separate platelets from plasma, which is accomplished by pelleting the platelets and discarding most of the PPP supernatant. To maximise platelet recovery and yield, a higher RCF and longer duration of centrifugation than used in the first spin were needed. However, we found that if the RCF time was too high, the recovery and yield were reduced due to platelet aggregation. Aggregated platelets were not resuspended in PPP, thus resulting in substantial platelet count reduction. The blood analyser detects aggregated platelets in PRP2; although the actual numbers of platelets were not decreased, as aggregated (activated) platelets release growth factors during the preparation process, the amount of growth factors in the final product was found to decrease. We concluded that the optimal combination was 1000 g for 5 min for the first spin and 1500 g for 15 min for the second spin.

The RCFs we found to be optimal for preparation of PRP from canine blood were higher than those found for human blood, although the centrifugation times were similar [20, 21]. This may be related to haematologic difference between human and dog blood. Canine mean corpuscular volume and mean corpuscular haemoglobin values are lower than human values [27, 28]. These means dog RBCs are smaller and less dense than human RBCs, so relatively higher centrifugal force is required to separate canine blood components.

The optimised protocol increased platelet concentration was 6- to 7-fold relative to the initial concentration in whole blood (Table 2), and final platelet concentration was 1748 ± 193 × 10^3 platelets μL^{-1} (Table 3). The

American Red Cross defines PRP as 5.5×10^{10} platelets/ 50 mL (1100×10^3 platelets μL^{-1}) [29]. Furthermore, accumulated data suggests that the PRP products must have at least 300×10^3 platelets μL^{-1} to be therapeutically effective, which is 4- to 5-fold higher concentration than whole blood [30–34]. These recommendations may not be appropriate to every situation; however, because this protocol produces a high yield of platelets, the concentration can adjusted as necessary by manipulating the ratio of PPP to PRP. Franklin et al. [25] recently conducted a study in which they used five commercially available kits to prepare PRP from canine whole blood. The yield and compositions of the canine PRP prepared using these kits varied considerably. The concentration of platelets in the canine PRP prepared using our optimised protocol was higher than the concentrations achieved with any of the commercial systems. Frye et al. [35] also showed PRP, with platelet and leukocyte concentrations similar to ours through the double-spin method using commercial kits, but its disadvantage was that it was expensive.

Using differential centrifugation to prepare platelet concentrates completely free of other blood cell types is impossible because the specific gravities of the various components slightly overlap [36]. However, our optimised protocol resulted in PRP with negligible number of RBCs compared with other studies [20, 21], and only $8.18 \pm 0.98\%$ of total blood WBC counts were contained in PRP1. Also, the WBC concentration in the final product was 2-fold lower than the normal range. In particular, the recovery rate of lymphocytes and monocytes from PRP1 obtained with the first spin was higher than that of neutrophils because the lymphocyte and monocyte weights were relatively light and were located in the upper layer near the platelets after centrifugation.

The role of WBC in PRP therapy remains a matter of disagreement in the literature. Some studies have suggested that increased WBC concentrations in PRP can impede tissue regeneration and healing. The presence of WBC in PRP has been associated with increased scar tissue and collagen degradation ex vivo. High WBC concentration may affect negatively with matrix production in tendons [37–39]. To prevent potential negative effects, it has been suggested that platelet preparations only be transfused if they contain fewer than 5×10^5 WBC/μL [40]. However, some research has suggested that some WBC contamination may be beneficial because WBC can increase growth factor secretion. PRP that contained enough number of WBCs was recommended as another therapeutic purpose because WBC triggered growth factor secretion by the tissue being treated with the PRP [41, 42]. There is not enough data in the literature to determine whether WBCs are beneficial to PRP therapy [29]. Additional studies will be necessary to optimise PRP with regard to their WBC content. Previously, Perazzi et al. [23] performed PRP preparation study using the double-centrifugation method, which is similar to ours. In their study, platelet concentration at least four times the baseline was obtained in 10 out of 12 dogs (83.3% of cases), but WBC concentration was also higher than that at the baseline. Furthermore, they did not measure growth factor concentration in PRP from their protocol; thus, it remained unknown that high platelet number represented high growth factor concentration in PRP.

Among the numerous growth factors present in platelet α granules, PDGF-BB was selected as an index of activated platelets in this study because it is only secreted by activated platelets and not contained in plasma. Thus, its concentration represented the extent to which platelets were activated. PDGF-BB concentration was highest in PRP prepared by the optimised method. Although the PRP that had the highest platelet concentration also had the highest PDGF-BB level, platelet concentration is not the only determinant of growth factor concentration. The type of anticoagulant used during blood collection, the ratio of blood to anticoagulant, the type of activating agent and the activation protocol can all have an influence of the concentration of growth factor in PRP [20]. A previous study showed that platelets released the highest PDGF-BB when they were activated with $CaCl_2$ [43]. Further, the amount of TGF-β released by platelets activated by thrombin or $CaCl_2$ was similar [43]. In addition, the process of obtaining autologous thrombin is complicated, but activation using $CaCl_2$ is inexpensive and easy. Therefore, we used $CaCl_2$ to activate platelets. However, we did not measure whether platelets were fully activated in the present study. Among the PRPs with the same number of platelets, the amount of growth factors will depend on the number of activated platelets. To activate as much platelets as possible, various agonist (collagen, ADP and thrombin, etc.) and ratio between PRP and agonist should be further studied.

One potential limitation of using centrifugation to prepare PRP is that there is a risk for bacterial contamination during transfers between tubes. However, this risk can be greatly reduced if transfers are conducted in a laminar flow hood under sterile conditions. Despite this potential drawback, the protocol we have described in this study does not require particularly expensive equipment or high technical ability and can readily be carried out in a veterinary clinical setting.

Conclusions

The PRP therapy, research and associated-industry are burgeoning fields in veterinary medicine. For the effective and reliable clinical application of PRP in veterinary medicine, more studies are needed with regard to PRP characteristics as well as patient factors that influence the effectiveness of PRP. Our protocol meets the guideline of The American Red Cross and recommendations of other articles associated with the number of platelets in PRP. The PRP from our optimised protocol may produce consistently reproducible results and it will help advance comparative research and therapeutic use of PRP-related products in veterinary medicine.

Abbreviations

ACD: Acid citrate dextrose; EGF: Epidermal growth factor; MCH: Mean corpuscular haemoglobin; MCV: Mean corpuscular volume; PDGF-BB: Platelet-derived growth factor-BB; PPP: Platelet-poor plasma; PRP: Platelet-rich plasma; RBC: Red blood cell; RCF: Relative centrifugal force; TGF: Transforming growth factor; VEGF: Vascular endothelial growth factor; WBC: White blood cell

Acknowledgements

Not applicable

Funding

This work was supported by Basic Science Research Program through the National Research Foundation of Korea (NRF), which is funded by the Ministry of Science, ICT & Future Planning (NRF-2015R1C1A1A01051759) and 2015 Research Grant from Kangwon National University (No. 520150508).

Authors' contributions

HSS, HMW and BJK conceived the study and performed its design and coordination. HSS performed the experiment and conducted data analysis. BJK participated in data analysis and interpretation and performed statistical analysis. HMW and BJK proofread the manuscript and gave final approval of the version to be published. All authors read and approved the final manuscript.

Authors' information

This manuscript is part of a MS thesis submitted by Dr. Shin to the College of Veterinary Medicine, Kangwon National University.

Consent for publication

Not applicable

Competing interests

The authors declare that they have no competing interests.

References

1. Eppley BL, Woodell JE, Higgins J. Platelet quantification and growth factor analysis from platelet-rich plasma: implications for wound healing. Plast Reconstr Surg. 2004;114(6):1502–8.
2. Kaplan DR, Chao FC, Stiles CD, Antoniades HN, Scher CD. Platelet alpha granules contain a growth factor for fibroblasts. Blood. 1979;53(6):1043–52.
3. Assoian RK, Komoriya A, Meyers CA, Miller DM, Sporn MB. Transforming growth factor-beta in human platelets. Identification of a major storage site, purification, and characterization. J Biol Chem. 1983;258(11):7155–60.
4. Drago L, Bortolin M, Vassena C, Taschieri S, Del Fabbro M. Antimicrobial activity of pure platelet-rich plasma against microorganisms isolated from oral cavity. BMC Microbiol. 2013;13(1):1.
5. Fortier LA, Mohammed HO, Lust G, Nixon AJ. Insulin-like growth factor-I enhances cell-based repair of articular cartilage. J Bone Joint Surg Br. 2002;84(2):276 88.
6. Bendinelli P, Matteucci E, Dogliotti G, Corsi MM, Banfi G, Maroni P, et al. Molecular basis of anti-inflammatory action of platelet-rich plasma on human chondrocytes: mechanisms of NF-κB inhibition via HGF. J Cell Physiol. 2010;225(3):757–66.
7. Mazzocca AD, McCarthy MBR, Intravia J, Beitzel K, Apostolakos J, Cote MP, et al. An in vitro evaluation of the anti-inflammatory effects of platelet-rich plasma, ketorolac, and methylprednisolone. Arthroscopy: The Journal of Arthroscopic & Related Surgery. 2013;29(4):675–83.
8. Everts PA, Hoffmann J, Weibrich G, Mahoney C, Schönberger J, Van Zundert A, et al. Differences in platelet growth factor release and leucocyte kinetics during autologous platelet gel formation. Transfus Med. 2006;16(5):363–8.
9. Marx RE, Carlson ER, Eichstaedt RM, Schimmele SR, Strauss JE, Georgeff KR. Platelet-rich plasma: growth factor enhancement for bone grafts. Oral Surg Oral Med Oral Pathol Oral Radiol Endod. 1998;85(6):638–46.
10. Alio JL, Abad M, Artola A, Rodriguez-Prats JL, Pastor S, Ruiz-Colecha J. Use of autologous platelet-rich plasma in the treatment of dormant corneal ulcers. Ophthalmology. 2007;114(7):1286–1293. e1.
11. Savarino L, Cenni E, Tarabusi C, Dallari D, Stagni C, Cenacchi A, et al. Evaluation of bone healing enhancement by lyophilized bone grafts supplemented with platelet gel: a standardized methodology in patients with tibial osteotomy for genu varus. J Biomed Mater Res B Appl Biomater. 2006;76(2):364–72.
12. Eppley BL, Pietrzak WS, Blanton M. Platelet-rich plasma: a review of biology and applications in plastic surgery. Plast Reconstr Surg. 2006;118(6):147e–59e.
13. Carter CA, Jolly DG, Worden CE, Hendren DG, Kane CJ. Platelet-rich plasma gel promotes differentiation and regeneration during equine wound healing. Exp Mol Pathol. 2003;74(3):244–55.
14. Souza TF, Andrade AL, Ferrreira G, Sakamoto SS. Albuquerque VBd, Bonfim S, Luvizotto MCR, Louzada MJQ: healing and expression of growth factors (TGF-β and PDGF) in canine radial ostectomy gap containing platelet-rich plasma. Vet Comp Orthop Traumatol. 2012;25(6):445.
15. Iacopetti I, Perazzi A, Ferrari V, Busetto R. Application of platelet-rich gel to enhance wound healing in the horse: a case report. Journal of Equine Veterinary Science. 2012;32(3):123–8.
16. Weibrich G, Kleis WK, Hafner G, Hitzler WE. Growth factor levels in platelet-rich plasma and correlations with donor age, sex, and platelet count. J Cranio-Maxillofac Surg. 2002;30(2):97–102.
17. Weibrich G, Hansen T, Kleis W, Buch R, Hitzler W. Effect of platelet concentration in platelet-rich plasma on peri-implant bone regeneration. Bone. 2004;34(4):665–71.
18. Kawasumi M, Kitoh H, Siwicka KA, Ishiguro N. The effect of the platelet concentration in platelet-rich plasma gel on the regeneration of bone. J Bone Joint Surg Br. 2008;90(7):966–72.
19. Kakudo N, Minakata T, Mitsui T, Kushida S, Notodihardjo FZ, Kusumoto K. Proliferation-promoting effect of platelet-rich plasma on human adipose-derived stem cells and human dermal fibroblasts. Plast Reconstr Surg. 2008;122(5):1352–60.
20. Araki J, Jona M, Eto H, Aoi N, Kato H, Suga H, et al. Optimized preparation method of platelet-concentrated plasma and noncoagulating platelet-derived factor concentrates: maximization of platelet concentration and removal of fibrinogen. Tissue Engineering Part C: Methods. 2011;18(3):176–85.
21. Amable PR, Carias RBV, Teixeira MVT, da Cruz Pacheco Í, do Amaral RJFC, Granjeiro JM, et al. Platelet-rich plasma preparation for regenerative medicine: optimization and quantification of cytokines and growth factors. Stem Cell Res Ther. 2013;4(3):1.
22. Fukaya M, Ito A. A new economic method for preparing platelet-rich plasma. Plast Reconstr Surg Glob Open. 2014;2(6):e162.
23. Perazzi A, Busetto R, Martinello T, Drigo M, Pasotto D, Cian F, Patruno M, Iacopetti I. Description of a double centrifugation tube method for concentrating canine platelets. BMC Vet Res. 2013;9:146–6148-9-146.
24. Argüelles D, Carmona J, Pastor J, Iborra A, Viñals L, Martínez P, et al. Evaluation of single and double centrifugation tube methods for concentrating equine platelets. Res Vet Sci. 2006;81(2):237–45.
25. Franklin SP, Garner BC, Cook JL. Characteristics of canine platelet-rich plasma prepared with five commercially available systems. Am J Vet Res. 2015;76(9):822–7.

26. Brodniewicz-Proba T. Human plasma fractionation and the impact of new technologies on the use and quality of plasma-derived products. Blood Rev. 1991;5(4):245–57.
27. ASTM Committee F-4 on Medical and Surgical Materials and Devices, ASTM Committee F-4 on Medical and Surgical Materials and Devices. Subcommittee F04. 04 on Cardiovascular Implants and Materials: Vascular graft update: safety and performance. In Edited by Anonymous ASTM International; 1986:169–179.
28. Prothero JW: The Design of Mammals. In Edited by Anonymous Cambridge University Press; 2015;93–102.
29. Ehrenfest DMD, Rasmusson L, Albrektsson T. Classification of platelet concentrates: from pure platelet-rich plasma (P-PRP) to leucocyte-and platelet-rich fibrin (L-PRF). Trends Biotechnol. 2009;27(3):158–67.
30. Marx RE. Platelet-rich plasma: evidence to support its use. J Oral Maxillofac Surg. 2004;62(4):489–96.
31. Anitua E, Andia I, Ardanza B, Nurden P, Nurden AT. Autologous platelets as a source of proteins for healing and tissue regeneration. Thromb Haemost. 2004;91(1):4–15.
32. Everts P, Overdevest EP, Jakimowicz JJ, Oosterbos CJ, Schönberger J, Knape JT, et al. The use of autologous platelet–leukocyte gels to enhance the healing process in surgery, a review. Surg Endosc. 2007;21(11):2063–8.
33. Monteiro SO, Lepage OM, Theoret CL. Effects of platelet-rich plasma on the repair of wounds on the distal aspect of the forelimb in horses. Am J Vet Res. 2009;70(2):277–82.
34. Maia L, de Souza MV, Júnior JIR, de Oliveira AC, Alves GES, dos Anjos Benjamin L, et al. Platelet-rich plasma in the treatment of induced tendinopathy in horses: histologic evaluation. Journal of equine veterinary science. 2009;29(8):618–26.
35. Frye CW, Enders A, Brooks MB, Struble AM, Wakshlag JJ. Assessment of canine autologous platelet-rich plasma produced with a commercial centrifugation and platelet recovery kit. Vet Comp Orthop Traumatol. 2016;29(1):14–9.
36. Kurita M, Aiba-Kojima E, Shigeura T, Matsumoto D, Suga H, Inoue K, et al. Differential effects of three preparations of human serum on expansion of various types of human cells. Plast Reconstr Surg. 2008;122(2):438–48.
37. Schnabel LV, Mohammed HO, Miller BJ, McDermott WG, Jacobson MS, Santangelo KS, et al. Platelet rich plasma (PRP) enhances anabolic gene expression patterns in flexor digitorum superficialis tendons. J Orthop Res. 2007;25(2):230–40.
38. McCarrel T, Fortier L. Temporal growth factor release from platelet-rich plasma, trehalose lyophilized platelets, and bone marrow aspirate and their effect on tendon and ligament gene expression. J Orthop Res. 2009;27(8):1033–42.
39. McCarrel TM, Minas T, Fortier LA: Optimization of leukocyte concentration in platelet-rich plasma for the treatment of tendinopathy. J Bone Joint Surg Am. 2012;94(19):e143(1–8).
40. Misso S, Feola B, Marotta C, Graziano D, Fratellanza A, Minerva V, et al. Sottopopolazioni leucocitarie in concentrati piastrinici da aferesi e da plasma ricco di piastrine. La trasfusione del sangue. 2001;46(4):258–62.
41. Zimmermann R, Reske S, Metzler P, Schlegel A, Ringwald J, Eckstein R. Preparation of highly concentrated and white cell-poor platelet-rich plasma by plateletpheresis. Vox Sang. 2008;95(1):20–5.
42. Castillo TN, Pouliot MA, Kim HJ, Dragoo JL. Comparison of growth factor and platelet concentration from commercial platelet-rich plasma separation systems. Am J Sports Med. 2011;39(2):266–71.
43. Textor JA, Tablin F. Activation of equine platelet-rich plasma: comparison of methods and characterization of equine autologous thrombin. Vet Surg. 2012;41(7):784–94.

9

Effects of isoflurane, sevoflurane, propofol and alfaxalone on brain metabolism in dogs assessed by proton magnetic resonance spectroscopy (^{1}H MRS)

Franz Josef Söbbeler[1*], Inés Carrera[2], Kirby Pasloske[3], Millagahamada Gedara Ranasinghe[3], Patrick Kircher[2] and Sabine Beate Rita Kästner[1]

Abstract

Background: The purpose of this study was to determine the effects of isoflurane, sevoflurane, propofol and alfaxalone on the canine brain metabolite bioprofile, measured with single voxel short echo time proton magnetic resonance spectroscopy at 3 Tesla. Ten adult healthy Beagle dogs were assigned to receive isoflurane, sevoflurane, propofol and alfaxalone at 3 different dose rates each in a randomized cross-over study design. Doses for isoflurane, sevoflurane, propofol and alfaxalone were F_E'Iso 1.7 vol%, 2.1 vol%, 2.8 vol%, F_E'Sevo 2.8 vol%, 3.5 vol% and 4. 7 vol%, 30, 45 and 60 mg kg^{-1} h^{-1} and 10, 15 and 20 mg kg^{-1} h^{-1} respectively. A single voxel Point Resolved Spectroscopy Sequence was performed on a 3 T MRI scanner in three brain regions (basal ganglia, parietal and occipital lobes). Spectral data were analyzed with LCModel. Concentration of total N-acetylaspartate (tNAA), choline, creatine, inositol and glutamine and glutamate complex (Glx) relative to water content was obtained. Plasma concentration of lactate, glucose, triglycerides, propofol and alfaxalone were determined. Statistics were performed using repeated measures ANOVA or Wilcoxon Sign Rank test with alpha = 5%.

Results: Plasma glucose increased with isoflurane, sevoflurane and alfaxalone but decreased with propofol. Plasma lactate increased with all anesthetics (isoflurane > sevoflurane > propofol > alfaxalone). Cerebral lactate could not be detected. Only minor changes in cerebral metabolite concentrations of tNAA, choline, inositol, creatine and Glx occurred with anesthetic dose changes.

Conclusion: The metabolomic profile detected with proton magnetic resonance spectroscopy at 3 Tesla of canine brain showed only minor differences between doses and anesthetics related to tNAA, choline, creatine, inositol and Glx.

Keywords: Anesthesia, Lactate, Glucose, MRI, Cerebral, PRESS, Plasma, LcModel, Canine

Background

Injectable as well as volatile anesthetics influence cerebral metabolism. The classic paradigm that neuronal activity ≈ metabolism ≈ blood flow has been used to study the effect of anesthetics on brain metabolism. Positron Emission Tomography studies with 2-deoxy-2(^{18}F)fluoro-D-glucose to determine the cerebral metabolic rate of glucose (CMRglu) as an indirect measure of neuronal activity [1] found a consistent suppression of CMRglu under isoflurane, sevoflurane and propofol with varying impact on different brain regions in man [2–6]. Cerebral metabolic rate of oxygen is also reduced by sevoflurane, propofol, isoflurane and also Althesin® (a combination of 9 mg mL^{-1} alfaxalone- and 3 mg mL^{-1} alfadolone acetate) [7–9]. In microdialysis studies in rodents [10, 11] volatile anesthetics led to a rapid and dose-dependent increase in cerebral lactate levels without changes in cerebral glucose levels. Ketamine/xylazine, and chloral hydrate moderately increased cerebral lactate, but cerebral glucose levels rose markedly. Both propofol and pentobarbital did not affect

* Correspondence: franz.josef.soebbeler@tiho-hannover.de
[1]Small Animal Clinic (Söbbeler, Kästner), University of Veterinary Medicine Hanover Foundation, Bünteweg 9, 30559 Hannover, Germany
Full list of author information is available at the end of the article

cerebral lactate levels and only propofol led to a minor increase in cerebral glucose.

Brain metabolism can also be investigated by magnetic resonance spectroscopy (MRS), which is a non-invasive magnetic resonance imaging technique that allows the determination of the biochemical composition of the brain in vivo for accurate identification and quantification of metabolites in localized brain regions [12–14]. With proton magnetic resonance spectroscopy (^{1}H MRS) at 3 Tesla several metabolites can be identified in the normal brain, such as N-acetylaspartate (NAA), choline, creatine, myo-inositol, and sum of glutamate and glutamine (Glx) [15–18]. At > 7 Tesla, the spectral differentiation between the glutamine and glutamate is complete, and other smaller metabolites like glucose and GABA are well depicted [19, 20].

Several ^{1}H MRS studies have been performed to investigate metabolism within the brain under general anesthesia in rodents [21, 22], monkeys [23], humans [24] and dogs [25]. The main findings of these studies [21–24] were the increase in cerebral lactate under the dose-dependent influence of volatile anesthetics independent of plasma lactate [21–23]. They also found increases in other cerebral metabolites, especially glutamate, alanine and creatine. These changes have been shown to be fully reversible within minutes after completion of the anesthesia [21]. On the other hand, the injectable anesthetics and premedication drugs ketamine/medetomidine, medetomidine, pentobarbital, fentanyl, diazepam and propofol did not influence cerebral lactate concentration [21, 22].

In veterinary medicine, clinical MRI can only be performed under general anesthesia. Recently, relative metabolite concentrations and their ratios in the brain of healthy beagle dogs under general anesthesia have been published [15–17], as well as a few clinical studies [26, 27] using different anesthetic protocols. Since the influence of anesthetics on the canine brain bioprofile at 3 Tesla is actually not known, the purpose of the study reported here was to determine the possible effects of the commonly used anesthetics isoflurane, sevoflurane, propofol and alfaxalone on canine brain bioprofile assessed with single voxel short echo time proton magnetic resonance spectroscopy at a field strength of 3.0 Tesla. Secondary aim of this study was to evaluate the possible effects of the anesthetics on plasma levels of lactate and glucose.

Our hypothesis was that volatile anesthetics isoflurane and sevoflurane, but not the injectable anesthetics propofol and alfaxalone, cause a dose-dependent increase in cerebral lactate. Furthermore, we hypothesized an increase in cerebral levels of creatine and glutamate under influence of volatile anesthetics compared to the injectable anesthetics propofol and alfaxalone. Regional differences in cerebral metabolites were anticipated to be independent of anesthetics.

Methods

All animal procedures were performed according to the German animal protection law after review and approval by the ethical committee for animal experimentation of the Federal State Office for Consumer Protection and Food Safety of Lower Saxony, Germany (3392 42,502–04-13/1252).

Animals

Ten purpose-bred (purpose bred at our own institution) adult Beagle dogs (8 neutered males and 2 spayed females) were included in the study. Age ranged from 32 to 91 month (mean ± SD, 50.7 ± 22.2 months) and the weight ranged from 11 to 21.8 kg (mean ± SD, 16.5 kg ± 3.2).

The dogs were housed in groups of 5 to 6 dogs per group with daily periods in enriched outside runs and regular walking by veterinary students. Ambient temperature is regulated to 18–21 °C. The dogs received commercial dog food (Hills VetEssentials Canine adult) according to body weight, twice daily except on study days.

Health status of the dogs was confirmed by a clinical and neurological examination and complete blood count and blood chemistry. Physical status was classified according to the American Society of Anesthesiologists (ASA) physical status classification system as ASA I.

Study design

The study was performed as a randomized, experimental trial in a complete cross-over design with four treatments [isoflurane (I), sevoflurane (S), propofol (P), alfaxalone (A)] and a wash out period of at least 14 days between treatments.

Instrumentation

All dogs were fasted overnight, water was available until the trial started. Blood was drawn from the jugular vein for analysis of blood gases, electrolytes, plasma lactate, plasma glucose and plasma triglycerides. A peripheral venous catheter was placed into the cephalic or lateral saphenous vein for induction and maintenance of anesthesia (treatment P and A) and cardiovascular support (treatment I, S, P, A). A central venous catheter was placed into the right or left jugular vein for blood sampling. All dogs were wrapped in self-made bubble wrap vests equipped with 41 °C warm gel heat pads for temperature management. Earplugs were used for noise protection.

Anesthetic protocol

In treatment I and S dogs were induced by mask with 5% isoflurane (Isofluran CP®, CP-Pharma) or 6% sevoflurane (SevoFlo®, EcuPhar GmbH) in 100% oxygen with a flow of 8 L min^{-1}. In treatment P and A, induction took place with 10 mg kg^{-1} propofol (Narcofol®, 10 mg mL^{-1}, CP Pharma) or 3 mg kg^{-1} alfaxalone

(Alfaxan®, 10 mg mL^{-1}, Jurox Pty Ltd) injected over a period of 60 s. Isoflurane, sevoflurane, propofol and alfaxalone were administered in three different doses. At each dose, proton magnetic resonance spectroscopic measurements were performed. A 30 min equilibration period was allowed before each measurement was conducted. The order and doses for isoflurane, sevoflurane were 2.1 vol%/2.8 vol%/1.7 vol% and 3.5 vol%/4.7 vol%/2.8 vol%, respectively, representing 1.5 MAC, 2 MAC and 1.2 MAC (1 MAC_{ISO} = 1.39 vol% and 1 MAC_{SEVO} = 2.36 vol% according to T Kazama and K Ikeda [28], values above are calculated and rounded, respectively). For propofol and alfaxalone, doses were 30 mg kg^{-1} h^{-1}, 45 mg kg^{-1} h^{-1}, 60 mg kg^{-1} h^{-1} and 10 mg kg^{-1} h^{-1}, 15 mg kg^{-1} h^{-1}, 20 mg kg^{-1} h^{-1}, respectively (Fig. 1). These anesthetics were administered as an incremental increase in dose rate to try and avoid period to period interaction with the possible accumulation of the injectable anesthetics.

After induction, intubation and instrumentation the animals were placed in sternal recumbency in the MRI scanner and the first equilibration phase started (in treatment I and S additional time was needed to adjust the end-expiratory concentration before each equilibration phase). Volume-controlled intermittent positive pressure ventilation was adjusted to maintain end tidal CO_2 in the eucapnic range of 35 and 45 mmHg. Measurements included pulse rate, SpO_2, $P_E'CO_2$, respiratory rate, inspiratory and expiratory isoflurane-, sevoflurane- and oxygen concentrations and body temperature.

For cardiovascular support a buffered balanced electrolyte solution (Sterofundin®) and 6% HES 130/0.42 (Venofundin® 6% HES) at a rate of 5 mL kg^{-1} h^{-1} dobutamine 3 μg kg^{-1} min^{-1} was administered to support cardiac output. Infusion rates of Sterofundin® were reduced with increasing infusion volume of injectable anesthetics, respectively.

The dogs were recovered in a quiet environment and warmed until physiologic body temperature was reached. They were returned into their group on the following day.

Blood sampling

Blood samples for plasma lactate, plasma triglycerides, blood gases and plasma glucose were taken after each measurement period via the central venous catheter. In Treatment P and A, additional blood was taken for plasma concentrations of propofol and alfaxalone at the

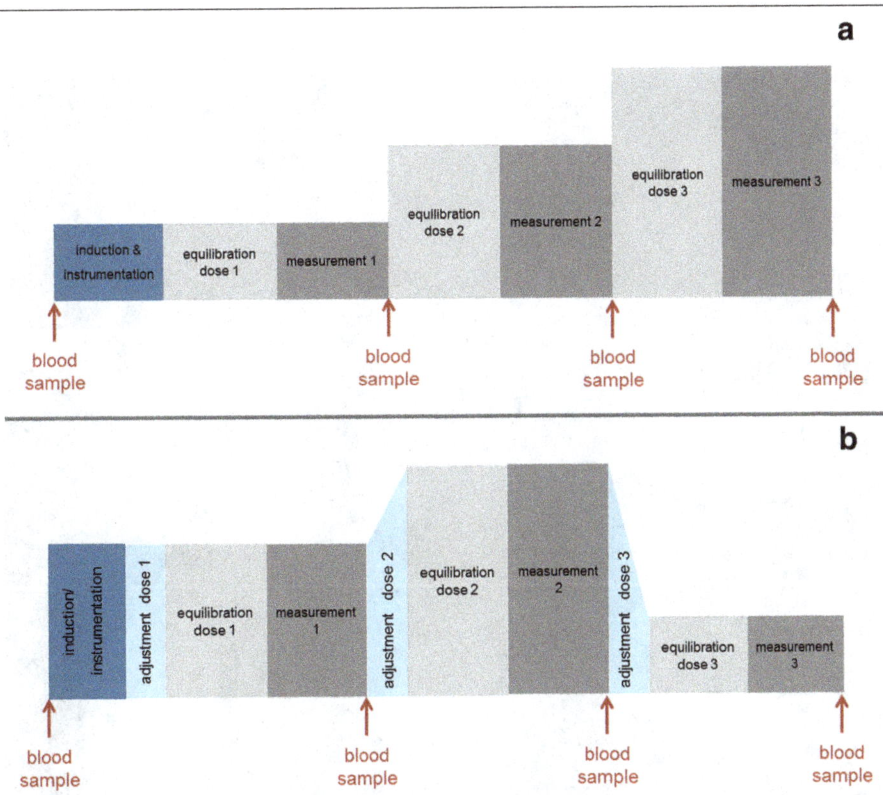

Fig. 1 Schematic timeline for propofol and alfaxalone (**a**) and isoflurane and sevoflurane (**b**) The 30 min equilibration phase was followed by a measurement period of approximately 30 min where a total of three measurements were performed (BG, PL and OL). For treatment I and S the end expiratory concentration had to be adjusted before each equilibration phase. Jugular venous blood samples were taken for serum glucose, lactate and plasma concentrations of propofol and alfaxalone

end of each measurement period before increasing the dose rate (Fig. 1). Plasma glucose concentration (Reflovet® Plus – Roche; reflexionphotometric measurement) and blood gases (ABL80 FLEX – Radiometer GMBH; amperometric/potentiometric measurement) were measured immediately whereas blood samples for plasma lactate, plasma triglycerides and plasma concentrations of propofol and alfaxalone were centrifuged at 11,800 rpm for 2 min, plasma was separated and immediately stored at – 82 °C until analyzed. Plasma lactate and plasma triglycerides were analyzed via absorption photometric measurement (cobas c311 – Roche Hitachi). Propofol plasma concentrations were quantified by means of gas chromatography - mass spectrometry (GC/MS) after solid-phase extraction and alfaxalone plasma concentrations were determined with liquid chromatography – tandem mass spectrometry (LC/MS) after solid phase extraction [29].

Imaging protocol

Magnetic resonance imaging was performed with a 3.0 T Philips Achieva MRI scanner (Philips MedicalSystems, Best, the Netherlands) with a 8-channel receive-transmit knee coil (Philips MedicalSystems, Best, the Netherlands). For morphological imaging of the brain, transverse, dorsal, and sagittal turbo spin echo T2-weighted images were performed. Scan parameters were as follow: echo time, 80 milliseconds; repetition time, 3000 milliseconds; turbo spin factor, 15; matrix, 256 × 204; slice thickness, 3 mm; number of signal averages, 1. These images were performed during the first 30 min equilibration phase to reduce total time of anesthesia.

Single voxel ^{1}H MRS was performed by one of the investigators (FS) by use of short-echo time point resolved technique (PRESS) with voxels graphically prescribed from the T2-weighted images. Volume samples were performed over various regions of the brain parenchyma, including left basal ganglia (voxel of interest 1.5 cm^3), left parietal lobe (voxel of interest 1.95 cm^3), and midline occipital lobe (voxel of interest 1.5 cm^3) (Fig. 2). Only the left hemisphere was analyzed, based on a previously reported study, in which differences in the metabolite concentration between left and right hemispheres were not found in the canine brain [15]. Parameters for the ^{1}H MRS technique were as follow: echo time, shortest possible (32–34 milliseconds – usually 32 milliseconds in occipital lobe and 33 milliseconds in basal ganglia and parietal lobe); repetition time, 2000 milliseconds; number of sample averages, 256; bandwidth, 2000 Hz. Care was taken to avoid cerebrospinal fluid and peripheral soft and bony tissues to prevent lipid contamination. Before each ^{1}H MRS acquisition, field homogeneity was

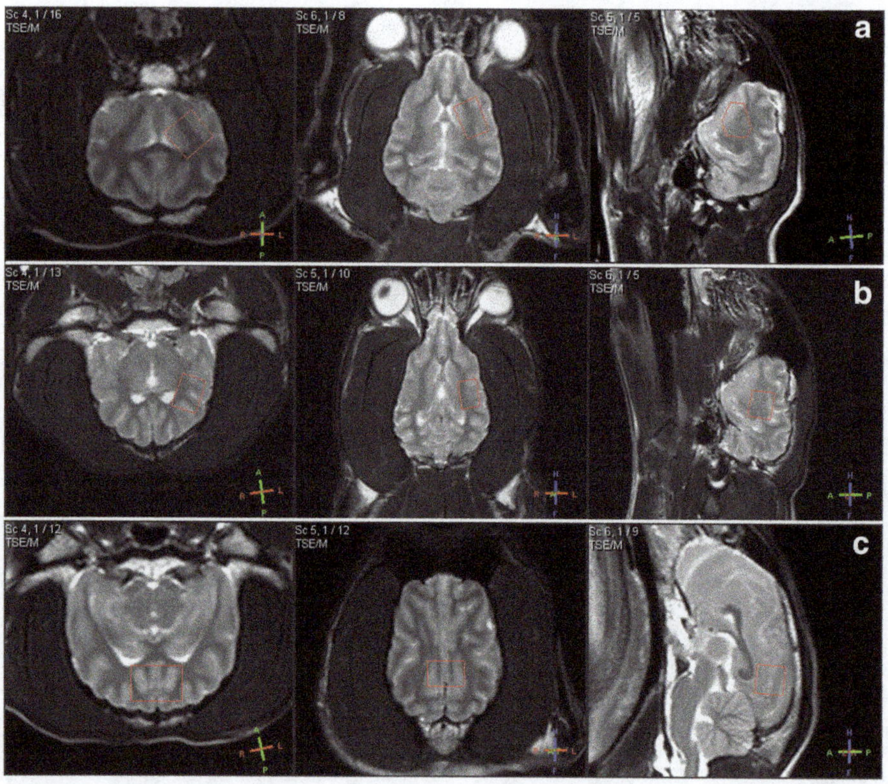

Fig. 2 T2 weighted images of the brain of one beagle dog. Transversal (left), dorsal (middle), parasagittal (right; **a** and **b**) or sagittal (right; **c**) view; The red rectangles display the ^{1}H MRS voxels of interests (VOI) for left basal ganglia (**a**), left parietal lobe (**b**) and midline occipital lobe (**c**)

optimized with a second-order automatic pencil-beam shim, which was followed by water suppression techniques (excitation). A water-unsuppressed image was also acquired to serve as a concentration reference for quantifying metabolite concentrations. In addition to a typical shim time of 2 min, each examination was acquired in 8 min and 36 s. Rejection criteria for the ^{1}H MRS data were presence of an unstable baseline, line width > 10 Hz, signal-to-noise ratio < 6, presence of artifacts, or presence of lipid contamination.

Data processing

Metabolite concentrations were estimated with an automated data processing spectral fitting (linear combination model) algorithm (LCModel). The software automatically adjusted the phase and chemical shift of the spectra, estimated the baseline, and performed eddy current correction. Relative metabolite concentrations and their uncertainties were estimated by fitting the spectrum to a basis set of spectra acquired from individual metabolites in solution. Seventeen metabolites were included in the linear combination model (alanine, aspartate, glucose, creatine, phosphocreatine, glutamine, glutamate, glycerophosphocholine, phosphocholine, lactate, lipids, myoinositol, N-acetylaspartate, *N*-acetylaspartylglutamate, scylloinositol, glutathione, and taurine). Only those metabolites with CRLBs < 20% were evaluated in this study.

One investigator (FS) reviewed MRI and ^{1}H MRS images. The MRI images were assessed for abnormalities such as changes in signal intensity of the gray and white matter, presence of space-occupying lesions, mass effect, or ventriculomegaly. Metabolite concentrations relative to water and metabolite ratios with creatine as a reference were calculated from the ^{1}H MRS data.

Statistical analysis

No comparable study on cerebral has been performed in dogs, so that a priori power analysis for calculation of sample size was based on the effect size from Jacob et al. 2012 performed in humans using a power of 90% and an alpha of 0.05.

Data were analyzed with aid of statistical software SAS Enterprise Guide (Version 6.1 M1, for Windows, SAS Institute Inc., Cary, NC, USA). Kolmogorov-Smirnov Test and Q-Q plots were used to test distribution of the data. Effect on cerebral metabolite concentrations were analyzed using a repeated measure ANOVA. This was performed for metabolite concentration relative to brain water content itself as well as for calculated metabolite ratios with creatine as internal reference metabolite.

Pearson's correlations were performed to investigate the possible effect of plasma concentrations on metabolite concentrations and the effect of plasma sodium concentration on total NAA and inositol. Arithmetic mean of metabolite concentrations of the three doses for each anesthetic was calculated followed by a repeated measure ANOVA for determination of anesthetic effect. For differences of cerebral metabolite concentrations between investigated brain regions a repeated measures ANOVA for first measurement (equivalent to the second dose) in treatment S was performed. Wilcoxon Signed Rank Test was used for pulse rate, body temperature, plasma levels of lactate, glucose and triglycerides blood gas values as well as plasma drug concentrations. Bonferroni alpha adjustment for correction of alpha-error accumulation was applied when appropriate. Level of significance was set at alpha = 5%. Data are presented as mean ± standard deviation (SD).

Results

The T2-weighted images revealed no morphological abnormalities. Out of 360 planned measurements (10 dogs × 4 treatments × 3 doses × 3 brain regions) 348 spectra were obtained. Inadequate anesthesia led to abortion of trial in three dogs (two dogs receiving isoflurane 1.7 vol% (1.2 MAC) and in one dog receiving propofol only measurements at a rate of 45 mg kg^{-1} h^{-1} could be performed). Four spectroscopic measurements were discarded from isoflurane treatment due to insufficient signal-to-noise ratio (BG 2.8 vol% & 1.7 vol% and OL 2.1 vol% & 2.8 vol% - 4 measurements). In total, 344 spectra were included in the study. All spectra included were of good quality with a signal-to-noise-ratio (mean ± SD) of 14.07 ± 5.66 and linewidths (mean ± SD) of 4.75 ± 2.37 Hz. Example spectra of all three brain regions of one dog undergoing treatment I are shown in Fig. 3.

Changes in metabolite concentration relative to brain water content between the investigated brain regions followed the same trend with all anesthetics and are exemplary listed for the first measurement (equivalent to second Dose) in treatment S only (mean ± SD displayed in Tables 1, 2, 3, 4 and 5). Creatine concentration differed between all three brain regions. The lowest concentration in parietal lobe differed to the highest in occipital lobe ($p <$ 0.0001) and to basal ganglia ($p = 0.0001$). Occipital lobe differed also to basal ganglia ($p = 0.00156$). Glx was lower in parietal lobe compared to basal ganglia ($p = 0.0045$) and occipital lobe ($p = 0.041$). N-acetylaspartate is lowest in basal ganglia being significant to the highest concentration in occipital lobe ($p = 0.0445$). The ratio to creatine was higher in parietal lobe compared to basal ganglia ($p < 0.0001$) and occipital lobe ($p < 0.0001$). Total choline was higher in in basal ganglia compared to parietal ($p < 0.0001$) and occipital lobes ($p < 0.0001$) but the ratio in occipital lobe was lowest compared to basal ganglia (p < 0.0001) and parietal lobe ($p < 0.0001$). Myoinositol

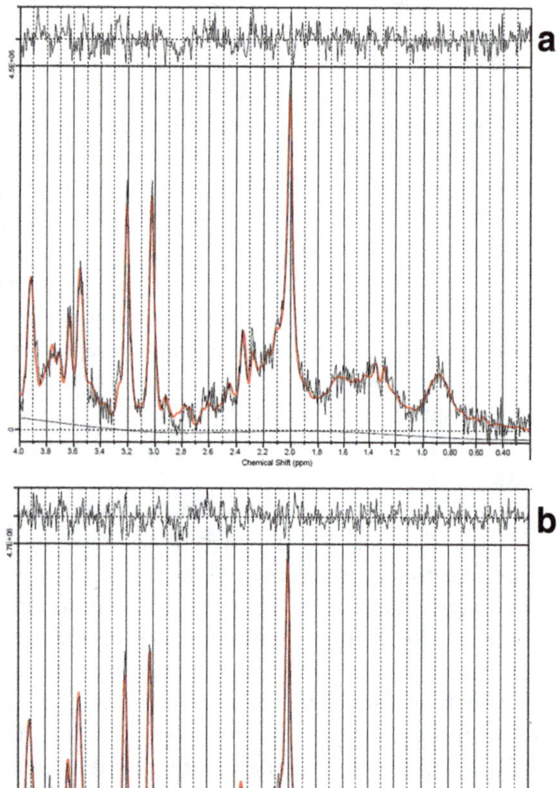

Fig. 3 Example ^{1}HMRS spectra of basal ganglia (**a**) parietal lobe (**b**) and occipital lobe (**c**) in one dog receiving 1.5 MAC (2.1 vol%) isoflurane. The x-axis represents the chemical shift in ppm of each metabolite and the y-axis represents the signal intensity

ratios to creatine were higher in parietal lobe compared to basal ganglia ($p = 0.0064$) and occipital lobe ($p = 0.0002$).

A lactate signal was not detected at any time. Few changes in cerebral metabolite concentrations relative to brain water content were found among the doses of the four anesthetics. Significant differences were detected for Glx in treatment I in parietal lobe but these changes did not coincide with either time or dose (Table 1). The total NAA (tNAA) concentration relative to water content in basal ganglia increased in a dose- or time-dependent manner in treatment A to reach a significant level between the first and third dose. Significant differences in tNAA were detected in treatment P in basal ganglia but these changes did not coincide with either time or dose (Table 2). Total choline concentration relative to brain water content decreased over time with both volatile anesthetics being significant in all brain regions except for treatment I in the occipital lobe (Table 3). Cerebral concentration of inositol revealed no significant differences (Table 4). Creatine concentration relative to cerebral water decreased with treatment S time-dependently (Table 5).

Metabolite ratios were calculated with creatine as internal reference metabolite. Total NAA to creatine ratio in treatment P in the occipital lobe showed significant differences between doses without relationship to dose or time (Table 2). A reduction in total choline to creatine ratio over time was detected for treatment I in the occipital lobe only (Table 3).

For comparison of the four anesthetics metabolite concentrations and their ratios with creatine as the denominator were arithmetically averaged over the three doses of each anesthetic. In treatment I higher levels of Glx were detected compared to injectable anesthetics in the parietal lobe (Table 1). Total choline was lower with isoflurane compared to treatment A in the basal ganglia and treatment P in the occipital lobe (Table 3) and creatine was lower with isoflurane compared to treatment A in the basal ganglia (Table S5). Metabolite ratios to creatine revealed no significant differences between anesthetics (Tables 1, 2, 3, 4 and 5).

Plasma concentrations of alfaxalone and propofol showed a wide individual range. Mean plasma concentrations increased with infusion rate with a statistically significant differentiation between the low dose and the middle and high dose, but not between the middle and the high dose for both injectable anesthetics (Fig. 4). Pearson's correlation asserted no interdependence of plasma concentration of propofol and alfaxalone on metabolite concentration and of sodium levels on total NAA and inositol.

In Treatment P, blood pH, HCO_3^- and sBE decreased. Plasma levels of glucose showed a mild increase in Treatment I but stayed within clinical reference. Plasma lactate increased dose-dependently with both volatile anesthetics and plasma triglycerides increased with administration of propofol (Table 6).

Body temperature decreased over time in treatments I, S and A. In treatment P, body temperature started to

Table 1 Mean ± SD of Glx concentrations (mmol L-1 of brain water) and Glx/tCr ratios

			Dose 1 Mean ± SD	Dose 2 Mean ± SD	Dose 3 Mean ± SD	Arithmetic mean Mean ± SD
GLX	BG	Isoflurane	13.568 ± 1.196	13.017 ± 1.037	13.039 ± 1.703	13.146 ± 1.003
		Sevoflurane	12.532 ± 1.369	12.931 ± 1.156	13.226 ± 1.266	12.896 ± 1.005
		Propofol	12.388 ± 1.066	12.730 ± 1.191	12.839 ± 1.582	12.760 ± 1.105
		Alfaxalone	12.941 ± 1.353	13.133 ± 1.670	13.423 ± 1.756	13.166 ± 1.233
	PL	Isoflurane	11.831 ± 2.167^{AB}	13.119 ± 1.695^{A}	11.821 ± 1.911^{B}	12.345 ± 1.674^{1}
		Sevoflurane	11.189 ± 1.375	10.632 ± 1.301	10.767 ± 0.888	10.863 ± 0.997^{12}
		Propofol	10.201 ± 1.818	10.165 ± 1.669	10.481 ± 2.286	10.295 ± 1.722^{2}
		Alfaxalone	10.087 ± 2.052	10.766 ± 2.084	10.315 ± 1.418	10.390 ± 1.353^{2}
	OL	Isoflurane	12.957 ± 1.341	12.263 ± 1.648	13.083 ± 1.845	12.913 ± 1.463
		Sevoflurane	12.869 ± 2.277	12.311 ± 1.752	12.700 ± 1.539	12.627 ± 1.694
		Propofol	12.043 ± 0.400	12.135 ± 0.809	12.587 ± 1.289	12.223 ± 0.646
		Alfaxalone	12.555 ± 1.586	12.320 ± 1.075	12.609 ± 1.055	12.495 ± 1.032
GLX/tCr	BG	Isoflurane	2.326 ± 0.136	2.118 ± 0.144	2.215 ± 0.416	2.196 ± 0.214
		Sevoflurane	2.082 ± 0.221	2.032 ± 0.185	2.117 ± 0.180	2.077 ± 0.127
		Propofol	2.082 ± 0.199	2.109 ± 0.153	2.136 ± 0.216	2.119 ± 0.141
		Alfaxalone	2.045 ± 0.182	2.082 ± 0.232	2.091 ± 0.290	2.073 ± 0.175
	PL	Isoflurane	2.177 ± 0.365	2.353 ± 0.352	2.110 ± 0.342	2.224 ± 0.306
		Sevoflurane	2.064 ± 0.265	1.908 ± 0.240	1.932 ± 0.178	1.968 ± 0.197
		Propofol	1.826 ± 0.385	1.858 ± 0.388	1.931 ± 0.516	1.865 ± 0.396
		Alfaxalone	1.857 ± 0.365	2.001 ± 0.451	1.915 ± 0.242	1.924 ± 0.272
	OL	Isoflurane	1.964 ± 0.302	1.800 ± 0.243	2.028 ± 0.278	1.984 ± 0.287
		Sevoflurane	1.914 ± 0.353	1.810 ± 0.300	1.870 ± 0.240	1.864 ± 0.282
		Propofol	1.777 ± 0.063	1.838 ± 0.147	1.834 ± 0.156	1.839 ± 0.131
		Alfaxalone	1.868 ± 0.280	1.839 ± 0.213	1.922 ± 0.193	1.877 ± 0.220

Mean ± SD for the three different doses and the arithmetic mean of the three doses for isoflurane, sevoflurane, propofol and alfaxalone in basal ganglia (BG), parietal lobe (PL) and occipital lobe (OL). Different alphabetical superscripts differ significantly ($p < 0.05$) between different doses of each anesthetic and different numerical superscripts differ significantly between arithmetic mean Glx concentrations of each anesthetic. For treatment I and S: Dose 1 ≙ time 3; Dose 2 ≙ time 1; Dose 3 ≙ time 2

increase during second measurement to reach baseline values again after the third measurement (Table 7).

Recovery from Anaesthesia

All dogs in Treatment I and S were extubated within 2–5 min after discontinuing anesthesia and recovery was uneventful. The first dog in treatment A and the first dog in treatment P developed myoclonia and reverse sneezing. Therefore, isoflurane was given for 30 min after discontinuing the constant rate infusion of alfaxalone or propofol to avoid myclonia. After discontinuation of isoflurane the recovery period was uneventful with time to extubation from 23 to 68 min.

Discussion

Using ^{1}H MRS at 3 T we found no evidence of increased intracerebral concentration of lactate with isoflurane, sevoflurane, propofol or alfaxalone in the canine brain. There were only minor differences between doses and anesthetics related to tNAA, Choline, Creatine, Inositol and Glx.

Cerebral lactate, formerly seen only as a waste product of anaerobe glycolysis is nowadays considered a beneficial metabolite serving as an energy substrate amongst others during hypoglycemia [10, 30]. Cerebral levels of lactate were increased upon exposure to volatile anesthetics in rodents in a reversible manner [11, 21, 22]. This effect was independent of blood lactate concentration. By performing a linear regression analysis of brain lactate measured by ^{1}H MRS and blood lactate concentration no relationship was determined in rats [22]. Isoflurane was also shown to enhance neuroprotective effects of exogenously administered lactate in an experimental stroke model [10]. As isoflurane led to a 6-fold increase in cerebral lactate in mice, we expected to be able to detect a sufficient lactate resonance in canine brain at 3 T. However, at this field strength we were not able to quantify cerebral lactate. In comparison to our

Table 2 Mean ± SD of tNAA concentrations (mmol L-1 of brain water) and tNAA/tCr ratios

			Dose 1	Dose 2	Dose 3	Arithmetic mean
			Mean ± SD	Mean ± SD	Mean ± SD	Mean ± SD
tNAA	BG	Isoflurane	6.911 ± 0.753	7.318 ± 0.425	6.955 ± 0.387	7.094 ± 0.339
		Sevoflurane	7.100 ± 0.548	7.297 ± 0.554	7.219 ± 0.512	7.205 ± 0.509
		Propofol	7.288 ± 0.484^{AB}	7.007 ± 0.466^{A}	7.524 ± 0.618^{B}	7.226 ± 0.444
		Alfaxalone	7.104 ± 0.472^{A}	7.499 ± 0.410^{AB}	7.724 ± 0.541^{B}	7.442 ± 0.376
	PL	Isoflurane	7.485 ± 0.585	7.692 ± 0.379	7.575 ± 0.360	7.583 ± 0.321
		Sevoflurane	7.664 ± 0.490	7.631 ± 0.690	7.673 ± 0.526	7.656 ± 0.540
		Propofol	7.622 ± 0.538	7.592 ± 0.617	7.667 ± 0.528	7.595 ± 0.516
		Alfaxalone	7.681 ± 0.364	7.704 ± 0.376	7.805 ± 0.449	7.730 ± 0.282
	OL	Isoflurane	7.725 ± 0.309	7.898 ± 0.497	7.599 ± 0.934	7.696 ± 0.556
		Sevoflurane	7.788 ± 0.642	7.907 ± 0.496	7.837 ± 0.492	7.844 ± 0.494
		Propofol	7.859 ± 0.393	7.741 ± 0.490	7.628 ± 0.398	7.687 ± 0.432
		Alfaxalone	7.680 ± 0.472	7.675 ± 0.559	7.426 ± 0.724	7.594 ± 0.498
tNAA/tCr	BG	Isoflurane	1.187 ± 0.126	1.195 ± 0.095	1.212 ± 0.108	1.203 ± 0.095
		Sevoflurane	1.183 ± 0.125	1.148 ± 0.108	1.157 ± 0.086	1.163 ± 0.099
		Propofol	1.229 ± 0.100	1.166 ± 0.117	1.255 ± 0.102	1.205 ± 0.107
		Alfaxalone	1.126 ± 0.098	1.272 ± 0.238	1.202 ± 0.105	1.200 ± 0.110
	PL	Isoflurane	1.381 ± 0.100	1.377 ± 0.103	1.349 ± 0.071	1.365 ± 0.065
		Sevoflurane	1.416 ± 0.134	1.369 ± 0.108	1.381 ± 0.083	1.389 ± 0.095
		Propofol	1.361 ± 0.151	1.382 ± 0.172	1.404 ± 0.174	1.370 ± 0.159
		Alfaxalone	1.419 ± 0.135	1.429 ± 0.134	1.450 ± 0.130	1.433 ± 0.119
	OL	Isoflurane	1.167 ± 0.078	1.158 ± 0.047	1.170 ± 0.053	1.175 ± 0.066
		Sevoflurane	1.157 ± 0.093	1.158 ± 0.052	1.153 ± 0.069	1.156 ± 0.063
		Propofol	1.160 ± 0.054^{AB}	1.171 ± 0.060^{A}	1.113 ± 0.052^{B}	1.156 ± 0.054
		Alfaxalone	1.137 ± 0.076	1.144 ± 0.089	1.127 ± 0.064	1.136 ± 0.064

Mean ± SD for the three different doses and the arithmetic mean of the three doses for isoflurane, sevoflurane, propofol and alfaxalone in basal ganglia (BG), parietal lobe (PL) and occipital lobe (OL). Different alphabetical superscripts differ significantly ($p < 0.05$) between different doses of each anesthetic

results the previously reported rodent studies [21, 22] were able to reliably detect lactate levels with a field strength of 9.4 T. Jacob et al. [24] published 2-fold higher cerebral lactate values in children with sevoflurane compared to propofol detected at 3 T. However, these data included metabolite concentrations with associated CRLB values of "80% or fewer in 80% of the scans" and thus are not reliable. Uncertainties in metabolite concentrations in LcModel are expressed in CRLBs and in general only values of 20% or less are of acceptable reliability [31]. Lactate resonances in ^{1}H MRS are only detectable during neuronal stimulation [32] and in pathologic conditions such as neoplastic or inflammatory lesions [12, 14] also in canine brain [27]. Under these circumstances lactate can reliably be detected also at 3 T. In various species and with different measuring techniques it has been shown that halogenated volatile anesthetics increase cerebral levels of lactate [11, 21–23]. As we did not detect lactate under influence of isoflurane and sevoflurane administered at a dose of 2 MAC we can conclude that halogenated volatile anesthetics do not have an effect on cerebral levels of lactate in dogs. However, technical difficulties such as coupling effects of the lactate doublet [33] and overlapping resonances of lactate and lipids resonating at the same region of the spectrum at this field strength cannot be excluded.

Increased serum lactate with volatile anesthetics can be explained by increased lactate production or decreased hepatic lactate clearance. Volatile anesthetics dose dependently decrease blood pressure by venodilation and reduced myocardial contractility. This could potentially lead to reduced peripheral perfusion with an increase in lactate production and a reduction in hepatic blood flow, thereby, decreasing hepatic clearance. In contrast, desflurane and propofol were shown to even increase peripheral perfusion index in a clinical study in humans by means of a new generation pulse oximeter [34]. Measurement of cardiac output was not performed. In dogs, 1.85 MAC isoflurane tended to increase hepatic blood flow [35]. Various studies have shown effects of

Table 3 Mean ± SD of tCh concentrations (mmol L-1 of brain water) and tCh/tCr ratios

			Dose 1	Dose 2	Dose 3	Arithmetic mean
			Mean ± SD	Mean ± SD	Mean ± SD	Mean ± SD
tCh	BG	Isoflurane	1.887 ± 0.112^{A}	2.079 ± 0.110	1.932 ± 0.166^{A}	1.969 ± 0.089^{1}
		Sevoflurane	1.971 ± 0.109^{A}	2.107 ± 0.145^{B}	2.068 ± 0.128^{AB}	2.049 ± 0.103^{12}
		Propofol	2.034 ± 0.118	2.015 ± 0.109	2.010 ± 0.139	2.026 ± 0.090^{12}
		Alfaxalone	2.069 ± 0.103	2.082 ± 0.105	2.108 ± 0.123	2.086 ± 0.080^{2}
	PL	Isoflurane	1.805 ± 0.180^{A}	1.885 ± 0.129^{B}	1.841 ± 0.132^{AB}	1.843 ± 0.134
		Sevoflurane	1.721 ± 0.107^{A}	1.806 ± 0.100^{B}	1.747 ± 0.133^{AB}	1.758 ± 0.101
		Propofol	1.843 ± 0.117	1.773 ± 0.233	1.788 ± 0.204	1.768 ± 0.218
		Alfaxalone	1.854 ± 0.103	1.822 ± 0.107	1.814 ± 0.162	1.830 ± 0.112
	OL	Isoflurane	1.616 ± 0.288	1.805 ± 0.121	1.667 ± 0.202	1.653 ± 0.258^{1}
		Sevoflurane	1.707 ± 0.148^{A}	1.807 ± 0.094^{B}	1.768 ± 0.132^{AB}	1.761 ± 0.118^{12}
		Propofol	1.795 ± 0.122	1.831 ± 0.122	1.832 ± 0.116	1.823 ± 0.105^{2}
		Alfaxalone	1.812 ± 0.140	1.802 ± 0.102	1.789 ± 0.092	1.801 ± 0.097^{12}
tCh/tCr	BG	Isoflurane	0.324 ± 0.021	0.339 ± 0.017	0.331 ± 0.043	0.330 ± 0.027
		Sevoflurane	0.329 ± 0.033	0.332 ± 0.031	0.331 ± 0.020	0.330 ± 0.025
		Propofol	0.342 ± 0.017	0.335 ± 0.025	0.335 ± 0.024	0.337 ± 0.020
		Alfaxalone	0.328 ± 0.020	0.331 ± 0.018	0.328 ± 0.017	0.329 ± 0.016
	PL	Isoflurane	0.334 ± 0.039	0.338 ± 0.030	0.329 ± 0.029	0.332 ± 0.030
		Sevoflurane	0.318 ± 0.033	0.324 ± 0.021	0.313 ± 0.023	0.319 ± 0.022
		Propofol	0.329 ± 0.031	0.322 ± 0.047	0.325 ± 0.028	0.318 ± 0.043
		Alfaxalone	0.342 ± 0.032	0.337 ± 0.027	0.338 ± 0.040	0.339 ± 0.030
	OL	Isoflurane	0.242 ± 0.031^{A}	0.265 ± 0.010^{B}	0.257 ± 0.008^{AB}	0.251 ± 0.026
		Sevoflurane	0.253 ± 0.020	0.265 ± 0.015	0.260 ± 0.023	0.260 ± 0.018
		Propofol	0.265 ± 0.014	0.278 ± 0.028	0.268 ± 0.023	0.275 ± 0.027
		Alfaxalone	0.268 ± 0.018	0.268 ± 0.016	0.273 ± 0.019	0.270 ± 0.015

Mean ± SD for the three different doses and the arithmetic mean of the three doses for isoflurane, sevoflurane, propofol and alfaxalone in basal ganglia (BG), parietal lobe (PL) and occipital lobe (OL). Different alphabetical superscripts differ significantly ($p < 0.05$) between different doses of each anesthetic different numerical superscripts differ significantly between arithmetic mean tCh concentrations of each anesthetic

volatile anesthetics on mitochondria [36–39]. Interference of volatile anesthetics with mitochondrial oxidation of NADH to NAD and thus reduced oxidative phosphorylation resulting in a shift to lactate production was shown for rat liver and monkey kidney cells [40, 41]. Therefore, the observed increased serum lactate levels are more likely related to direct mitochondrial effects than malperfusion.

Differences in metabolite concentrations between different brain regions presented in this paper show a similar pattern as previously published for canine brain [15, 17] and were independent of the anesthetic used. In humans, comparison of brain metabolite concentrations measured with different scanners and techniques showed good agreement but absolute values differed [42]. Data from other institutions can only be used as reference but direct comparison of data acquired on scanners from other institutions is not recommended.

In basal ganglia tNAA was the only metabolite showing dose-dependent increase of 8% in dogs receiving alfaxalone, being significantly different ($p = 0.0036$) between the first and third dose. However, this increase might also be time associated as the dose in treatment P and A increased over time. In the parietal lobe a similar increase was detected but statistical significance was not reached. In the occipital lobe, no changes were noted. The detected increase in cerebral levels of tNAA is unexpected. In pathologic conditions associated with neuronal loss and dysfunction such as demyelinating and neurodegenerative disorders [43] tNAA is decreased. As we did not detect a decrease in tNAA there seems to be no neuronal degeneration or loss occurring during anesthesia. Increases in tNAA are rare and only described for canvan's disease in humans. Canvan's disease is an autosomal recessive leukodystrophy with absence of aspartoacylase resulting in lack of NAA-degradation [12] with increases in tNAA of about 50% or more [44, 45]. To the author's knowledge, this condition has not been reported in dogs and does not explain the detected changes during anesthesia.

15. Carrera I, Richter H, Meier D, Kircher PR, Dennler M. Regional metabolite concentrations in the brain of healthy dogs measured by use of short echo time, single voxel proton magnetic resonance spectroscopy at 3.0 tesla. Am J Vet Res. 2015;76(2):129–41.
16. Warrington CD, Feeney DA, Ober CP, Jessen CR, Steward SM, Armien AG, Fletcher TF. Relative metabolite concentrations and ratios determined by use of 3-T region-specific proton magnetic resonance spectroscopy of the brain of healthy beagles. Am J Vet Res. 2013;74(10):1291–303.
17. Ono K, Kitagawa M, Ito D, Tanaka N, Watari T. Regional variations and age-related changes detected with magnetic resonance spectroscopy in the brain of healthy dogs. Am J Vet Res. 2014;75(2):179–86.
18. Baker EH, Basso G, Barker PB, Smith MA, Bonekamp D, Horska A. Regional apparent metabolite concentrations in young adult brain measured by (1)H MR spectroscopy at 3 tesla. J Magn Reson Imaging. 2008;27(3):489–99.
19. Pradhan S, Bonekamp S, Gillen JS, Rowland LM, Wijtenburg SA, Edden RA, Barker PB. Comparison of single voxel brain MRS AT 3T and 7T using 32-channel head coils. Magn Reson Imaging. 2015;33(8):1013–8.
20. Tkac I, Oz G, Adriany G, Ugurbil K, Gruetter R. In vivo 1H NMR spectroscopy of the human brain at high magnetic fields: metabolite quantification at 4T vs. 7T. Magn Reson Med. 2009;62(4):868–79.
21. Boretius S, Tammer R, Michaelis T, Brockmoller J, Frahm J. Halogenated volatile anesthetics alter brain metabolism as revealed by proton magnetic resonance spectroscopy of mice in vivo. NeuroImage. 2013;69:244–55.
22. Makaryus R, Lee H, Yu M, Zhang S, Smith SD, Rebecchi M, Glass PS, Benveniste H. The metabolomic profile during isoflurane anesthesia differs from propofol anesthesia in the live rodent brain. J Cereb Blood Flow Metab. 2011;31(6):1432–42.
23. Valette J, Guillermier M, Besret L, Hantraye P, Bloch G, Lebon V. Isoflurane strongly affects the diffusion of intracellular metabolites, as shown by 1H nuclear magnetic resonance spectroscopy of the monkey brain. J Cereb Blood Flow Metab. 2007;27(3):588–96.
24. Jacob Z, Li H, Makaryus R, Zhang S, Reinsel R, Lee H, Feng T, Rothman DL, Benveniste H. Metabolomic profiling of children's brains undergoing general anesthesia with sevoflurane and propofol. Anesthesiology. 2012; 117(5):1062–71.
25. Lee SH, Kim SY, Woo DC, Choe BY, Ryu KN, Choi WS, Jahng GH, Yim SV, Kim HY, Choi CB. Differential neurochemical responses of the canine striatum with pentobarbital or ketamine anesthesia: a 3T proton MRS study. J Vet Med Sci. 2010;72(5):583–7.
26. Carrera I, Kircher PR, Meier D, Richter H, Beckman K, Dennler M. In vivo proton magnetic resonance spectroscopy for the evaluation of hepatic encephalopathy in dogs. Am J Vet Res. 2014;75(9):818–27.
27. Stadler KL, Ober CP, Feeney DA, Jessen CR. Multivoxel proton magnetic resonance spectroscopy of inflammatory and neoplastic lesions of the canine brain at 3.0 T. Am J Vet Res. 2014;75(11):982–9.
28. Kazama T, Ikeda K. Comparison of MAC and the rate of rise of alveolar concentration of sevoflurane with halothane and isoflurane in the dog. Anesthesiology. 1988;68(3):435–7.
29. Ferre PJ, Pasloske K, Whittem T, Ranasinghe MG, Li Q, Lefebvre HP. Plasma pharmacokinetics of alfaxalone in dogs after an intravenous bolus of Alfaxan-CD RTU. Vet Anaesth Analg. 2006;33(4):229–36.
30. Gladden LB. Lactate metabolism: a new paradigm for the third millennium. J Physiol. 2004;558(Pt 1):5–30.
31. Provencher S. LCModel & LCMgui User's Manual; LCModel Version 6.3–1. In: http://www.s-provencher.com/pub/LCModel/manual/manual.pdf Stephen Provencher Incorporated; April 28, 2013.
32. Prichard J, Rothman D, Novotny E, Petroff O, Kuwabara T, Avison M, Howseman A, Hanstock C, Shulman R. Lactate rise detected by 1H NMR in human visual cortex during physiologic stimulation. Proc Natl Acad Sci U S A. 1991;88(13):5829–31.
33. Sotak CH, Alger JR. A pitfall associated with lactate detection using stimulated-echo proton spectroscopy. Magn Reson Med. 1991;17(2):533–8.
34. Kowalczyk M, Fijalkowska A, Nestorowicz A. New generation pulse oximetry in the assessment of peripheral perfusion during general anaesthesia - a comparison between propofol and desflurane. Anaesthesiol Intensive Ther. 2013;45(3):138–44.
35. Hartman JC, Pagel PS, Proctor LT, Kampine JP, Schmeling WT, Warltier DC. Influence of desflurane, isoflurane and halothane on regional tissue perfusion in dogs. Can J Anaesth. 1992;39(8):877–87.
36. Hall GM, Kirtland SJ, Baum H. The inhibition of mitochondrial respiration by inhalational anaesthetic agents. Br J Anaesth. 1973;45(10):1005–9.
37. Brunner EA, Cheng SC, Berman ML. Effects of anesthesia on intermediary metabolism. Annu Rev Med. 1975;26:391–401.
38. Lee SL, Alto LE, Dhalla NS. Subcellular effects of some anesthetic agents on rat myocardium. Can J Physio Pharmacol. 1979;57(1):65–70.
39. Hanley PJ, Ray J, Brandt U, Daut J. Halothane, isoflurane and sevoflurane inhibit NADH:ubiquinone oxidoreductase (complex I) of cardiac mitochondria. J Physiol. 2002;544(Pt 3):687–93.
40. Brabec MJ, Bedows E, Davidson BA, Knight PR. Effect of general anesthetics and pressure on aerobic metabolism of monkey kidney cells. Anesthesiology. 1984;61(1):43–7.
41. Nahrwold ML, Lecky JH, Cohen PJ. The effect of halothane on mitochondrial permeability to NADH. Life Sci. 1974;15(7):1261–5.
42. Haga KK, Khor YP, Farrall A, Wardlaw JM. A systematic review of brain metabolite changes, measured with 1H magnetic resonance spectroscopy, in healthy aging. Neurobiol Aging. 2009;30(3):353–63.
43. van der Knaap MS, Jvd G, Luyten PR, JAD H, JJP N, Valk J. 1H and 31P magnetic resonance spectroscopy of the brain in degenerative cerebral disorders. Ann Neurol. 1992;31(2):202–11.
44. Wittsack HJ, Kugel H, Roth B, Heindel W. Quantitative measurements with localized 1H MR spectroscopy in children with Canavan's disease. J Magn Reson Imaging. 1996;6(6):889–93.
45. Marks HG, Caro PA, Wang ZY, Detre JA, Bogdan AR, Gusnard DA, Zimmerman RA. Use of computed tomography, magnetic resonance imaging, and localized 1H magnetic resonance spectroscopy in Canavan's disease: a case report. Ann Neurol. 1991;30(1):106–10.
46. Elliott KA, Swank RL, Henderson N. Effects of anesthetics and convulsants on acetylcholine content of brain. Am J Phys. 1950;162(2):469–74.
47. Modak AT, Weintraub ST, McCoy TH, Stavinoha WB. Use of 300-msec microwave irradiation for enzyme inactivation: a study of effects of sodium pentobarbital on acetylcholine concentration in mouse brain regions. J Pharmacol Exp Ther. 1976;197(2):245–52.
48. Ringer SK, Ohlerth S, Carrera I, Mauch J, Spielmann N, Bettschart-Wolfensberger R, Weiss M. Effects of hypotension and/or hypocapnia during sevoflurane anesthesia on perfusion and metabolites in the developing brain of piglets-a blinded randomized study. Paediatr Anaesth. 2016;26(9):909–18.
49. Brand A, Leibfritz D, Richter-Landsberg C. Oxidative stress-induced metabolic alterations in rat brain astrocytes studied by multinuclear NMR spectroscopy. J Neurosci Res. 1999;58(4):576–85.
50. Ni C, Li C, Dong Y, Guo X, Zhang Y, Xie Z. Anesthetic Isoflurane Induces DNA Damage Through Oxidative Stress and p53 Pathway. Mol Neurobiol. 2016:54(5):3591–605.
51. Acquaviva R, Campisi A, Murabito P, Raciti G, Avola R, Mangiameli S, Musumeci I, Barcellona ML, Vanella A, Li Volti G. Propofol attenuates peroxynitrite-mediated DNA damage and apoptosis in cultured astrocytes: an alternative protective mechanism. Anesthesiology. 2004;101(6):1363–71.
52. Do SH, Kamatchi GL, Washington JM, Zuo Z. Effects of volatile anesthetics on glutamate transporter, excitatory amino acid transporter type 3: the role of protein kinase C. Anesthesiology. 2002;96(6):1492–7.
53. Zuo Z. Isoflurane enhances glutamate uptake via glutamate transporters in rat glial cells. Neuroreport. 2001;12(5):1077–80.
54. Mcintosh JC, Cooper JR. Studies on the function of N-acetyl aspartic acid in brain. J Neurochem. 1965;12(9):825–35.
55. Strange K, Emma F, Paredes A, Morrison R. Osmoregulatory changes in myo-inositol content and Na+/myo-inositol cotransport in rat cortical astrocytes. Glia. 1994;12(1):34–43.
56. Haskins SC. Monitoring anesthetized patients. In: Tranquilli WJ, Thurmon JC, Grimm KA, editors. Lumb and Jones' veterinary Anaesthesia. 4th ed. Oxford UK: Blackwell Publishing Ltd; 2007. p. 533–58.
57. Kam PC, Cardone D. Propofol infusion syndrome. Anaesthesia. 2007;62(7): 690–701.
58. Camu F. Carbohydrate intolerance during halothane anesthesia in dogs. Acta Anaesthesiol Belg. 1973;24(3):177–88.
59. Camu F. Impaired early insulin response to glycemic stimulus during enflurane anesthesia in dogs. Acta Anaesthesiol Belg. 1976;27(suppl):267–71.
60. Diltoer M, Camu F. Glucose homeostasis and insulin secretion during isoflurane anesthesia in humans. Anesthesiology. 1988;68(6):880–6.
61. Saho S, Kadota Y, Sameshima T, Miyao J, Tsurumaru T, Yoshimura N. The effects of sevoflurane anesthesia on insulin secretion and glucose metabolism in pigs. Anesth Analg. 1997;84(6):1359–65.

62. Tanaka T, Nabatame H, Tanifuji Y. Insulin secretion and glucose utilization are impaired under general anesthesia with sevoflurane as well as isoflurane in a concentration-independent manner. J Anesth. 2005;19(4):277–81.
63. Kim JM, Shin JS, Yoon IH, Min BH, Jeong WY, Lee GE, Kim MS, Kim JE, Jang JY, Park CG. The effect of propofol on intravenous glucose tolerance test in rhesus monkey. J Med Primatol. 2014;43(4):242–6.
64. Muñoz KA, Robertson SA, Wilson DV. The effects of ketamine or midazolam on the intubation dose of alfaxalone, hemodynamic function, glucose and insulin concentrations in healthy dogs. [abstract]. Prague: AVA Autumn Meeting; 2016.
65. Eger EI 2nd, Saidman LJ, Brandstater B. Minimum alveolar anesthetic concentration: a standard of anesthetic potency. Anesthesiology. 1965;26(6):756–63.
66. Smith C, McEwan AI, Jhaveri R, Wilkinson M, Goodman D, Smith LR, Canada AT, Glass PS. The interaction of fentanyl on the Cp50 of propofol for loss of consciousness and skin incision. Anesthesiology. 1994;81(4):820–8. discussion 826A
67. Antognini JF, Schwartz K. Exaggerated anesthetic requirements in the preferentially anesthetized brain. Anesthesiology. 1993;79(6):1244–9.
68. Rampil IJ, Mason P, Singh H. Anesthetic potency (MAC) is independent of forebrain structures in the rat. Anesthesiology. 1993;78(4):707–12.

10

Safety pharmacology and subchronic toxicity of jinqing granules in rats

Xuerong Zhou†, Qian Rong†, Min Xu, Yuanli Zhang, Qi Dong, Yuanling Xiao, Qiji Liu, Helin Chen, Xiaoyu Yang, Kaisheng Yu, Yinglun Li*, Ling Zhao, Gang Ye, Fei Shi and Cheng Lv

Abstract

Background: Jinqing granules which are made of a mixture extract that contains Radix *Tinosporae* and *Canarii fructus* in proportions according to a longstanding formula have a good effect on the prevention and treatment of gastric ulcer disease. It has not been through safety through systematic toxicological studies, however. To provide basis for clinical application, we performed safety pharmacology and subchronic toxicity experiments in specific pathogen-free Sprague-Dawley rats.

Results: In safety pharmacology experiments, Jinqing granules had no evident adverse effects on the central nervous, cardiovascular, or respiratory systems. In subchronic toxicity study, 2–8 g/kg of Jinqing granules induced no evident adverse effects on Clinical signs, body weight changes, food and water intake, death daily, indicators of urine, hematological assay, serum biochemistry, organ coefficient and histopathological examination. However, the 16 g/kg dose was associated with slightly slowed weight growth, decreased number of sperm in seminiferous tubules and increased values of serum aspartate aminotransferase and bilirubin. During the 30-day feeding test, 3 rats that received the 16 g/kg dose died, but the deaths were most likely due to trauma of oral gavage, not to drug toxicity.

Conclusion: Jinqing granules given to Sprague-Dawley rats orally for 30 days at a dose of 8 g/kg or less appears safe, but higher doses were not proven safe. The significance of these observations with respect to animal usage of Jinqing granules deserves thorough investigation.

Keywords: Jinqing granules, Rats, Toxicity, Safety pharmacology, Subchronic toxicity

Background

China has a several-thousand year history of using traditional medicines in clinical practice. The invention and application of traditional Chinese medications, based on specific theoretical systems and patterns of use, reflect the characteristics of Chinese culture, with its long history and rich natural resources [1]. So far, there are about 12,000 kinds of Chinese traditional medicine used in clinical, mostly herbs implied [2]. The origins and development of Chinese medicine are life's practical experiences and medical practices of laboring people [3]. The World Health Organization [4] has reported that about 80% of the world's populations, especially people who live in developing countries, use natural medicines to treat disease. In recent years, with rapid global economic integration, China's pharmaceutical industry has moved strongly into the international medicine market [5]. However, the safety and effectiveness of many common Chinese traditional herbs have not been established [6, 7]. Therefore, in order to ensure the safety of prescribed traditional Chinese medicine, it is necessary that they undergo subchronic toxicity and pharmacological safety testing.

Radix Tinosporae is the root of *Tinospora sagittata (Oliv.)* Gagnep, or *Tcapillipes* Gagnep [8]. *Radix Tinosporae* is used for treating sore throat, carbuncle, furuncle, diarrhea, abdominal pain and other conditions [9–12]. *Canarii fructus,* the dry ripe fruit of *Canarium album* Raeusch, is used in the treatment of sore throat, cough and sputum viscosity [13].

Jinqing granules are made of a traditional Chinese medicine mixture extract that contains *Radix Tinosporae* and *Canarii fructus* in proportions according to a longstanding formula [14]. Jinqing granules were used in our application for a drug patent in 2014. In early trials,

* Correspondence: liyinglun01@163.com
†Equal contributors
College of Veterinary Medicine, Sichuan Agricultural University, Chengdu, Sichuan 611130, People's Republic of China

Radix Tinosporae was effective in the prevention and early treatment of *helicobacter pylori* [15]. The main active constituents of the granules are gallic acid and tetrahydropalmatine. According to literature reports on traditional Chinese medicines, *Canarium ablbum* Raeusch and *Tinospora capillipes* Ganep have favorable effects on gastric abscesses, diarrhea, and abdominal pain [8]. Even though Jinqing granules are used to treat a variety of diseases, their safety in long-term use is still questionable. About 10% of the world's population has gastric ulcers, and about 1% of the ulcers progress to gastric cancer [16]. Therefore, Jinqing granules may have a very large market.

In early acute toxicity experiments, we found that the lethal dose 50 (LD_{50}) of Jinqing granules is 5 g/kg in rats. On the basis of the LD_{50}, in this work, we have studied subchronic toxicity of Jinqing granules given orally to Sprague-Dawley (SD) rats in accordance with relevant Chinese standards.

Methods

Jinqing granules

Radix Tinosporae and *Canarii fructus* were both collected from Chengdu (Sichuan, China). The plants were identified and authenticated by Professor Qiao-jia Fan of the College of Veterinary Medicine, Sichuan Agricultural University, Chengdu, China. The mixture extract that contains *Radix Tinosporae* and *Canarii fructus* in proportions according to a longstanding formula add some excipients to make Jinqing granules. The granules were completely dissolved in sterilized distilled water and made into dosages of 16 g/mL, 8 g/mL, 4 g/mL, and 2 g/mL, according to the requirements of China's new-drug safety evaluation.

Animals

Healthy male and female SD rats, 4 and 8 weeks old, were purchased from the specific pathogen-free facility at Chengdu Dossy Experimental Animals Co., Ltd. [License no. SCXK (Sichuan) 2008–24]. All experimental procedures involving animals were approved by Sichuan Agricultural University Animal Care and Use Committee (registration No. SCAU2016061801). Based on the principles of the International Committee on Laboratory Animals, the rats were separated equally according to gender and maintained at 20–25 °C and relative humidity of 55 ± 5%. Artificial lighting was adjusted to 12 h of light (from 08:00 to 20:00) and 12 h of darkness from 20:00 to 08:00. Conventional laboratory feed was provided by the Chengdu Dashuo Biology Science and Technology Co., Ltd. The rats were allowed to drink water freely, and they acclimated for 7 days before experiments were begun.

Safety pharmacology experiments

Safety pharmacology experiments were performed according to guidelines of the Veterinary Drugs Control [17–20].

Fifty SD rats were randomly distributed into 5 groups (5 female and 5 male in each group). The five groups were: Group I, normal control group (sterile distilled water); Group II, 2 g/kg Jinqing granules; Group III, 4 g/kg Jinqing granules; Group IV, 8 g/kg Jinqing granules; and Group V, 16 g/kg Jinging granules. Animals were treated daily at 9 a.m. with gastric infusion in a volume of 10 ml/kg given for 7 days.

We observed the animals for behavior, posture, salivation, pupil change, muscle tremors, hair, and feces were observed from 10 a.m. to 16 p.m. continually for 14 days [17–20]. In order to prevent living animals from eating animals that had died due to accumulation of drug in the body, endangered or dead rats were autopsied promptly [21].

Before and 24 h after the last administration of control water or Jinqing granules, the rats were placed in the versatile recorder of rats' locomotor activity and allowed to adapt to the environment for 30 min. Their activity (number of movements in 1 min) was recorded by watching the rats' movements in order to determine if this aspect of the central nervous system was normal.

The climbing pole test was performed in order to evaluate the mobility of the rats after receiving the medication for various times. Twenty-four hours after the last administration, a smooth metal bar was erected vertically and fixed at the bottom. The rats were placed at the top of the metal bar and allowed to descend head first. Their ability to coordinate this activity was graded as: Level 0, normal step-by-step climbing down; Level 1, coasting down; Level 2, inability to hang from the lever; Level 3, discoordination over a period of time.

On the day before medication was given, the day after it was given, and the eighth day after being given, 3% pentobarbital sodium was injected intraperitoneally to anesthetize the rats [17–20]. The animals' heart rate, electrocardiogram, and the depth of breathing and respiratory rate were recorded with the BL-420F multi-channel physiological signal acquisition processing system.

Subchronic toxicity experiment

The toxicity experiments were conducted according to the Economic Cooperation and Development Guideline 407 [22].

One hundred-twenty rats were randomly distributed into 6 groups (10 female and 10 male rats in each group). The 6 groups were: Group I, normal group; Group II, saline control group; Group III, 2 g/kg; Group IV, 4 g/kg; Group V, 8 g/kg; Group VI, 16 g/kg in a volume of 10 ml/kg Jinging granules. Animals were treated daily at 9 a.m. with gastric infusion in a volume of 10 ml/kg given for 30 days. The determination of repeated dose 30-day oral toxicity was carried out according to the Organization for Economic Cooperation and Development Guideline 407 [22]. In order to avoid accumulation of drug that existed in the dead rats in the living body by eating, and analyzed the causes of death in rats, the dead rats were needed to anatomical analysis immediately. [21].

Daily from 10 a.m. to 16 p.m., we observed the rats' behavior, attitude, presence of saliva, pupillary change, muscle tremors, hair texture, food intake, water intake, feces, poisoning, and death, continually for 30 days. Weight was recorded every three days.

At the end of medication period, urine samples were collected from all animals. The samples were sent to Chengdu Lilai Biology Science and Technology Co., Ltd., for determination of pH, ascorbic acid, specific gravity, glucose, leukocyte counts, nitrite, protein, ketones, urobilinogen, and bilirubin.

About 2.0 mL of blood was collected in an anticoagulation tube containing sodium citrate to measured hematologic indices, and another 2.0 mL blood was collected in non-heparinized tubes to measured serum biochemistry.

Rats were sacrificed after blood was collected and were opened surgically for evaluation of possible pathological changes. The weights of liver, heart, spleen, lung, kidney, brain, ovaries, and testes were recorded. The relative weight of organs was calculated according to the formula: organ coefficient = organ weight / body weight ×100%) [23, 24].

Organs were soaked in 10% solution of buffered formalin (pH 7.4) for three days, followed by dehydration, embedding, sectioning, dewaxing, and staining with hematoxylin-eosin. Pathologic alterations were assessed with a Nikon 80i optical microscope. Photomicrographs were taken for reference.

Statistical analysis

Results were analyzed with SPSS 19.0 statistical software. The mean and standard deviation were expressed. One-way analysis of variance (ANOVA) and Newman-Keuls post hoc test were performed for statistical analyses. Statistically significant difference was defined as $p < 0.05$.

Table 1 Jinqing granules effect on autonomic activities in rats (n = 10)

Jinqing dose	Gender	Before dosing (times)	After dosing (times)
Control group	Male	160.00 ± 23.97	183.00 ± 11.18
	Female	175.00 ± 20.49	161.43 ± 17.82
2 g/kg	Male	153.00 ± 12.75	138.00 ± 52.99
	Female	168.00 ± 12.55	182.00 ± 27.29
4 g/kg	Male	145.00 ± 55.69	125.00 ± 63.54
	Female	161.00 ± 9.62	135.00 ± 33.73
8 g/kg	Male	179.00 ± 28.95	167.00 ± 54.04
	Female	156.00 ± 11.40	136.00 ± 23.82
16 g/kg	Male	170.00 ± 14.72	155.00 ± 39.37
	Female	178.75 ± 59.35	176.25 ± 14.36

Values represent means ± SD (N = 10). P values for all comparisons of before dosing and after dosing were ≥0.05.

Results

Safety pharmacology experiments

During the safety pharmacology experiments, no deaths occurred, and among all animals in all groups, no abnormalities in fur, posture, pupils, feces, salivation, or muscle tremors were noted. Each dose-group of rats was no evident abnormalities of behavior controlled by the central nervous system, e.g., posture, change in pupil size, salivation, gait, and muscle tremors.

The index for active movement in each dose group of animals receiving Jinqing granules revealed no differences from the index of the control group ($P > 0.05$). Thus, Jinqing granules had no evident effect on the rats' spontaneous activity. The results are shown in Table 1.

In the climbing pole test, the treatment groups and the control-group rats both climbed down step-by-step,

Table 2 The effects of Jinqing granules on the heart rate of rats (n = 10)

Jinqing dose	Gender	Before dosing	The second day after dosing	One week after dosing
Control group	Male	333.60 ± 25.96	372.40 ± 27.17	397.00 ± 36.92
	Female	387.60 ± 10.21	358.80 ± 70.38	406.40 ± 12.90
2 g/kg	Male	328.20 ± 23.30	369.40 ± 48.82	396.20 ± 10.64
	Female	392.20 ± 9.39	420.40 ± 25.31	342.60 ± 24.33
4 g/kg	Male	330.20 ± 28.96	336.40 ± 38.40	369.20 ± 57.80
	Female	389.20 ± 11.61	324.00 ± 16.55	382.20 ± 49.47
8 g/kg	Male	333.60 ± 25.96	308.60 ± 35.81	388.60 ± 35.41
	Female	387.60 ± 10.21	341.60 ± 48.69	362.00 ± 41.41
16 g/kg	Male	334.50 ± 21.89	371.25 ± 27.37	388.50 ± 13.96
	Female	372.25 ± 10.84	403.25 ± 74.22	367.25 ± 34.88

Values represent means ± SD (N = 10). P values for all comparisons of before dosing and after dosing were ≥0.05

Table 3 The effects of Jinqing granules on the respiratory rate of rats (n = 10)

Jinqing dose	Gender	Before dosing	The second day after dosing	One week after dosing
Control group	Male	96.00 ± 11.22	81.20 ± 11.63	91.80 ± 14.17
	Female	88.80 ± 12.30	94.20 ± 23.88	105.80 ± 29.45
2 g/kg	Male	96.00 ± 14.70	86.40 ± 13.89	93.80 ± 6.94
	Female	92.40 ± 15.06	80.00 ± 17.39	113.80 ± 5.76
4 g/kg	Male	96.80 ± 12.30	77.00 ± 9.43	84.80 ± 7.60
	Female	94.25 ± 13.01	74.40 ± 10.55	97.60 ± 17.42
8 g/kg	Male	91.20 ± 9.86	70.80 ± 9.18	94.20 ± 15.06
	Female	88.80 ± 12.30	68.20 ± 22.65	98.60 ± 15.55
16 g/kg	Male	96.00 ± 11.22	71.59 ± 13.30	80.00 ± 7.48
	Female	95.34 ± 14.70	87.75 ± 4.5	112.25 ± 22.40

Values represent means ± SD (N = 10). P values for all comparisons of before dosing and after dosing were ≥0.05

i.e., at level 0, which is evidence that Jinqing granules had no discernable effect on the animals' coordination.

The measurements of heart rate and respiratory rate on the day before administration of the medication, the day after administration, and the eighth day after administration revealed no significant differences between control-group rats and those who received Jinqing granules at any dose ($P > 0.05$). At the same time, at three different time points within the same group, there were no significant differences in heart rate and respiratory rate ($P > 0.05$). Thus, we conclude that Jinqing granules had no discernable significant effects on the cardiovascular and respiratory systems of the SD rats. The results are listed in Tables 2 and 3. Figure 1 illustrates time-breath curves of Jinqing granules' effect on the rats and Fig. 2 is time-heart curves.

Subchronic toxicity experiments

During the 30-day feeding test, 2 male and 1 female rats in Group VI died. Autopsy of these animals disclosed findings suggestive of improper oral lavage administration; no signs of Jinqing toxicity were found. Also, among the various groups of animals, no abnormalities were seen in fur, action, posture, pupillary change, diet, salivation, muscle tremors, and feces.

The rats' food and water consumption are shown in Table 4. Water consumption was not significantly different between groups that received Jinqing granules and those in the control group ($P > 0.05$). Food intake also was similar in the groups that received Jinqing granules and the control group, except that animals, both male and female, that had received 16 g/kg (Group VI) consumed slightly less food ($P < 0.05$).

Figure 3 illustrates the weight gain curves of the various groups of male rats, and Fig. 4 is female rats. No difference was recorded between the control group (Group I) and the saline group (Group II) ($P > 0.05$). The body weight gain of Groups III -V (2 g/kg to 8 g/kg Jinqing granules) also were not significantly different from the body weight gain of control animals ($P > 0.05$). However,

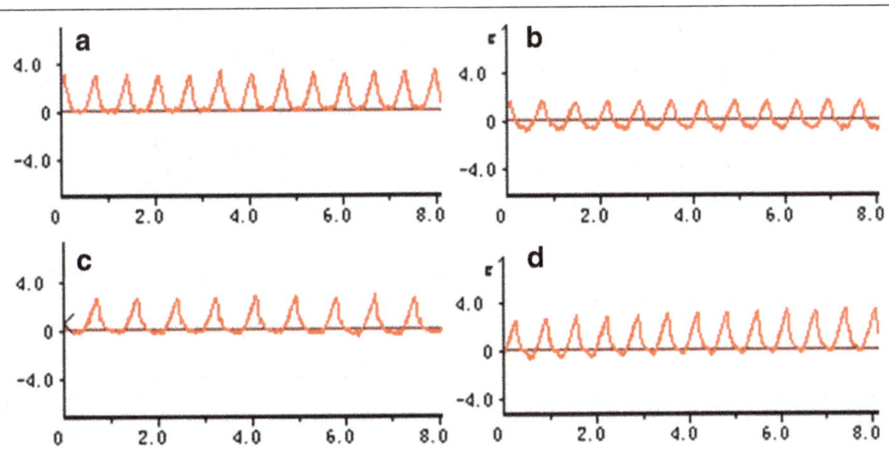

Fig. 1 The effect of Jinqing granules on breath rate of rats. **a** Control group; **b** The Group V before administration; **c** The Group V at the end of the second administration; **d** The Group V at a week after the last administration

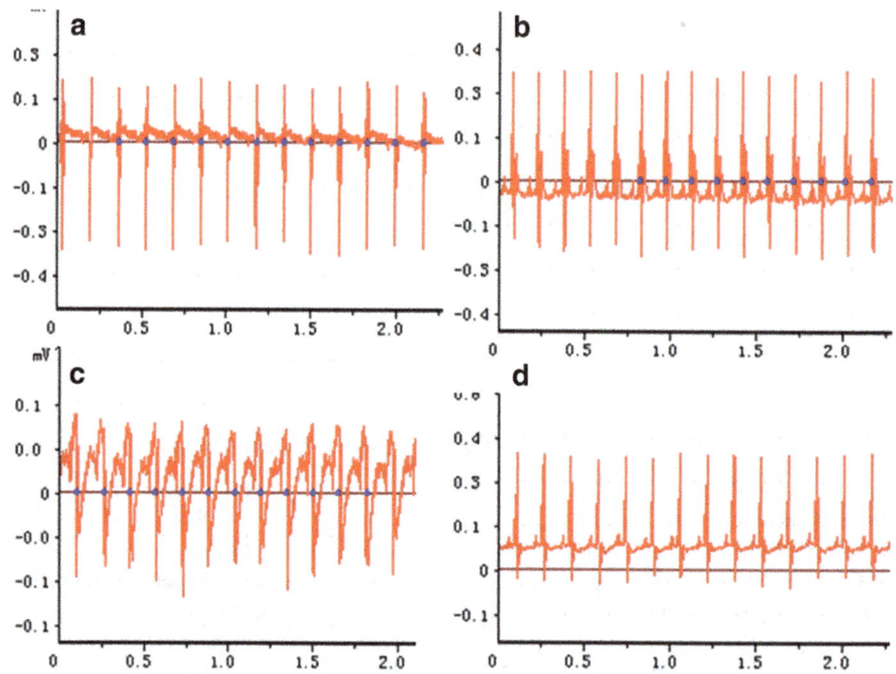

Fig. 2 The effect of Jinqing granules on heart rate of rats. **a** Control group; **b** The Group V before administration; **c** The Group V at the end of the second administration; **d** The Group V at a week after the last administration

the weight gain of Group VI (16 g/kg) male rats compared with weight gain of control rats was slightly less. Group VI female rats had a similar decline in weight gain, from the 19th to the 31st day.

Indicators of urine samples that, the ascorbic acid in the negative rate is up to 90%. Therefore, other indicators of false negative rate can be ignored. The values for pH, specific gravity, glucose, white blood cells, and nitrite were normal in all animals at all doses of Jinqing granules. The values for bilirubin was slightly increased in the 16 g/kg dose compared to control values ($p < 0.05$). The values of occult blood, protein, ketone, and urobilinogen were slightly increased but did not reach statistical significance ($P > 0.05$). Dataes is in Table 5.

Table 4 Mean food and water consumption of Sprague-Dawley rats orally administered Jinqing granules for 30 days ($n = 20$)

Jinqing dose	Gender	Diet (g/rat/day)	Water (ml/rat/day)
Control group	Male	20.5	31.7
	Female	20.1	31.4
Saline group	Male	21.0	31.6
	Female	20.7	31.8
2 g/kg	Male	20.3	31.3
	Female	20.2	31.0
4 g/kg	Male	20.1	30.9
	Female	19.8	31.5
8 g/kg	Male	19.5	31.2
	Female	19.4	30.6
16 g/kg	Male	17.6*	30.7
	Female	17.3*	30.3

*$P < 0.05$ significant difference from control

Table 6 presents the hematologic indices in the various groups of rats. The indices were not significantly different from control values at any dose of Jinqing granules, except for a slightly higher lymphocyte count at the 16 g/kg dose. Although some values in Groups III - VI were higher than in the control group, the differences were not statistically significant.

Serum biochemistry values of treated animals and controls are presented in Table 7. The only statistically significant differences in values between animals that received Jinqing granules and control animals was an increase in aspartate aminotransferase and total bilirubin at the 16 g/kg dose ($P < 0.05$).

Organ coefficients are presented in Table 8. Slightly higher values in the liver and ovaries of animals treated with 16 g/kg of Jinqing granules than in control animals were recorded ($p < 0.05$). Otherwise, no differences among the groups were found.

After the 30-day trial, the heart, liver, spleen, lung, kidney, stomach, intestines, brain, testis and ovary were taken from 3 rats of each group for histopathologic examination (Fig. 5). Tissue damage was seen only in animals that had received the 16 g/kg dose of Jinqing granules. In the heart, each group had a complete tegument and ventricular and ventricular muscle contour (Fig 5a),

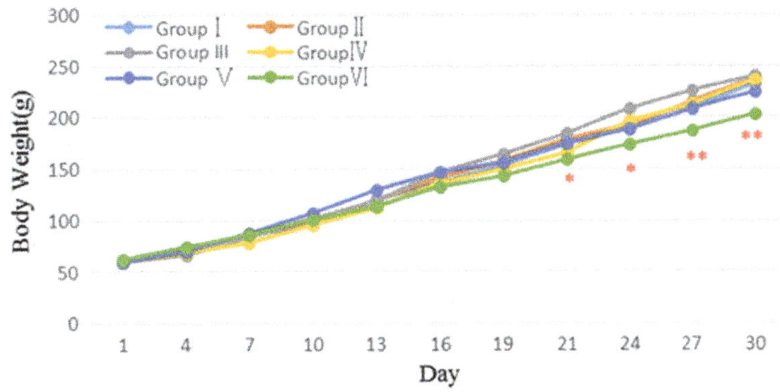

Fig. 3 Body weight changes of male rats during the sub-chronic toxicity study. Data are presented as the mean ± SD (5 rats/sex/group); *$p < 0.05$, **$p < 0.01$ Group VI vs. the Group I

with no evident pathological damage. In the liver, compared with the control group (Fig 5b), Group VI animals had expansion of liver sinusoids (Fig 5c), and various degrees of vacuolar degeneration in hepatocytes (Fig 5d). In the spleen, in control animals (Group I), the capsule was intact, the boundary between white pulp and red pulp was distinct, and the lymphocyte number was normal (Fig 5e). In contrast, in Group VI rats, the lymphocyte were decreased, and the number of macrophages was increased (Fig 5f). In the lung, the capsules of all groups were complete, and all levels of bronchi (primary bronchus, secondary bronchi, and tertiary bronchi) were neatly arranged in all animals (Fig 5g). In the kidney, pathological changes were not evident in any group. The renal capsule was intact; the boundary between cortex and medulla was clear; and the renal tubules and collecting ducts were arranged neatly, with normal density (Fig 5h). In the stomach, in Group I to Group VI, structural integrity of the simple columnar epithelium, muscularis mucosa and muscularis propria were maintained (Fig 5i). In the intestines, the mucosa, submucosa, muscular layer, and outer membrane layer structure were intact, and boundaries between these structures were distinct in all animal groups (Fig 5j). In brain, the nerve fiber layer, cerebral cortex, and hippocampus pyramidal cells were arranged neatly and tightly, without inflammatory infiltration or hemorrhagic foci (Fig 5k). In the ovary, from Group I to Group VI, the morphology and quantity of ovarian primordial follicles, proliferating follicles and mature follicles were normal compared with those features in the control animals (Fig 5l). In the testes, seminiferous tubules had a complete structure, and the spermatogenic cells resting in testicular tubules were arranged neatly and tightly (Fig 5m); however, compared with the control group, the number of sperm in seminiferous tubules appeared decreased in Group VI animals (Fig 5n).

Discussion

In this work, we conducted subchronic toxicity tests [20] and safety pharmacology experiments [17–20] in rats treated with Jinqing granules in order to assess the potential toxicity of this traditional Chinese medicine. Conventional laboratory food was chosen in order to

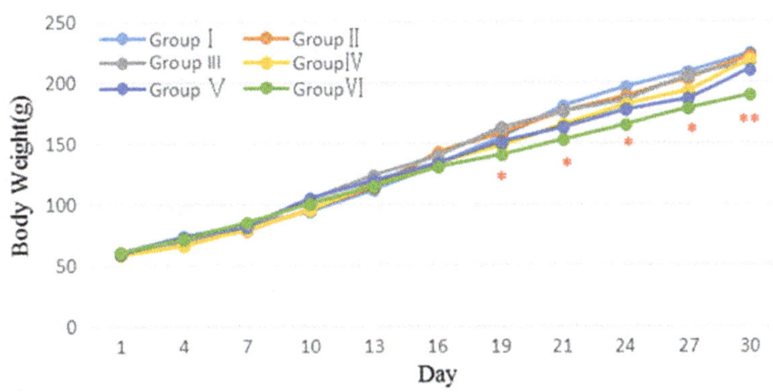

Fig. 4 Body weight changes of female rats during the sub-chronic toxicity study. Data are presented as the mean ± SD (5 rats/sex/group); *$p < 0.05$, **$p < 0.01$ Group VI vs. the Group I

Table 5 Effect of Jinqing granules on indicators of urine in rats ($n = 20$)

Parameters	GLU%				WBC%				NIT%			
	(–)	(+)	(++)	(+++)	(–)	(+)	(++)	(+++)	(–)	(+)	(++)	(+++)
Control group	100				100				100			
Saline group	100				100				100			
2 g/kg	100				100				100			
4 g/kg	100				100				100			
8 g/kg	100				100				100			
16 g/kg	100				100				100			
Control group	100				100				95	5		
Saline group	95		5		95		5		100			
2 g/kg	95	5			100				100			
4 g/kg	100				100				100			
8 g/kg	100				100				100			
16 g/kg	85	5	5	5	90	5	5		85	10		5
Control group	95	5			95		5		95	5		
Saline group	90	10			100				100			
2 g/kg	95			5	100				100			
4 g/kg	90	5		5	95	5			95	5		
8 g/kg	90		10		100				95	5		
16 g/kg	80*	10	5	5	85	10	5		100			

*$P < 0.05$ significant difference from control

GLU glucose, *WBC* white blood cells, *NIT* nitrite, *PRO* protein, *BLD* occult blood, *KET* ketone, *BIL* bilirubin, *URO* urobilinogen, V_C ascorbic acid

have a uniform diet without variation throughout the testing period.

Safety pharmacology is a pharmacological method used to study drugs given at the recommended treatment doses, or higher doses, which may exert harmful pharmacological effects or adverse drug reactions [25–27]. Safety pharmacology research can provide information for clinical research and safe drug use, and can be used for long-term toxicity testing as a reference for the design and development of new indications [28–30]. The present research, conducted according to safety pharmacology research technical guidelines for natural medicines, tested the effects of Jinqing granules on critical body functions, such as respiratory rate, heart rate, and central nervous system activities.

Because the central nervous system plays a vital role in the development of and the regulation of physiological behaviors, the rats' daily routine activities and the climbing pole test were used to detect effects of Jinqing granules on the central nervous system [31]. Treatment at all doses did not affect the animals' performance in these rudimentary tests. Although the possibility of subtle central nervous system effects was not excluded, the tests gave no evidence of gross damage.

Measurement of rats' heart rate also did not reveal an abnormal effect in the Jinqing-treated animals, which is

Table 6 Effect of subchronic administration of Jinqing granules on hematologic indices in rats ($n = 20$)

Parameters	WBC ($\times 10^9$/L)	RBC ($\times 10^{12}$/L)	PLT ($\times 10^9$/L)	HGB (g/L)	LYM% ($\times 10^9$/L)	GRAN ($\times 10^9$/L)	HCT %
Control group	7.82 ± 1.12	8.52 ± 0.82	1024.67 ± 141.96	159.80 ± 8.56	78.28 ± 3.70	1.71 ± 0.40	35.83 ± 3.18
Saline group	8.58 ± 0.75	9.14 ± 0.88	1313.29 ± 105.33	166.86 ± 8.73	80.75 ± 4.43	1.93 ± 0.41	36.01 ± 2.22
2 g/kg	7.59 ± 1.54	8.17 ± 0.72	1140.13 ± 266.16	157.87 ± 14.27	79.11 ± 3.41	1.89 ± 0.28	38.61 ± 4.47
4 g/kg	7.91 ± 1.17	8.56 ± 2.04	1105.07 ± 115.30	152.53 ± 8.63	81.75 ± 0.96	1.52 ± 0.27	37.59 ± 3.75
8 g/kg	7.93 ± 1.94	8.73 ± 1.02	1076.13 ± 98.33	155.67 ± 7.89	76.99 ± 1.78	1.57 ± 0.46	36.15 ± 4.50
16 g/kg	7.32 ± 2.07	9.19 ± 0.49	1297.10 ± 86.70	167.4 ± 12.15	82.07 ± 2.97*	1.82 ± 0.42	38.96 ± 1.48

Values represent mean ± SD

WBC white blood cell, *RBC* red blood cell, *PLT* blood platelet, *HGB* hemoglobin, *LYM* lymphocytes, *Gran* neutrophils, *HCT* red blood cell specific volume

*$P < 0.05$, significantly different from control values

Table 7 Effect of subchronic administration of Jinqing granules on serum biochemistry measurements in rats (n = 20)

Parameters	ALT(U/L)	AST(U/L)	TP(g/L)	TG(g/L)	GLU(mmol/L)	UREA(mmol/L)	CREA (mmol/L)	T-Bil(g/L)	ALB(g/L)
Control group	32.17 ± 5.59	105.58 ± 31.84	57.59 ± 4.12	0.34 ± 0.17	5.33 ± 1.77	5.64 ± 1.18	32.76 ± 3.95	2.32 ± 0.43	25.81 ± 4.46
Saline group	34.13 ± 3.90	111.45 ± 22.26	55.33 ± 5.57	0.43 ± 0.15	5.15 ± 2.67	5.51 ± 1.36	33.94 ± 6.81	2.36 ± 0.33	26.38 ± 4.14
2 g/kg	31.63 ± 3.84	119.03 ± 31.76	56.16 ± 3.64	0.32 ± 0.08	5.46 ± 1.77	5.66 ± 0.88	29.55 ± 8.76	2.87 ± 0.27	26.76 ± 4.67
4 g/kg	35.72 ± 5.99	119.78 ± 15.37	59.07 ± 5.52	0.33 ± 0.21	5.19 ± 1.64	5.46 ± 0.96	31.74 ± 7.14	2.44 ± 0.41	27.29 ± 5.33
8 g/kg	33.96 ± 3.97	125.76 ± 20.33	55.98 ± 3.73	0.34 ± 0.07	5.04 ± 1.44	6.02 ± 0.66	35.28 ± 6.94	3.15 ± 0.35	25.91 ± 4.58
16 g/kg	37.69 ± 3.03	137.63 ± 26.44*	58.45 ± 4.09	0.45 ± 0.09	4.88 ± 2.31	6.23 ± 1.07	36.66 ± 5.46	3.43 ± 0.42*	27.61 ± 8.61

Values represent means ± SD

ALT alanine aminotransferase, *AST* aspartate aminotransferase, *TP* total protein, *TG* triglycerides, *GLU* glucose, *UREA* blood urea nitrogen, *CREA* creatinine, *TC* total cholesterol, *ALB* albumin

*$P < 0.05$, significantly difference from control values

some evidence that the drug may have no adverse effect on the cardiovascular system [32, 33].

The subchronic toxicity testing is used to assess the long-term safety of exogenous substances [34]. In our 30-day clinical trial, two male and one female rats in Group VI died. Because autopsy of these animals disclosed signs of damage from improper oral lavage, and no other abnormalities were found at autopsy, we feel that toxic effects of Jinqing were not the cause of the deaths.

Changes in body weight can be used as indicators of general toxicity of drugs and chemicals [35–37]. In our study, Jinqing granules had only minimal effect on the rate of weight gain, and the effect was only statistically significant at the highest dose (Group VI; 16 g/kg) and not until 3 to 4 weeks of treatment. Whether this effect was due to effects of the medication is unknown.

Hematological analyses in humans and animals are a sensitive indicator of drug and chemical toxicity [38–40]. In analyses of blood indices, we found no abnormalities in several measurements in the Jinqing-treated animals (white blood cell count, red blood cell count, platelet count, hemoglobin, and neutrophil count), but a slight, statistically significant increase in lymphocyte counts (from 77 to 82 × 10 ^{9}/ml in Group IV animals) was found; we suspect this difference is of no clinical significance, because they were within normal physiological ranges [41–43].

As with other measurements, the biochemical tests revealed little abnormality in the Jinqing-treated animals, although aspartate aminotransferase and total bilirubin were modestly increased in Group VI animals. Aspartate aminotransferase is released into the blood [44], when liver-cell injury occurs, but an increase in serum aspartate aminotransferase value is not specific for liver disease [45]. Bilirubin is a breakdown product of normal heme catabolism [46]. With disease of the liver or biliary system, serum bilirubin values may rise [47], but increased values may be present in hematologic or other diseases as well. In our study, the combination of increased serum aspartate aminotransferase and total bilirubin raise the possibility of liver injury, but whether the mild abnormalities seen only with the highest doses of Jinqing are of clinical significance is unknown.

Table 8 Effect of subchronic administration of Jinqing granules on the organ coefficient (g/ g*100%) of male and female rats (n = 20)

Parameters	gender	Heart	Liver	Spleen	Lung	Kidney	Testis or Ovary
Control group	Male	0.35 ± 0.01	3.24 ± .024	0.30 ± 0.04	0.51 ± 0.05	0.79 ± 0.06	1.25 ± 0.12
	Female	0.37 ± 0.05	3.26 ± 0.19	0.31 ± 0.03	0.47 ± 0.02	0.76 ± 0.06	0.05 ± 0.01
saline group	Male	0.37 ± 0.03	3.36 ± 0.10	0.28 ± 0.04	0.53 ± 0.05	0.80 ± 0.04	1.27 ± 0.10
	Female	0.39 ± 0.03	3.45 ± 0.14	0.29 ± 0.03	0.52 ± 0.02	0.77 ± 0.05	0.04 ± 0.01
2 g/kg	Male	0.35 ± 0.02	3.37 ± 0.19	0.32 ± 0.05	0.54 ± 0.06	0.78 ± 0.04	1.24 ± 0.14
	Female	0.37 ± 0.04	3.37 ± 0.36	0.27 ± 0.06	0.55 ± 0.08	0.81 ± 0.11	0.05 ± 0.01
4 g/kg	Male	0.35 ± 0.01	3.39 ± 0.24	0.31 ± 0.05	0.52 ± 0.04	0.75 ± 0.06	1.21 ± 0.10
	Female	0.36 ± 0.02	3.27 ± 0.22	0.31 ± 0.07	0.50 ± 0.05	0.79 ± 0.04	0.05 ± 0.01
8 g/kg	Male	0.36 ± 0.04	3.44 ± 0.24	0.28 ± 0.04	0.54 ± 0.05	0.78 ± 0.06	1.28 ± 0.11
	Female	0.35 ± 0.02	3.32 ± 0.18	0.30 ± 0.03	0.52 ± 0.05	0.76 ± 0.02	0.05 ± 0.01
16 g/kg	Male	0.34 ± 0.05	3.49 ± 0.37*	0.26 ± 0.05	0.54 ± 0.13	0.83 ± 0.11	1.41 ± 0.13*
	Female	0.36 ± 0.03	3.52 ± 0.16*	0.26 ± 0.05	0.54 ± 0.04	0.80 ± 0.06	0.06 ± 0.01

Values represent means ± SD

*$P < 0.05$; sig.nificantly different from control

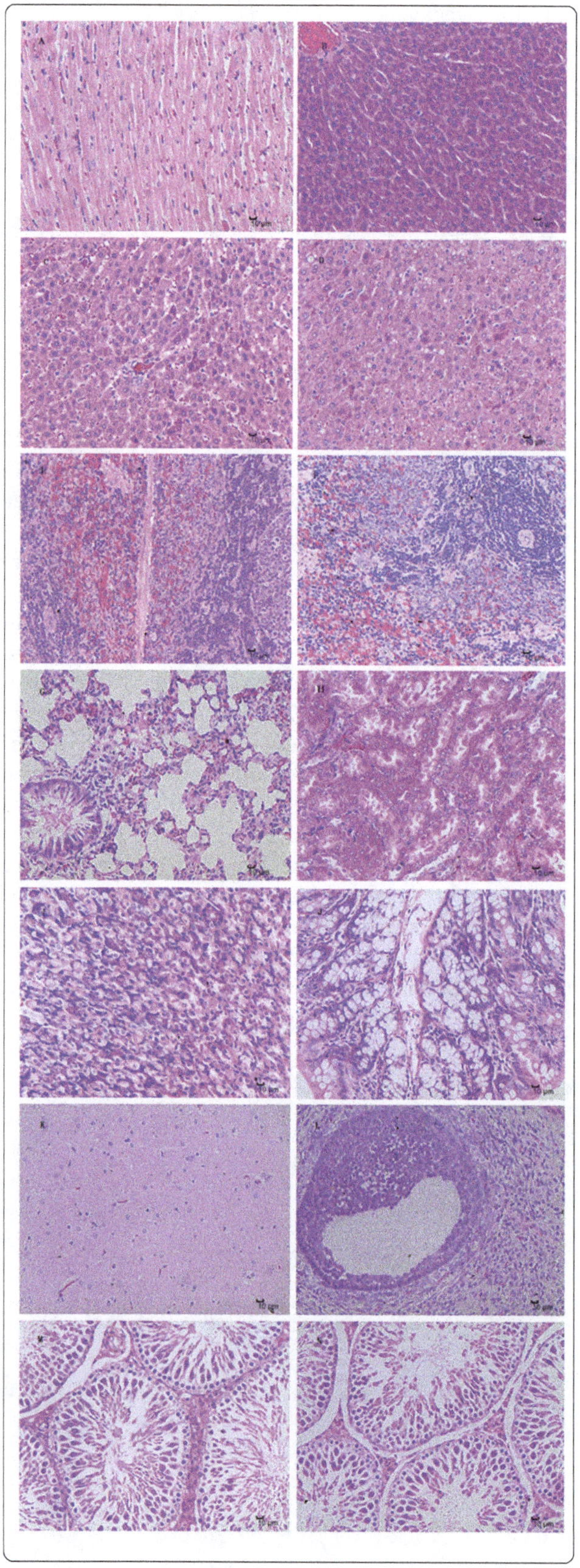

Fig. 5 H&E staining of the liver, kidney, brain, heart, lung, spleen from the rats used in the subchronic toxicity test. *N* = 3 per group, scale bar = 10 μm; 400×. **a** Representative section of heart tissue (Group I- VI), with no histological abnormality. **b** Liver, 0 g/kg, Group I, without histological abnormality. **c** Liver, Group VI animals, with expansion of liver sinusoids, **d** Liver, Group VI animals, with various degrees of vacuolar degeneration in hepatocytes. **e** Spleen, 0 g/kg (Group I), with no histological abnormality. **f** Spleen, Group VI rats, with decreased numbers of lymphocytes and increased numbers of macrophages. **g** Representative section of Lung, Group I-VI, with no histological abnormality. **h** Representative section of kidney, Group I-VI, with no histological abnormality. **i** Representative section of stomach, Group I-VI, with no histological abnormality. **j** Representative section of intestines, Group I-VI with not histological abnormality. **k** Representative section of brain, Group I-VI, with no histological abnormality. **l** Representative section of ovary, Group I- VI, with no histological abnormality. **m** Representative sections of testicle, Group I-V, with testicular tubules were arranged neatly and tightly. **n** Testicle, Group VI, with the number of sperm in seminiferous tubules appeared decreased

Serum creatinine is an important index of kidney function [48, 49], and blood urea nitrogen values can reflect glomerular filtration function [50]. That these tests were normal in our rats is evidence that Jinqing granules, even at high doses, did not adversely affect renal function. This conclusion is supported also by the normal urinary pH, specific gravity, and protein values in treated animals.

Organ coefficient is an important index in the evaluation of new-drug preclinical toxicity and effect on target organs [51, 52]. Studies have reported that the organ coefficient may be increased due to congestion, edema, hypertrophy, and other causes, and it may be decreased due to organ shrinking and degenerative changes [53, 54]. These effects may not be directly attributed to a direct effect of the drug being tested, and could be due a secondary change. In this study, no abnormalities in organ coefficient were found, except for slight but statistically significantly decreased values for the liver and testes at the 16 g/kg dose.

After the 30-day trial, histological examination of the heart, liver, spleen, lung, kidney, stomach, intestines, brain, testes and ovary found minimal changes, except for decreased number of sperm in seminiferous tubules of Group VI animals. Therefore, an adverse effect of Jinqing on reproductive capability and hepatotoxicity have to be considered.

Brain is a crucial organ for regulating mental development, and promotes endocrine release of human [55, 56]. The hippocampus and cortex play an absolutely essential role in learning and memory [57, 58]. Hypothalamus regulates a variety of functions, including sleep, body temperature, thirst and hunger. In this study, histopathological displayed a normal neuronal structure in the hippocampus, cortex and hypothalamus, without inflammatory infiltrate or hemorrhagic lesions. In addition, in the subchronic toxicity test the change of behavior was not observed. Tests have shown that Jinqing granules had no effect on rats' brain.

We acknowledge that our study has limitations. The most consequential may be the relatively short duration of Jinqing feeding; trials of longer-term administration of the medication are needed. Also, results of tests in Sprague-Dawley rats may not be applicable to other animal species or to humans. Finally, despite our extensive testing for adverse events associated with Jinqing feeding, the tests may not have been sufficiently sensitive or specific to detect all adverse events.

The doses of Jinquing granules we fed to rats are well above those usually used in the treatment or prevention of gastric ulcers. Thus, although our findings are not directly transferrable to porcine husbandry, they give some assurance about the safety of Jinqing feeding.

Conclusions

Extensive safety pharmacology and subchronic toxicity tests on rats fed ultra-high doses of Jinqing granules (up to 16 g/kg) revealed little evidence of toxicity on the animals' nervous, cardiovascular, respiratory, renal, and hematological systems. However, the highest dose was associated with slightly slowed weight growth and minor histologic changes of unknown significance, decreased numbers of sperm in seminiferous tubules, and increased values of serum aspartate aminotransferase and bilirubin. During the 30-day feeding test, 3 rats that received the 16 g/kg dose died, but the deaths were most likely due to trauma of oral gavage, not drug toxicity. Jinqing granules given to Sprague-Dawley rats orally for 30 days at a dose of 8 g/kg or less appears safe, but higher doses were not proven safe. The significance of these observations with respect to usage of Jinqing in animals, or possibly in humans, deserves thorough investigation.

Acknowledgments

This work was supported in part by a grant (2013NZ0019) from the Science and Technology Department of Sichuan Province, China. We thank the College of Veterinary Medicine, Sichuan Agricultural University, Cheng du 611130, China, for kindly providing facilities.

Funding

Supported in part by a grant (2013NZ0019) from Science & Technology Department of Sichuan Province, China.

Authors' contributions

XR and QR carried out most of the experiments and drafted the manuscript. YL, GY, LZ, FS and CL critically revised the experiment design and manuscript.

MX, YL, QD, YL, QJ, HL, XY and KS helped with the experiment. All authors read and approved the final manuscript.

Competing interests

The authors declare that they have no competing interests.

Consent for publication

Not applicable.

Ethics approval

All experimental procedures involving animals were approved by Sichuan Agricultural University Animal Care and Use Committee (registration No. SCAU2016061801).Based on the principles of the International Committee on Laboratory Animals, the rats were separated equally according to gender and maintained at 20–25 °C and relative humidity of 55 ± 5%. Artificial lighting was adjusted to 12 h of light (from 08:00 to 20:00) and 12 h of darkness from 20:00 to 08:00. The rats were allowed to drink water freely, and they acclimated for 7 days before experiments were begun.

References

1. Lin YH, Chen KK, Chiu JH. Coprescription of Chinese herbal medicine and western medications among prostate cancer patients: a population-based study in Taiwan. Evid Based Complement Alternat Med. 2012;1:147015.
2. Wang P, Zhou HL, Xue FZ, et al. Pattern recognition for traditional Chinese medicine nature of 60 kinds of herbal medicine based on high performance capillary electrophoresis fingerprint. J Chin Med Mat. 2013;36(9):1419–24.
3. Zhang XW, Jia HL. Origin and development of umbilical therapy in traditional Chinese medicine. Chinese Acupuncture & Moxibustion. 2014;34(6):607.
4. Parveen A, Parveen B, Parveen R. Challenges and guidelines for clinical trial of herbal drugs. J Pharm Bioallied Sci. 2015;7(4):329.
5. Ntie-Kang F, Onguéné PA, Lifongo LL, et al. The potential of anti-malarial compounds derived from African medicinal plants, part II: a pharmacological evaluation of non-alkaloids and non-terpenoids. Malar J. 2014;13(1):81.
6. Lai JN, Tang JL, Wang JD. Observational studies on evaluating the safety and adverse effects of traditional chinese medicine. Evid Based Complement Alternat Med. 2013;2013(18):697893.
7. CA Smith, Ros Priest et al. The ethics of traditional chinese and western herbal medicine research: views of researchers and human ethics committees in Australia. Evid Based Complement Alternat Med. 2011 (1741-427X):256915. Article ID 256915. doi:10.1155/2011/256915.
8. Chinese Pharmacopoeia Committee. Pharmacopoeia of the People's Republic of China. Beijing: Chinese medical science and technology press; 2015. p. 217.
9. Yan SK, Lin ZY, Dai WX, et al. Chemometrics-based approach to modeling quantitative composition-activity relationships for Radix Tinosporae. Interdiscip Sci. 2010;2(3):221–7.
10. Khan MA, Gray AI, Waterman PG. Tinosporaside, an 18-norclerodane glucoside from Tinospora cordifolia. Phytochemistry. 1989;28(1):273–5.
11. Wei L, Kazuo K, Lijuan L, et al. New lignan glucosides from the stems of Tinospora sinensis. Chem Pharm Bull. 2004;52(5):638–40.
12. Qin NB, Wang AL, Li DH, et al. Cytotoxic clerodane furanoditerpenoids from the root of Tinospora sagittata. Phytochem Lett. 2015;12:173–6.
13. He C. *Canarium album* (Lour.) Raeusch.(Qingguo, Chinese Olive). Diet Chin Herbs. 2015;5(17):307–13.
14. Rong Q, Li Y L, Xu M, et al. A formulation for the treatment of gastric ulcer drugs and its preparation method. Chin, CN 105287732 A, 2016-2-03.
15. Rong Q, Xu M, Dong Q, et al. In vitro and in vivo bactericidal activity of Tinospora sagittata (Oliv.) Gagnep. var. craveniana (S.Y.Hu) Lo and its main effective component Palmatine against Helicobacter pylori from pig. BMC Complement Altern Med. 2016;16(1):331.
16. Swaby H, Gregory NG. A note on the frequency of gastric ulcers detected during post-modem examination at a pig abattoir. Meat Sci. 2012;90:269–71.
17. China Institute of Veterinary Drugs Control, 2011. Test no.1596: safety pharmacology research technical guidelines of veterinary medicine, natural medicine.
18. Duan WL, Liang X. Technical guidelines assembly of veterinary medicine research. Beijing: Chemical Industry Press; 2011.
19. Pugsley MK, Authier S, Curtis MJ, et al. Principles of safety pharmacology. Br J Pharmacol. 2008;154(7):1382–99.
20. Lindgren S, Bass A, BriscoeBenchmarking R K, et al. safety pharmacology regulatory packages and best practice. J Pharmacol Toxicol Methods. 2008; 58(2):99–109.

21. Xiang F, Yin ZQ, Jia RY, et al. Acute and subchronic toxicity as well as evaluation of safety pharmacology of Galla chinensis solution. J Ethnopharmacol. 2014;162:181–90.
22. OECD. Guideline for testing of chemicals: repeated dose 28-day oral toxicity in rodents. Test no. 407, adopted in 1981, and revised method adopted 3 October 2008. Paris: OECD; 2008a.
23. Yan L, Gao H, Sun JJ. Research on body weight and reference value of main organ of wistar rats. Pract Prev Med. 2009;16(6):1708–11.
24. Ihongbe JC, Salisu AA, Bankole JK. A study on the effect of Mondia Whitei on organ and body weight of wistar rats. Int J Herbs Pharmacol Res. 2012; 1(1):18–23.
25. Shi L, Lv YP, Qian BC. Discussion on basic request and standardization in safety pharmacology. Chin J Clin Pharmac Ther. 2005;10:961–5.
26. Guth BD, Siegl PKS. Safety pharmacology assessment. Pharm Med. 2007; 21(5):357–61.
27. JM Korth-Bradley, et al. Pharmacokinetics and safety of a single intravenous dose of the antibiotic tigecycline in patients with cirrhosis. J Clin Pharmacol. 2010;51(1): 93–101.
28. Mandhane DSN, Ayer UB, Midha AS. Preclinical efficacy and safety pharmacology of SUN-1334H, a potent orally active antihistamine agent. Drugs in R & D. 2008;9(2):93–112.
29. Huang FH. General pharmacology study of new drug of TCM technical requirement and the analysis of common problems. J Tradit Chin Med. 2007;32:82–4.
30. Broichhausen C, Riquelme P, Ahrens N, et al. In question: the scientific value of preclinical safety pharmacology and toxicology studies with cell-based therapies. Mol Ther Methods Clin Dev. 2014;1(1):14026.
31. Zaciraglc A, Nakas-icindic E, Hadzovic A, Avdagic N. Average values of electrocardiograph parameters in healthy, adult Wistar rats. Med Arh. 2004; 58:268–70.
32. Bonilha AMM, Saraiva RM, Kanashiro RM, Portes LA, Antonio EL, Tucci PJF. A routine electrocardiogram cannot be used to determine the size of myocardial infarction in the rat. Braz J Med Biol Res. 2005;38:615–9.
33. Pratt DS, Kaplan MM. Evaluation of abnormal liver-enzyme results in asymptomatic patients. N Engl J Med. 2000;342:1266–71.
34. Aniagu SO, Nwinyi FC, Akumka DD, et al. Toxicity studies in rats fed nature cure bitters. Afr J Biotechnol. 2005;4:72–8.
35. Raza M, Al-Shabanah OA, El-Hadiyah TM, et al. Effect of prolonged vigabatrin treatment on hematological and biochemical parameters in plasma, liver and kidney of Swiss albino mice. Sci Pharm. 2002;70:135–45.
36. Tan PV, Mezui C, Enow-Orock G, et al. Teratogenic effects, acute and sub chronic toxicity of the leaf aqueous extract of ocimum suave Wild (Lamiaceae) in rats. J. Ethnopharmacol. 2008;115:232–7.
37. Teo S, Stirling D, Thomas S, et al. A 90-day oral gavage toxicity study of D-methylphenidate and D, L-methylphenidate in Sprague-Dawley rats. Toxicology. 2002;179:183–96.
38. Adeneye AA, Ajagbonna OP, Adeleke TI, et al. Preliminary toxicity and phytochemical studies of the stem bark aqueous extract of Musanga cecropioides in rats. J Ethno Pharmacol. 2006;105:374–9.
39. Liju VB, Jeena K, Kuttan R. Acute and subchronic toxicity as well as mutagenic evaluation of essential oil from turmeric (*Curcuma longa*). Food Chem Toxicol. 2013;53:52–61.
40. Rahman ME, Siddiqui MK, Jamil K. Effects of vepacide (*Azadirachta indica*) on aspartate and alanine aminotransferase profiles in a subchronic study with rats. Hum Exp Toxicol. 2001;20:243–9.
41. Alemán CL, Más RM, Rodeiro I, et al. Reference database of the main physiological parameters in Sprague–Dawley rats from 6 to 32 months. Lab Anim. 1998;32:457–66.
42. Petterino C, Argentino-Storino A. Clinical chemistry and haematology historical data in control Sprague–Dawley rats from pre-clinical toxicity studies. Exp Toxicol Pathol. 2006;57:213–9.
43. Han ZZ, Xu HD, Kim KH, et al. Reference data of the main physiological parameters in control Sprague–Dawley rats from pre-clinical toxicity studies. Lab Anim Res. 2010;26:153–64.
44. Han YD, Song SY, Lee JH, Lee DS, Yoon HC. Multienzyme-modified biosensing surface for the electrochemical analysis of aspartate transaminase and alanine transaminase in human plasma. Anal Bioanal Chem. 2011;400:797–805.
45. Ozer J, Ratner M, Shaw M, Bailey W, Schomaker S. The current state of serum biomarkers of hepatotoxicity. Toxicology. 2008;245:194–205.
46. Vítek L. The role of bilirubin in diabetes, metabolic syndrome, and cardiovascular diseases. Front Pharmacol. 2012;3:55.
47. Green RM, Flamm S. AGA technical review on the evaluation of liver chemistry tests. Gastroenterology. 2002;123:1367–84.
48. Remuzzi G, Bertani T. Pathophysiology of progressive nephropathies. N Engl J Med. 1998;339:1448–56.
49. Lameire N, Van Biesen W, Vanholder R. Acute renal failure. Lancet. 2005;365: 417–30.
50. Wang SL. Veterinary clinical diagnostics (third edition). Beijing: China Agriculture; 2006.
51. Yuan BL. The significance and shortcoming of organ or body weight ratio used in drug safety evaluation. Chin New Drug J. 2003;12:960–3.
52. Gu LJ, Yang XH, Chen QJ, Sun JX, Xiao Y, Le JY, et al. Study on the normal reference values of organs' weight and organ/body coefficients in SD rats. J Labour Med. 2005;22:453–4.
53. Wei J, Wu XG, Lin H. A further observation on the serum biochemical values of chickens infected with Eimeriatenella or E. acervulina and the discussion on the pathological lesions. Chin J Prev Vet Med. 2002;32:25–7.
54. Kristiansen E, Madsen C. Induction of protein droplet (α 2μ-globulin) nephropathy in male rats after short-term dosage with 1, 8-cineole and l-limonene. Toxicol Lett. 1995;80:147–52.
55. Biran J, Tahor M, Wircer E, Levkowitz G. Role of developmental factors in hypothalamic function. Front Neuroanat. 2015;9(7):47.
56. Machluf Y, Gutnick A, Levkowitz G. Development of the zebrafish hypothalamus. Ann N Y Acad Sci. 2011;1220(1):93–105.
57. O'Reilly RC, Rudy JW. Conjunctive representations in learning and memory: principles of cortical and hippocampal function. Psychol Rev. 2001;108(2): 311–45.
58. Witter MP, Naber PA, Haeften T, et al. Cortico-hippocampal communication by way of parallel parahippocampal-subicular pathways. Hippocampus. 2000;10(4):398–410.

11

Antiepileptic drugs' tolerability and safety – a systematic review and meta-analysis of adverse effects in dogs

Marios Charalambous[1*], Sara K. Shivapour[2], David C. Brodbelt[3] and Holger A. Volk[4]

Abstract

Background: The safety profile of anti-epileptic drugs (AEDs) is an important consideration for the regulatory bodies, owners and prescribing clinicians. Information on their adverse effects still remains limited. A systematic review including a meta-analytic approach was designed to evaluate existing evidence for the safety profile of AEDs in canine patients. Electronic searches of PubMed, CAB Direct and Google scholar were carried out without date or language restrictions. Conference proceedings were also searched. Peer-reviewed full-length studies reporting adverse effects of AEDs in epileptic and healthy non-epileptic dogs were included. Studies were allocated to three groups based on their design. Individual studies were evaluated based on the quality of evidence (study design, study group sizes, subject enrolment quality and overall risk of bias) and the outcome measures reported (proportion of specific adverse effects for each AED, prevalence and 95 % confidence interval of the affected population in each study and comparative odds ratio of adverse effects for AEDs).

Results: Ninety studies, including six conference proceedings, reporting clinical outcomes of AEDs' adverse effects were identified. Few studies were designed as blinded randomised controlled clinical trials. Many studies included low canine populations with unclear criteria of subject enrolment and short treatment periods. Direct comparisons suggested that imepitoin and levetiracetam might have a better safety profile than phenobarbital, whilst the latter might have a better safety profile than potassium bromide. However, none of these comparisons showed a statistically significant difference. Comparisons between other AEDs were not possible as a considerable amount of studies lacked power calculations or adequate data to allow further statistical analysis. Individual AED assessments indicated that levetiracetam might be one of the safest AEDs, followed by imepitoin and then phenobarbital and potassium bromide; these findings were all supported by a strong level of evidence. The safety profile in other AEDs was variable, but weak evidence was found to permit firm conclusions or to compare their safety to other AEDs.

Conclusions: This systematic review provides objective evaluation of the most commonly used AEDs' adverse effects. Adverse effects usually appeared mild in all AEDs and subsided once doses and/or serum levels were monitored or after the AED was withdrawn. Although phenobarbital might be less safe than imepitoin and levetiracetam, there was insufficient evidence to classify it as an AED with a high risk of major adverse effects. It is important for clinicians to evaluate both AEDs' effectiveness and safety on an individual basis before the selection of the appropriate monotherapy or adjunctive AED therapy.

Keywords: Systematic review, Meta-analysis, Epilepsy, Canine, Antiepileptic drugs, Safety, Side effects

* Correspondence: marios.charalambous.15@ucl.ac.uk
[1]Faculty of Brain Sciences, UCL Institute of Neurology, University College London, London WC1E 6BT, UK
Full list of author information is available at the end of the article

Background

In human medicine, a plethora of new antiepileptic drugs (AEDs) have been developed over the years for use either as monotherapy or adjunctive therapy [1]. Many of these drugs are now also used in veterinary medicine. This has led to an increase in the arsenal of AEDs used to treat canine epilepsy. As a rule, AEDs are evaluated on the grounds of their effectiveness and safety through clinical trials and experimental laboratory studies before they are approved for use in patients by the regulatory authorities, e.g. the European Medicines Agency (EMA) or the US Food and Drug Administration (FDA) [2]. The safety profile of drugs is an important consideration for their approval by the authorities and use by prescribing clinicians on their clients' animals [2, 3]. It affects clinicians' decisions to prescribe specific AED(s), as serious adverse effects can lead to chronic complications or even death. Less serious, but nonetheless important, adverse effects can significantly impact quality of life, leading to systematic illness which may increase the overall cost of treatment [3, 4]. Ultimately, the benefits of an effective AED may be outweighed by its adverse effects, and the latter should be always taken into consideration.

Many potential adverse effects for AEDs have been reported, but the evidence behind the severity of these effects or the likelihood of their occurrence has not been systematically compiled [5, 6]. Randomised clinical trials (RCTs) are a considerable source of evidence for some common or expected adverse effects [4]. However, information about serious, rare, and/or long-term adverse effects can typically be found in studies such as case reports, case series and observational studies [7, 8]. Consequently, the clinician will need to search for information from sources other than RCTs [7, 8]. Identification of all relevant studies can be time-consuming and for a busy practitioner it may be more effective to review this information via a systematic review. Systematic reviews are one of the most powerful and reliable tools to assess the severity and the probability of occurrence of AEDs' adverse effects across the spectrum of primary literature [9–12].

Although evidence for AEDs' efficacy has been recently reported and evaluated in a systematic review [13], it has been suggested that, apart from the efficacy, the selection of the appropriate AED should be also largely influenced by its safety profile [14]. To our knowledge there is only one systematic review in the field of canine epilepsy which evaluated the safety profile of a single AED, potassium bromide, across species and aetiology of seizures [15]. However, a systematic review of the adverse effects observed during treatment with any AED(s) in dogs, as well as AEDs' safety profile comparisons, has not been reported. The aim of this systematic review was to perform an objective analysis of AEDs' adverse effects in dogs, in order to provide evidence-based information on AEDs' safety profiles.

Methods

Search strategy

The literature search aimed to identify all studies assessing or reporting the adverse effects of an AED in dogs. Specifically, studies were evaluated based on the inclusion criteria below:

- Criterion 1-Type of study: Peer-reviewed studies in English (or translated). Experimental laboratory animal studies, clinical trials, observational and descriptive studies were included.
- Criterion 2-Case definition: For the clinical studies, dogs with IE were included as previously defined [13]. Briefly this required dogs within a certain age range, unremarkable interictal neurological status and diagnostic investigation for seizures. For the experimental laboratory animal studies (ELAS), healthy non-epileptic dogs were also included; for the latter a clear diagnostic investigation or health statement should have been reported in the study to exclude the possibility of underlying diseases.
- Criterion 3-Treatment: Dogs treated with any AED available used in canine IE were included. Doses and serum concentrations of AEDs, frequency of drug administration and treatment period were considered important information to record. Dogs treated with methods other than pharmacological intervention, e.g. homoeopathy methods, surgery, food trials, nerve stimulation, were excluded.
- Criterion 4-Outcome: Studies had to assess or report adverse effects following administration of AED(s) in canine subjects. Studies were conducted either to specifically assess or report AED(s)' safety (primary evidence studies) or to assess an outcome other than AED(s)' safety (i.e. efficacy), while also reporting adverse effects (supportive evidence studies). Assessment of the adverse effects should have been performed by the investigators or owner.

Search strategies included use of electronic search engines for publication databases, searching of reference lists of published papers and proceedings of relevant scientific conferences. Electronic databases used were Pub Med (www.ncbi.nlm.nih.gov/PubMed), CAB Abstracts (www.cabdirect.org) and Google Scholar (www.scholar.-google.com). Final electronic searches were carried out on 30 February 2015 by the primary and the second author independently, with no date or language restrictions. The search terms used in both search engines were as follows: (dog OR dogs OR canine) AND [(phenobarbital OR phenobarbitone OR primidone OR PBr OR KBr OR potassium bromide OR bromide OR nimodipine OR zonisamide OR ELB138 OR imepitoin OR levetiracetam OR verapamil OR gabapentin OR gaba OR topiramate OR felbamate OR pregabalin) OR [(treatment OR management) AND (epilepsy OR seizures)] OR (anti-convulsant OR anti-seizuring OR anti-epileptic OR AED) AND (safety OR safe OR adverse-effect OR adverse-effect OR effect OR undesirable effect OR tolerability OR toxicity OR drug toxicity OR reactions OR disease). Hand searching for articles from the reference lists of publications and searching major veterinary neurology conference meeting proceedings from 1970 to 2015 and relative textbook chapters was carried out by the primary and second authors independently. Conference proceedings were searched for the Annual Congresses of the European Society and College of Veterinary Neurology (ESVN / ECVN) and the American College of Veterinary Internal Medicine (ACVIM). Other conference proceedings were searched only if the reference list of identified publications indicated this. All items returned by the search engines, hand searches and correspondence were recorded and entered into the screening process.

Study selection

Restrictions based on publication date or language were not imposed. Studies written in non-English language were assessed initially based on an English translation (Google Translate software) and then verified by a veterinarian fluent in the language of publication.

A two-stage screening process was used [13] and the process was performed by the primary author. Firstly, studies of relevance to the systematic review objectives were identified (stage 1) and, secondly, studies likely to provide evidence of the highest available quality and sufficient detail for assessing the outcome measures and methodology were selected (stage 2). Stage 1 of the screening process identified from the total search results any studies that: (a) fulfilled inclusion criterion 1 and (b) reported findings related to the adverse effects and safety of AEDs administered in dogs. Stage 1 assessment evaluated the retrieved papers' titles and abstracts only. At stage 2, papers were selected for full data extraction according to the inclusion criteria 2, 3 and 4 and were evaluated in detail on the grounds of the quality of evidence and outcomes by MC.

Assessment of quality of evidence

Blinded RCTs (bRCTs) and blinded randomised ELAS (bRELAS) were considered most likely to produce higher quality evidence, followed by non-blinded RCTs (nbRCTs) and non-blinded randomised ELAS (nbRELAS), then non-randomised clinical trials (NRCTs) and non-randomised ELAS (NRELAS), uncontrolled clinical trials (UCTs) and uncontrolled ELAS (UELAS), cohort, case–control and cross sectional studies and lastly case series and reports [16–18]. Accordingly, the studies were allocated based on their design to one of three groups, i.e. bRCTs, bRELAS, nbRCTs and nbRELAS (first group), NRCTs, NRELAS, UCTs, UELAS, cohort, case–control and cross-sectional studies (second group) and case series and reports (third group).

As a general rule, the studies in the first group (bRCTs and bELAS in particular) were considered to provide higher quality evidence, followed by the studies in the second and third group. In addition, a three-part system of evidence quality assessment to indicate the strengths and weaknesses of each study within each group was used [13, 19]: (a) study group sizes, (b) subject enrolment quality and (c) overall risk of bias based on Cochrane [20] and Syrcle's [21] 'risk of bias' assessment tool in order to provide an indicator of confidence associated with the findings of each study. For instance, bRCTs or bRELAS with large group sizes, clear inclusion criteria, thorough diagnostic investigations and low overall risk of bias were considered to provide the highest available quality of evidence.

Study group sizes

This characteristic was categorized for each study using the following system [13, 19]: (a) >50 subjects per group ('good' number of subjects), (b) 20–50 subjects per group ('moderate' number), (c) 10–19 subjects per group ('small' number) and (d) <10 subjects per group ('very small' number).

Assessment of subject enrolment quality

Data on investigations to reach the diagnosis of IE were retrieved to evaluate the quality of subject enrolment in each study as 'well characterized', 'fairly characterized', 'poorly characterized' or 'unclear.' Well characterized diagnoses were defined as diagnostic investigations that included clinical signs and thorough test results consistent with the diagnosis of IE; specifically, the signalment, the absence of neurological deficits between the ictal phases, unremarkable routine biochemical and haematological blood tests and imaging results (including brain MRI and/or CT) and/or normal cerebrospinal fluid (CSF) analysis for all cases of the study. Fairly characterized, used for intermediate situations, were defined as diagnostic investigations that were based on signalment, clinical examination and basic diagnostic investigation (i.e. blood tests only), with only some study cases having had advanced brain imaging and/or CSF analysis. Poorly characterized were defined as diagnostic investigations that were based on signalment, clinical examination and/or basic diagnostic investigation (i.e. blood tests) only. Unclear related to reports where the approach to diagnosis of IE was not clearly stated (e.g. when clinical signs were not stated and insufficient or no details of diagnostic tests were provided or when dogs with IE were included without reporting details on diagnostic investigation).

For the ELAS, which included non-epileptic healthy animals, 'clearly characterized' were the studies that defined diagnostic investigations and thorough test results to exclude any systemic illness; 'unclear' were characterized when diagnostic investigations to rule out diseases were not clearly stated or when dogs were included and considered healthy without reporting details on diagnostic procedures.

Assessment of overall risk of bias

The overall risk of bias in the clinical trials was assessed based on the criteria of the Cochrane 'risk of bias' assessment tool [20]. Syrcle's 'risk of bias' assessment tool [21] was used to assess the overall risk of bias in ELAS. The latter tool is an adapted version of the Cochrane one and was designed to facilitate critical appraisal of evidence from ELAS.

Each of the following study components was categorized as presenting a 'high', 'low' or 'unclear' risk of introducing bias to the study findings: random sequence generation, allocation concealment, blinding of participants and personnel, blinding of outcome assessment, completeness of outcome data, selective reporting of outcomes and other sources of bias. For ELAS, two further components-random housing and baseline characteristics of dogs - were also assessed and mentioned as part of the "other sources of bias" section. Case series and reports as well as observational studies were considered to be of high overall risk of bias.

Level of the studies' evidence

The level of evidence provided for the safety profile of each AED was based on the overall quality of evidence of the studies. The level of evidence was allocated according to a previous similar system [13, 19] which was extensively modified for the needs of the current study: 'strong' evidence was provided for the safety profile when at least one bRCT and/or bRELAS reported or assessed the adverse effects of an AED; 'weak' evidence was provided for the safety profile when bRCTs and/or bRELAS were not available.

Assessment of outcome measures

The outcome measure of this study was the evaluation of the safety profile of AED(s) administered in dogs. The adverse effects were organized by body system (e.g. neurological, gastro-intestinal, dermatological, etc.) and types, including type I (dose dependent and predictable) and type II (idiosyncratic-dose independent and unpredictable). Different terms used by the studies but describing the same adverse effects (e.g. drowsiness and somnolence, wobbly gait and ataxia, lethargy and sedation, etc.) were considered synonymous and only one term was selected for use in the analysis. The outcome measure was assessed according to the methods below:

Proportion of specific adverse effects for each AED

This was expressed as a percentage and calculated for each AED by dividing the number of studies that reported a specific adverse effect by the total number of the studies for this AED. If an AED was used as a monotherapy and adjunctive therapy, further calculations were also performed for each sub-category.

Prevalence and 95 % confidence interval of the affected population in each study

Prevalence was expressed as a percentage and calculated for each study by dividing the number of subjects that developed adverse effects during the specified study period by the total size of the study population. The 95 % confidence interval (95 % CI) of the proportion of study animals that developed adverse effects related to the AED(s) was calculated by standard methods [22]. This was used as a further indicator of an AED's safety profile. If the 95 % CI of affected dogs (based on 95 % CI calculations) were ≥ 50 %, then it was considered that the majority of the study population experienced adverse effects.

For each study, the period of treatment, AED's doses and serum levels were reported with the aim to evaluate the association of these values with the prevalence of each AED's adverse effects.

Statistical analysis

For the comparison groups' studies, a further approach was conducted to identify statistical differences between studies with regards to reported adverse effects. For each AED study, the total number of patients experiencing adverse effects and/or the number of patients experiencing specific adverse effects (e.g. sedation, ataxia, polyuria, etc.) in all therapeutic groups were retrieved. The odds ratio (OR) was then estimated in order to indicate the increased or decreased odds of observing a specific adverse effect(s) in total for an AED compared to its control group (comparison AED or placebo or untreated animals). Statistical analysis was undertaken following the guidelines of the Handbook of the Cochrane Collaboration 5.0. The OR for dichotomous data was calculated using the random-effects model in Review Manager 5.3. Heterogeneity between studies was calculated using the Chi square test and was considered to be heterogeneous when $P \leq 0.1$. I^2 values of no more than

25, 26 to 74 % and no less than 75 % were considered as "low", "moderate" and "high" heterogeneity, respectively. Associations were considered to be statistically significant at $P < 0.05$. P values between 0.05 and 0.1 were considered as statistical trends of potential interest.

Results

Description of studies

By 29 December 2015, the search strategy had identified a total of 368 unique citations; 347 from the electronic searches of PubMed, CAB Abstracts, Google Scholar and manual searches from the publications' reference lists, 16 from manual searching of major conference proceedings and 6 unpublished studies included as part of published data. Two hundred ninety two items fulfilled stage 1 screening criteria. Of these, 90 final studies (published between 1981 and 2015) also fulfilled stage 2 selection criteria and were thus selected for review.

The vast majority of studies were allocated in the second (i.e. non-blinded, non-randomised and uncontrolled studies) and third (i.e. retrospective case series and reports) group. A few studies included more than one sub-study (i.e. a clinical trial and/or ELAS and/or retrospective case series part); accordingly, such studies were included in more than one group. Therefore, study designs represented were five bRCT [23–27], two nbRCT [28, 29] and seven nbRELAS [25, 30–35] in the first group, six NRCTs [36–41], 11 NRELAS [42–52], 22 UCTs [44, 48, 53–71], six UELAS [34, 72–76] and one cross sectional study [3] in second group, and 19 retrospective case series [77–95] and 16 case reports [96–111] in the third group. In addition, five unpublished studies described adverse effects and were reported briefly in EMA report; thus all these were considered as one study [112] and were not included in any category as there was insufficient information as far as their design was concerned.

Overall, the 90 selected studies reported 12 AEDs. In all studies but one [43], the AEDs were orally administered. Within each study, one or more AEDs were evaluated as a monotherapy and/or adjunct to other AEDs.

Disease characterisation

In the majority of the studies, the inclusion criteria for diagnosing IE were not well characterized. According to the described grading system for subject enrolment quality, 16 studies [27, 33, 53, 61, 63, 64, 68, 80, 81, 90, 96, 97, 100, 101, 110, 111] enroled treatment groups of well characterized IE, 13 studies [3, 44, 48, 54–57, 62, 66, 67, 77–79] enroled treatment groups of fairly characterized IE, and 14 studies [23–26, 39, 58, 59, 65, 74, 82, 84, 88, 108, 109] enroled treatment groups of poorly characterized IE. In 26 studies [28, 29, 36–38, 50, 60, 69, 70, 75, 83, 85–87, 89, 91–94, 98, 99, 102–106], the diagnostic procedures for enrolment of cases with IE were unclear.

As far as the ELAS including healthy animals were concerned, eight [31, 36, 45, 46, 50–52, 73] enroled treatment groups of clear and 14 [25, 30, 32, 34, 35, 37, 38, 42, 43, 47, 49, 72, 76] enroled treatment groups of unclear or unknown diagnostic investigation for ruling out other diseases. In one report, a dog was non-epileptic and was treated with phenobarbital and chlomipramine due to anxiety and aggression, but the diagnostic investigation for this was unclear [107].

Study group sizes

The vast majority of studies reported the total number of dogs evaluated. The majority of studies evaluated small or very small study size groups. Thirteen studies [25, 26, 40, 50, 62, 69–71, 75, 82, 88, 90, 113] evaluated groups with a good number of dogs, 13 studies [23, 24, 32, 37, 39, 65, 74, 77, 79, 80, 91, 94, 95] evaluated groups with a moderate number of dogs, 26 studies [3, 28, 34, 36, 38, 44–46, 48, 53, 54, 56–61, 63, 64, 66, 70, 75, 81, 83, 84, 114] evaluated groups with a small number of dogs and 38 studies [33–35, 39, 42, 43, 51–53, 55, 67, 68, 72, 73, 76, 78, 85, 87, 89, 92, 93, 96–100, 102–111, 115, 116] evaluated groups with a very small number of dogs. In two studies, the study group size was unclear [47, 49].

Signalment and baseline characteristics of study subjects

Baseline characteristics (such as breed, age and sex) of total enroled dogs were reported to some extent for all 90 studies. Clear presentation of statistical comparison of intervention groups with respect to signalment and baseline disease characteristics was not commonly encountered.

In all studies reporting baseline data, the recruited dogs represented multiple breeds, both sexes and a wide range of ages at study entry (median 5, mean 4, range 0.5-7 years). Major affected breeds were crossed-breeds and pure breeds such as Labrador and Golden Retrievers followed by German Shepherd dogs, Beagles, Boxers and Poodles. In the majority of the studies more males were affected compared to females, though these differences were not evaluated statistically.

Methodological quality of included studies

The vast majority of studies revealed high and/or unclear risk of bias for all the components (Fig. 1). As stated in the methods, retrospective case series and reports were not included in the methodological quality assessment as these were considered to be at an overall high risk of bias.

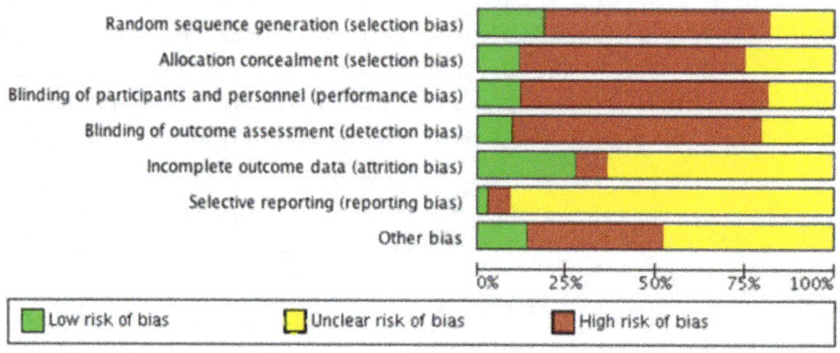

Fig. 1 Risk of bias. Risk of bias assessment presented as percentages across all included studies

Randomization and allocation concealment

Studies in group A used randomization to allocate the dogs and were considered to provide a low risk of bias. Eight studies [25, 28, 29, 32–35, 68] did not offer enough detail to confirm that allocation concealment was performed. Five studies stated that randomization was concealed without further details. Two studies [23, 27] assigned by random blocking (random allocation to blocks of 10 and 6 respectively). One study [27] used pre-defined randomization lists under double-blinded conditions. One study [31] used drawing lots and two studies [24, 30] used a computer-generated list of random numbers.

Blinding of outcome assessment

Only in five studies [23–27], in group A, blinding was clearly described; these were also considered to be at low risk. In these five studies, blinding was applied to all participants, personnel and outcome assessment. In one of them [23] all but the primary investigator were blinded.

Incomplete outcome data

Ten studies presented outcome data from all enroled dogs in the treatment group to which they were originally allocated and there were no losses between enrolment and evaluation [30, 33, 42, 51, 53, 59, 61, 67, 73, 78]. The same studies were considered to be at low risk of bias. In two studies, it was unclear whether all dogs completed the study, as inadequate information was provided [60, 64]. Across the remaining studies, there were dogs that were euthanized or excluded due to poor seizure control, owner request or for unidentified reasons; thus there were losses between the initial study populations and the final number of the dogs.

Selective reporting

It was difficult to assess selective reporting as study protocols were not sought beyond the information published. In two reports [29, 112] further information was attempted to be retrieved but complete protocols were never obtained.

Acknowledgment of other sources of bias

Twelve studies reported financial support [24, 26–28, 41, 44, 53, 58, 61, 68, 73, 79] but there was not adequate evidence to support whether this biased the results. One study [54] clearly mentioned that there was no financial support, while the remaining studies failed to report financial support.

In two studies [28, 78] the statistical analysis was not clarified. In one study [25], many dogs were excluded from both groups mainly for treatment-related reasons (post-randomisation bias). Six studies [29, 49, 60, 64, 70, 86] were conference abstracts, thus no further information could be retrieved. One dog in one study [66] and two dogs in two studies [28, 63] were diagnosed with symptomatic epilepsy (i.e. a cause was identified); this could potentially affect the final results on AED safety profile. Conflict of interest was clearly stated in one study [25].

In the ELAS, specifically, nine studies [25, 30, 33, 34, 42, 44, 51, 52, 68] reported details for the experimental dogs' housing. Random housing of the dogs occurred in all but nine studies [34, 35, 37, 42–44, 49, 72, 73]. The baseline characteristics of the dogs were reported in nine studies [25, 30, 33, 42, 44, 51, 52, 68, 73] and were similar for all the experimental groups in seven studies [25, 30, 33, 42, 44, 51, 52].

AEDs safety profile

A) Safety profile for each AED individually

Proportions of adverse effects for each AED are summarized in the text and presented in Figs. 2, 3, 4, 5, 6, 7, 8, 9, 10, 11. Details of doses and serum concentrations of AED(s), period of treatment as well as prevalence of adverse effects and 95 % CI of the proportion of affected cases (included type and most frequently occurred) for each study are summarized in the text and provided in detail in Tables 1, 2, 3, 4, 5, 6, 7.

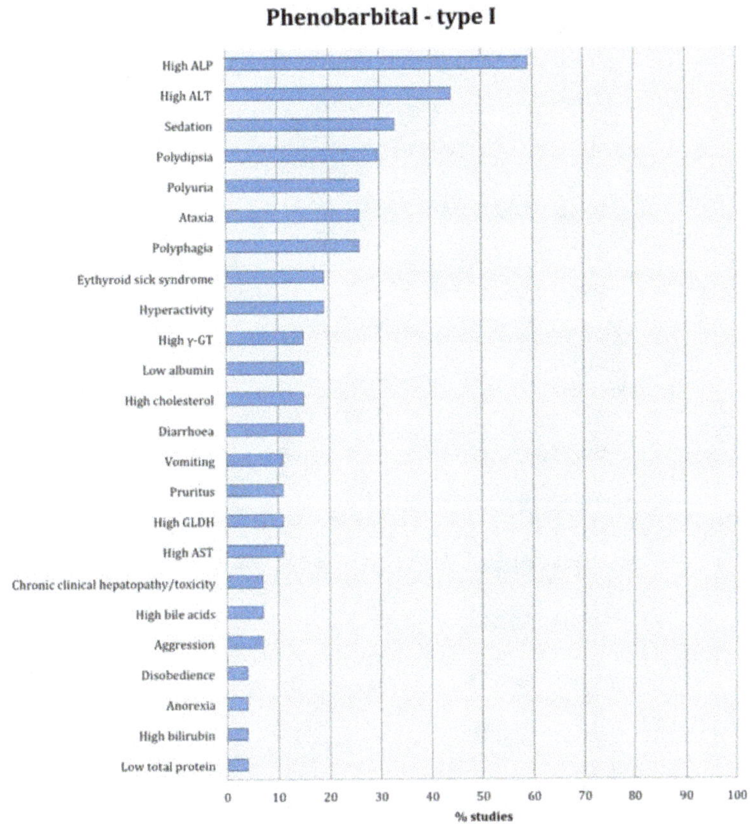

Fig. 2 Proportion of specific type I adverse effects for phenobarbital. Each adverse effect represents the percentage of studies that reported this specific adverse effect for phenobarbital monotherapy

Phenobarbital

There was an overall strong level of evidence provided for the phenobarbital safety profile. Forty-three studies [3, 23, 25, 27–29, 31, 33, 36–40, 42, 43, 45, 46, 49, 50, 52, 53, 60, 69, 71, 74–76, 79–81, 83–85, 87, 93–95, 98, 100, 103, 107, 109, 111] presented data about the safety profile of phenobarbital as a monotherapy agent, giving a combined sample size of 1003 dogs.

Twenty-seven studies reported type I adverse effects (dose dependent/predictable), including neurological signs and clinical pathological findings as the most common (Table 1). Specifically, these adverse effects most

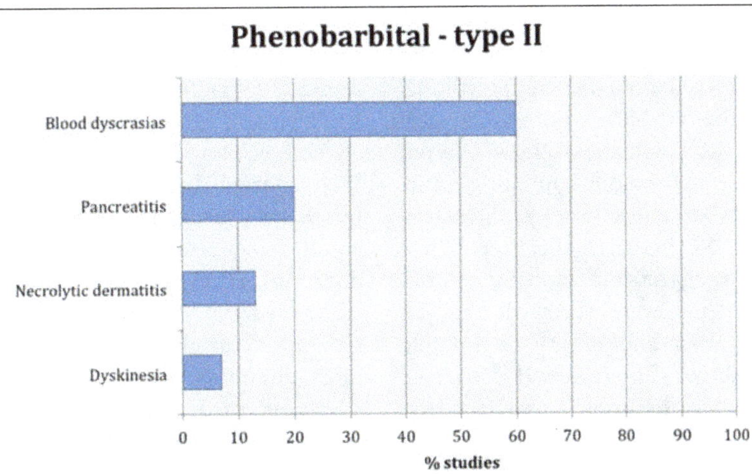

Fig. 3 Proportion of specific type II adverse effects for phenobarbital. Each adverse effect represents the percentage of studies that reported this specific adverse effect for phenobarbital monotherapy

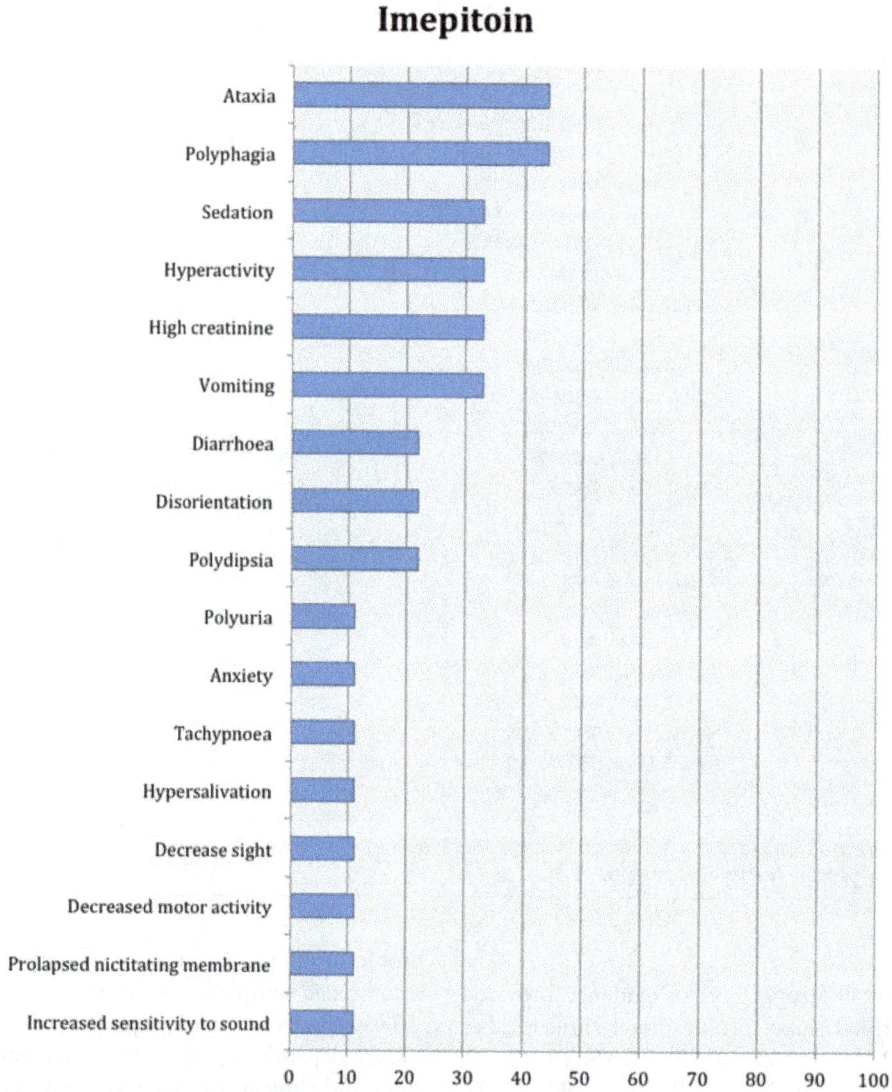

Fig. 4 Proportion of type I adverse effects for imepitoin. Each adverse effect represents the percentage of studies that reported this specific adverse effect for imepitoin monotherapy

commonly included increased serum ALP activity and ALT activity followed by sedation, ataxia, polydipsia, polyuria, polyphagia, euthyroid sick syndrome, hyperactivity, increased serum γ-GT activity, decreased serum albumin and diarrhoea. Less commonly, vomiting, pruritus, chronic clinical hepatopathy/toxicity, increased serum GLDH activity, AST activity, cholesterol, bile acids and bilirubin activity, aggression, anorexia and decreased serum total proteins were reported (Fig. 2). Twenty studies reported alterations in one or multiple liver enzymes, but only three of them reported chronic clinical hepatopathy/toxicity. The occurrence of euthyroid sick syndrome and asymptomatic/subclinical pancreatitis may have been underestimated because only a very few studies included the relevant diagnostic tests to evaluate these disorders. Two studies [31, 33] evaluated the effect of phenobarbital on adrenal function and found no significant effect. The same studies reported no adverse effects, although they focused on reporting adverse effects related to adrenal function. One study [71] reported that adrenal function might have been affected by phenobarbital (i.e. altered ACTH stimulation and dexamethasone suppression tests despite normal endogenous ACTH concentrations).

Fifteen studies reported type II adverse effects (idiosyncratic/unpredictable) with hematological signs as the most common (Table 1). Specifically, the most commonly reported adverse effects included blood dyscrasias (i.e. anemia, thrombocytopenia, leucopenia and/or pancytopenia) followed by pancreatitis, superficial necrolytic dermatitis and lastly dyskinesia (i.e. twitching episodes) (Fig. 3). In one study [50] elevated serum canine

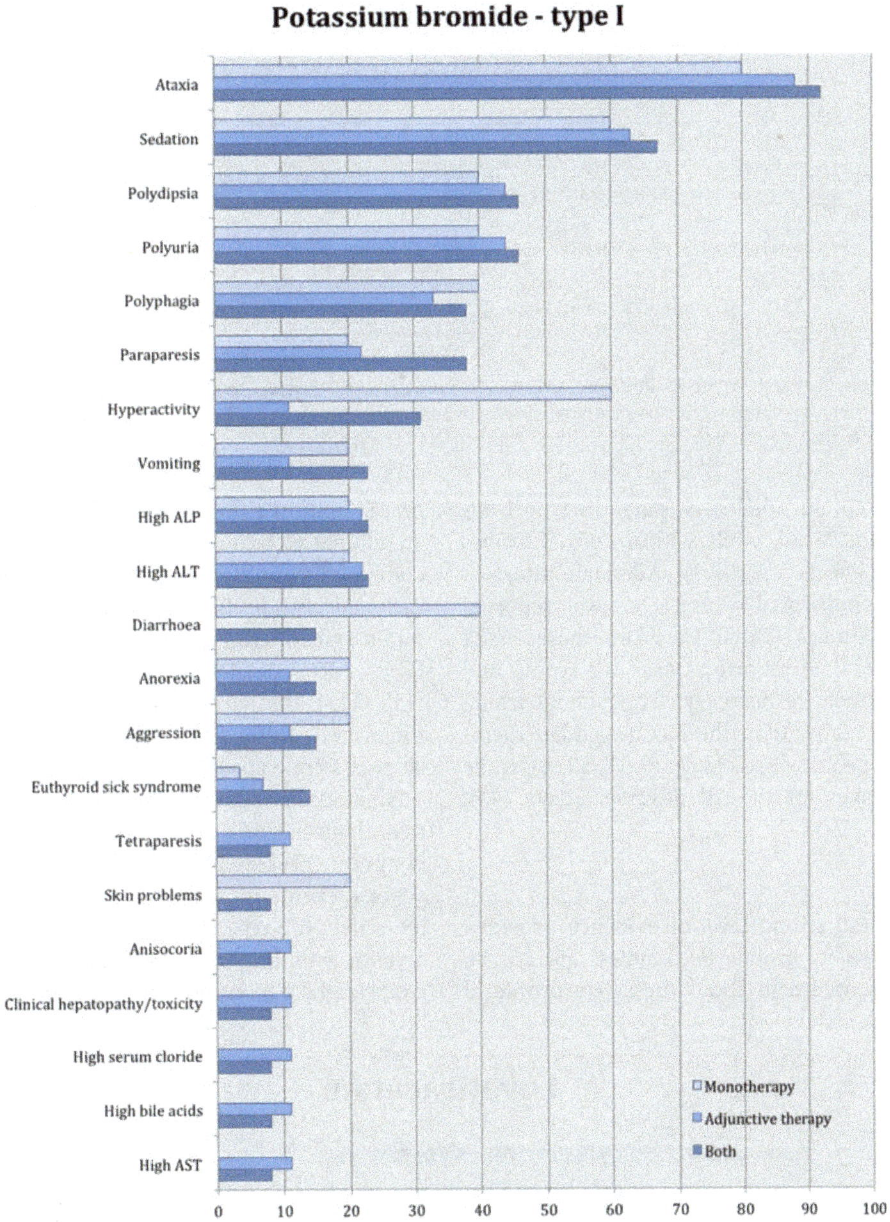

Fig. 5 Proportion of specific type I adverse effects for potassium bromide. Each adverse effect represents the percentage of studies that reported this specific adverse effect for potassium bromide monotherapy and adjunctive therapy

pancreatic lipase immunoreactivity (cPLI) concentration was detected in some dogs, but further diagnostic tests and clinical evaluation was not performed; thus, it is unknown if the dogs had developed clinical pancreatitis. In addition, in one study [81], 212 dogs with IE treated with phenobarbital monotherapy or combined therapy were evaluated and only 9 were found to have phenobarbital-induced blood dyscrasias, giving a prevalence of 4.2 % (95 % CI: 1.5–7.0 %).

Adequate data to allow calculations of the prevalence of adverse effects was reported in 25/43 (58 %) of the studies (Table 1). From these, 13/25 (52 %) showed >50 % prevalence of at least one adverse effect for the specific period of treatment they were conducted. Based on the 95 % CI, the majority of the study populations experienced at least one adverse effect in 11/25 (44 %) studies (Table 1).

Adequate information about the treatment period was reported in 34/43 (79 %) (Table 1). From these, in 10/34 (29 %) the treatment period was relatively short (<6 months). Adequate information about the dose was provided in 28/43 (65 %) studies (Table 1). From these, 19/28 (68 %) and 9/28 (32 %) reported type I and type II adverse effects respectively. The maintenance doses were

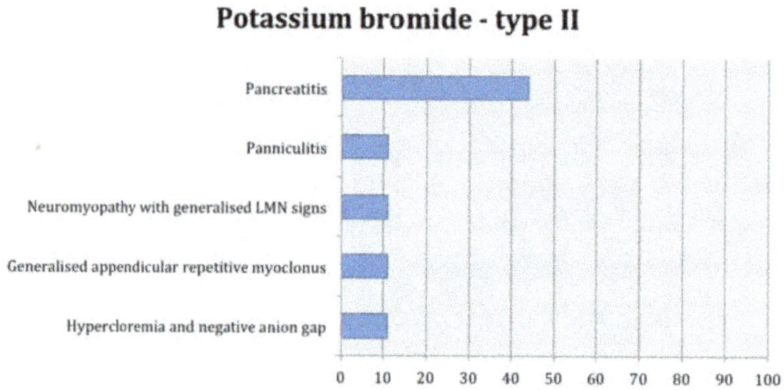

Fig. 6 Proportion of specific type II adverse effects for potassium bromide. Each adverse effect represents the percentage of studies that reported this specific adverse effect for potassium bromide monotherapy and/or adjunctive therapy

higher than the recommended dose range in type I adverse effects (11/19, 58 %), while within normal ranges for type II adverse effects (7/9, 78 %). Adequate information about the phenobarbital serum levels was reported in 24/43 (56 %) studies (Table 1). From these 17/24 (71 %) and 4/24 (17 %) reported doses for type I and type II adverse effects respectively. The phenobarbital serum levels were higher than the recommended therapeutic ranges in type I adverse effects (9/17, 53 %), while within normal ranges for type II adverse effects (4/4, 100 %).

Imepitoin

There was an overall strong level of evidence provided for the imepitoin safety profile. Six studies [25, 26, 44, 48, 112, 113] presented data about the safety profile of oral imepitoin either as monotherapy (all studies) and/or an adjunct to other AEDs (two studies) [44, 48], giving a combined sample size of 458 dogs. Two studies [25, 44] included both a clinical trial and ELAS part. EMA imepitoin assessment report [112] included two unpublished GLP toxicity studies and three unpublished clinical trials [117–119]; the latter three studies were not clearly distinguished in the EMA report and thus they were considered as one study.

Nine studies reported type I adverse effects including neurological and gastro-intestinal signs as the most common (Table 2). Specifically, the most common adverse events included ataxia and polyphagia, followed by sedation, hyperactivity, increased serum creatinine activity, vomiting and diarrhoea, disorientation and polydipsia. Less commonly, polyuria, anxiety, tachypnea,

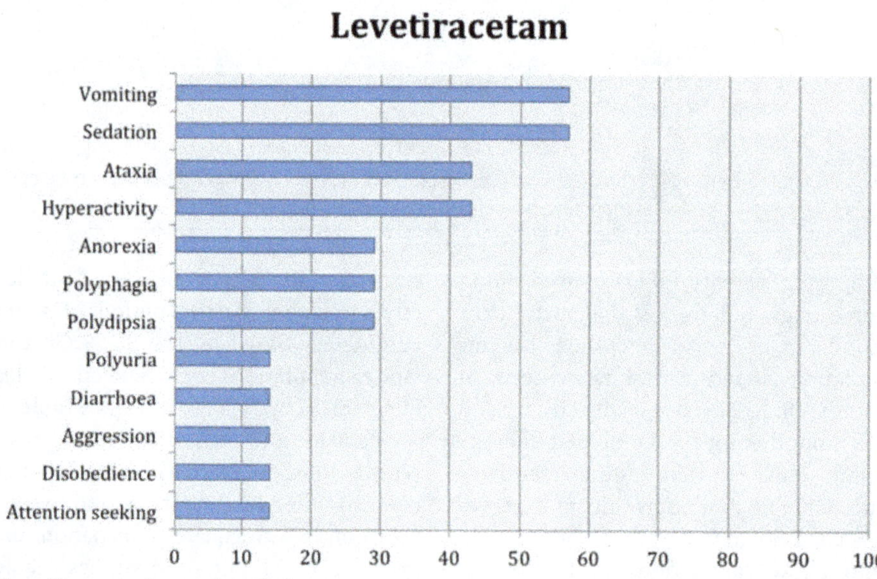

Fig. 7 Proportion of specific type I adverse effects for levetiracetam. Each adverse effect represents the percentage of studies that reported this specific adverse effect for levetiracetam monotherapy and/or adjunctive therapy

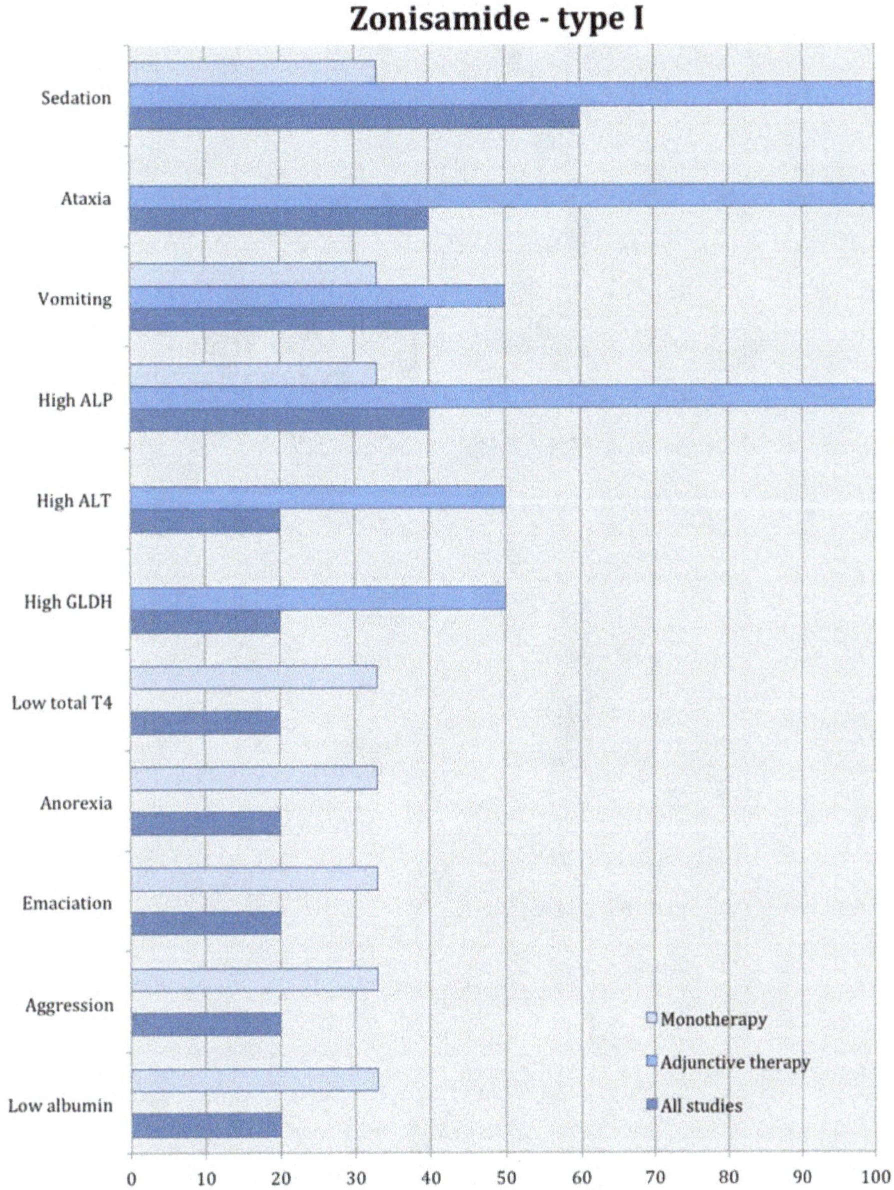

Fig. 8 Proportion of specific type I adverse effects for zonisamide. Each adverse effect represents the percentage of studies that reported this specific adverse effect for zonisamide monotherapy and adjunctive therapy

hypersalivation, decrease in sight and motor activity, prolapsed nictitating membrane and increased sensitivity to sound were reported (Fig. 4).

It is worth mentioning that the two GLP toxicity studies [112] and the ELAS part of one study [25] reported a few further adverse effects. However, these specific adverse effects were not included in the assessment above (see Table 2 for details) because higher than therapeutic doses were administered (3X, 5X or higher the recommended dose) which intended to evaluate the potential toxicity and tolerability of the drug. The same studies showed no adverse effects when imepitoin was administered in the recommended doses (≤30 mg/kg) apart from vomiting, hypersalivation and prolapsed nictitating membrane (as described above).

Adequate data to allow calculations of the prevalence of adverse effects was reported in 5/9 (55 %) of the studies (Table 2). From these, only two studies showed >50 % prevalence of adverse effects for the specific treatment periods within which they were conducted. However, one of the studies included a group of dogs receiving imepitoin adjunctive therapy to phenobarbital or primidone and therefore the prevalence may have been overestimated in these. Based on the 95 % CIs, the majority of the combined study populations experienced adverse effects in only one study (Table 2).

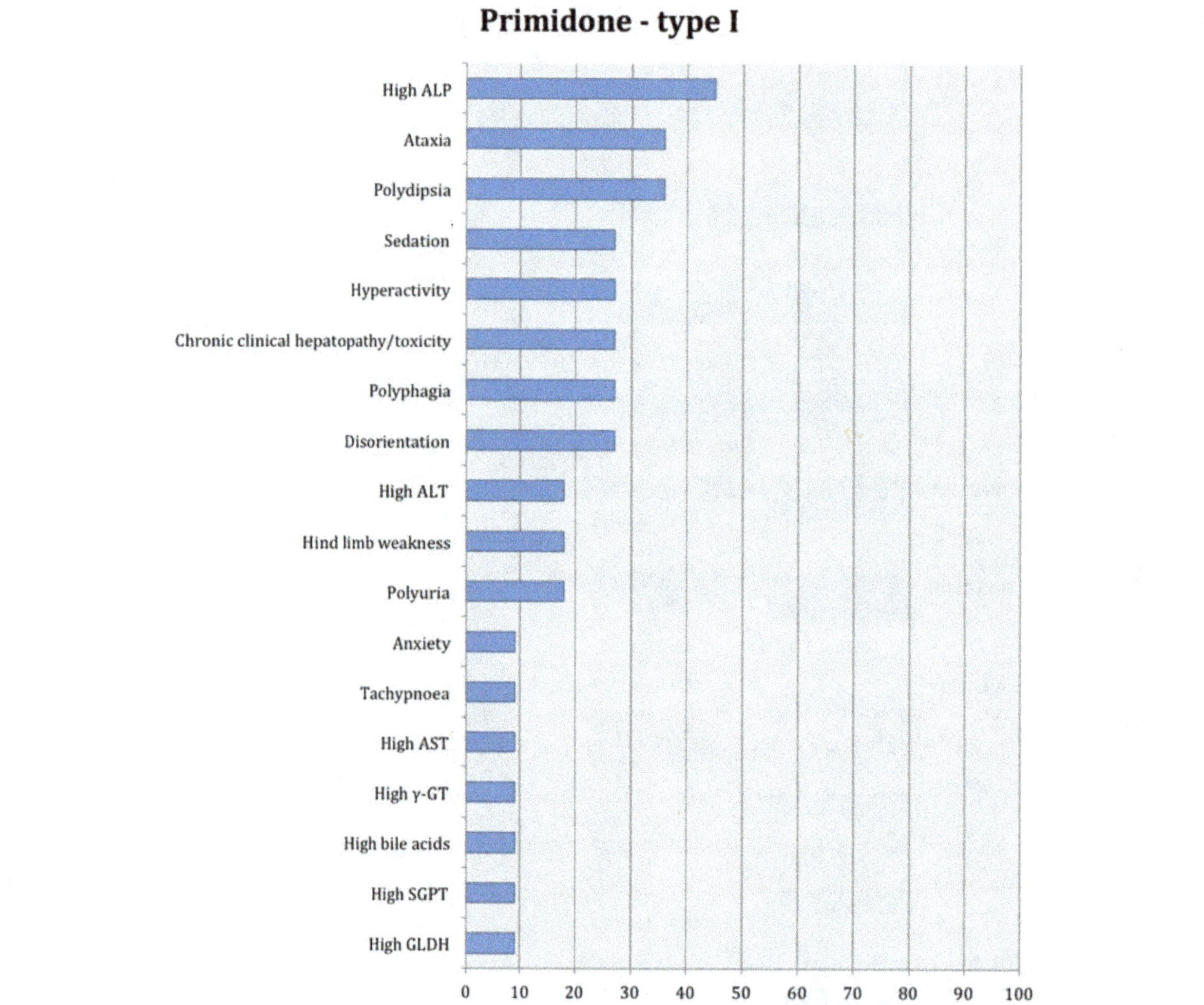

Fig. 9 Proportion of specific type I adverse effects for primidone. Each adverse effect represents the percentage of studies that reported this specific adverse effect for primidone monotherapy

Adequate information about the treatment period was reported in 7/9 (78 %) (Table 2). From these, in 6/7 (86 %) the treatment period was relatively short (<6 months). Adequate information about the doses was provided in all studies (Table 2). The imepitoin maintenance doses were mainly at the higher recommended dose, but the toxicology studies in which higher than recommended doses were used. Adequate information about the imepitoin serum levels was reported in 2/9 (22 %) studies (Table 2), but no correlation was detected between imepitoin serum levels and adverse effects.

Potassium bromide

There was an overall strong level of evidence provided for potassium bromide safety profile as monotherapy and weak as an adjunctive therapy. Twenty-one studies [3, 23, 29, 39, 51, 53, 66, 67, 73, 75, 77, 86, 88, 93, 96, 101, 102, 106, 110, 116] presented data about the safety of potassium bromide either as monotherapy (8 studies) [3, 23, 29, 39, 50, 51, 73, 86] or adjunctive therapy to phenobarbital and/or other AEDs (16 studies) [3, 39, 50, 53, 66, 67, 75, 77, 88, 93, 96, 101, 102, 106, 110, 116], giving a combined sample size of 1940 dogs.

Fifteen studies reported type I adverse effects, including neurological signs as the most common (Table 3). From these, 7/15 (47 %) and 10/15 (67 %) studies reported type I adverse effects for potassium bromide monotherapy and adjunctive therapy, respectively. Specifically, in all the studies, the adverse effects most commonly reported were ataxia followed by sedation, polyuria, polydipsia, polyphagia, paraparesis, hyperactivity, vomiting, increased serum ALP and ALT activity. Less commonly, diarrhoea, anorexia, aggression and then tetraparesis, skin issues, euthyroid sick syndrome, anisocoria, chronic clinical hepatopathy/toxicity, and lastly increased serum chloride, bile acids and AST

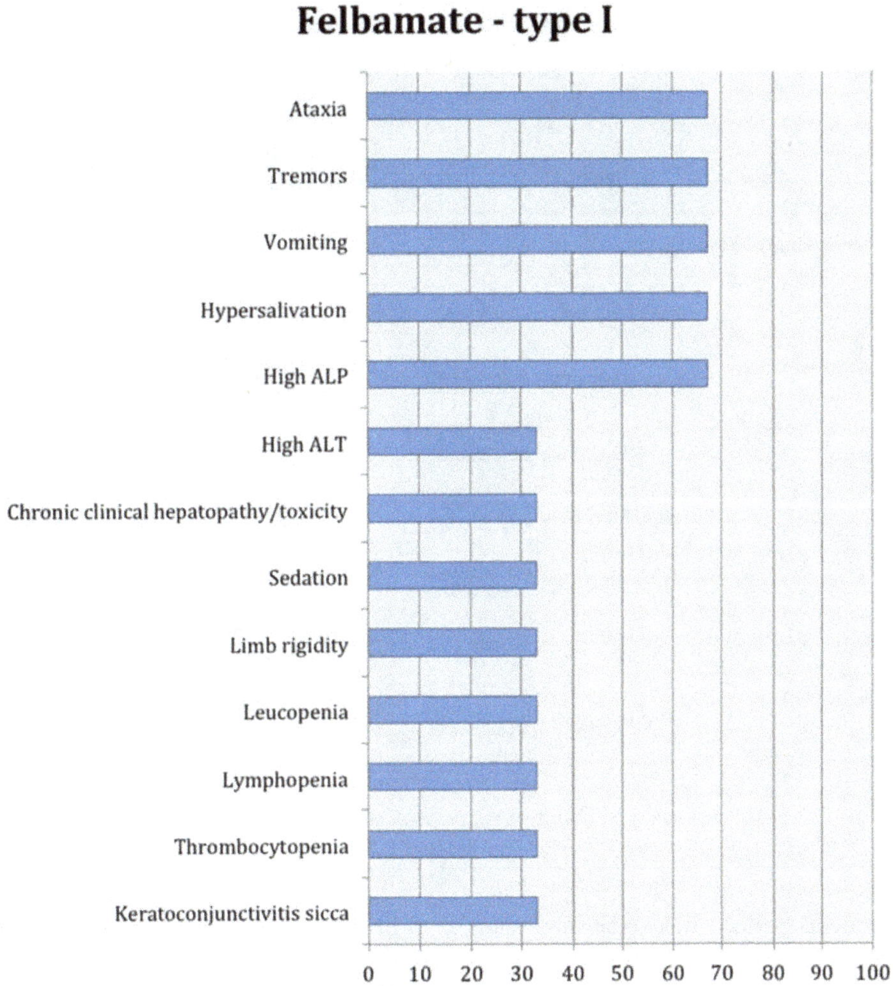

Fig. 10 Proportion of specific type I adverse effects for felbamate. Each adverse effect represents the percentage of studies that reported this specific adverse effect for felbamate monotherapy and/or adjunctive therapy

activity were reported. A similar pattern was shown in the adjunctive therapy studies; diarrhoea, skin conditions and increased amylase and lipase were not reported. In the monotherapy studies, the most common adverse effects were ataxia, sedation and hyperactivity followed by polyuria, polydipsia, polyphagia and diarrhoea; clinical hepatopathy/toxicity, tetraparesis, anisocora, euthyroid sick syndrome, increased serum bile acids and AST activity were not reported (Fig. 5). In one study [51], euthyroid sick syndrome was detected in both potassium bromide-treated and placebo group, indicating that this AED might not affect thyroid function. In another study [39], potassium bromide monotherapy did not affect the thyroxin serum levels.

Nine studies reported type II adverse effects, including gastro-intestinal signs as the most common (Table 3). Specifically, pancreatitis was most commonly reported, followed by panniculitis, generalized appendicular repetitive myoclonus, neuromyopathy with generalized lower motor signs and hyperchloraemia with negative anion gap (Fig. 6). The latter was detected in a dog, two days after a loading dose (200 mg/kg BID orally) of potassium bromide was given, but not after regular maintenance doses. In one study [50], although clinical pancreatitis due to potassium bromide or the phenobarbital/potassium bromide combination was suspected, it was not confirmed as the history and clinical status of the dogs were unknown.

Adequate data to allow calculations of the prevalence of adverse effects was reported in 14/21 (67 %) of the studies (Table 3). From these, 7/15 (47 %) showed >50 % prevalence of adverse effect for the specific period of treatment they were conducted. Based on the 95 % CI, the majority of the combined study population experienced at least one adverse effect in 7/15 (47 %) studies (Table 3).

Adequate information about the treatment period was reported in 17/21 (81 %) (Table 3). From these, in 5/17

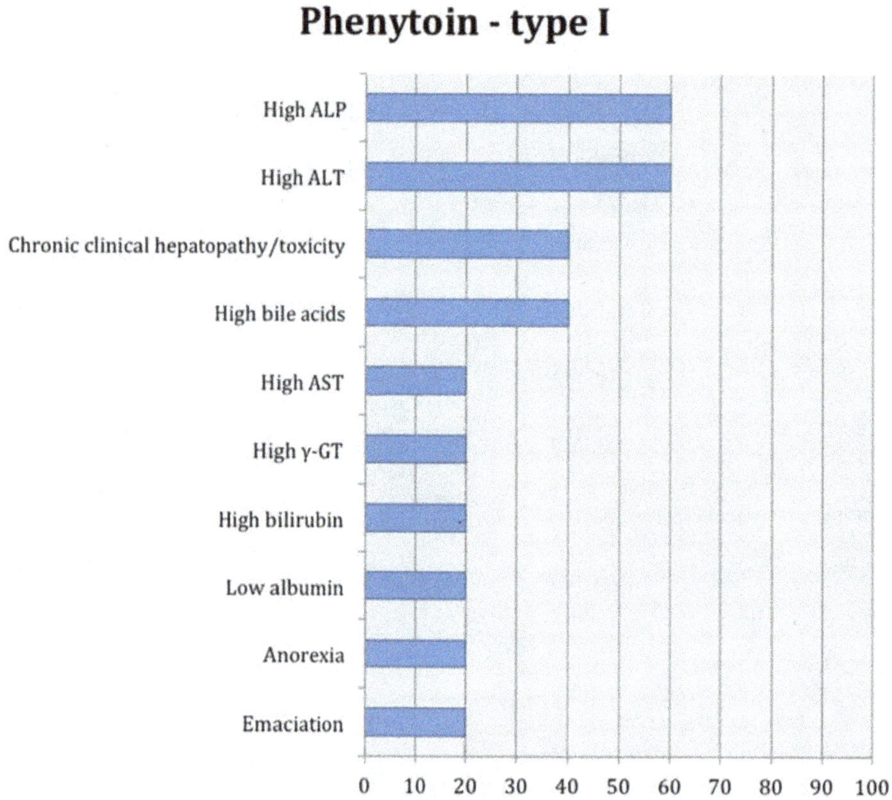

Fig. 11 Proportion of specific type I adverse effects for phenytoin. Each adverse effect represents the percentage of studies that reported this specific adverse effect for phenytoin monotherapy and/or adjunctive therapy

(29 %) the treatment period was relatively short (<6 months). Adequate information about the doses was provided in 13/21 (62 %) studies (Table 3). From these 9/13 (69 %) and 4/13 (31 %) reported doses for type I and type II adverse effects respectively. The maintenance doses were within the recommended dose margins in all but one study. Adequate information about the potassium bromide serum levels was reported in 16/21 (76 %) studies (Table 3). From these, 12/16 (75 %) and 6/16 (37 %) reported serum levels for type I and type II adverse effects respectively. The potassium bromide serum levels were higher than the recommended margins in type I adverse effects (7/12, 58 %), while within normal ranges for type II adverse effects (4/6, 67 %).

Levetiracetam

There was an overall strong level of evidence provided for the levetiracetam safety profile as monotherapy and adjunctive therapy. Six studies [24, 27, 53, 60, 72, 90] presented data about the safety profile of levetiracetam as monotherapy [27, 72] or adjunct to other AEDs (four remaining studies), giving a combined sample size of 129 dogs. One study [53] included both a clinical trial and retrospective case series part.

All the studies reported only type I adverse effects including neurological and gastro-intestinal signs as the most common (Table 4). Specifically, adverse effects most commonly included were vomiting and sedation followed by ataxia and hyperactivity. Less commonly, anorexia, polyphagia, polydipsia followed by polyuria, diarrhoea, aggression, disobedience and attention seeking were reported (Fig. 7). In the monotherapy study, only one episode of vomiting occurred. In one study, no adverse effects were reported.

Adequate data to allow calculations of the prevalence of adverse effects was reported in all studies (Table 4). From these, only two showed >50 % prevalence of adverse effects for the specific period of treatment during which it was conducted. Based on the 95 % CI, the majority of the population experienced adverse effects in none of the studies (Table 4).

Adequate information about the treatment period was reported in all of the studies (Table 4). From these, in 3/7 (43 %) the treatment period was relatively short (<6 months). Adequate information about the doses was provided in all of studies (Table 4). The maintenance doses exceeded the recommended dose range in two studies. Adequate information about the levetiracetam serum levels was reported in 2/7 (29 %) studies (Table 4),

Table 1 Details of number of dogs, 95 % CI affected cases, AED doses and serum levels, treatment period and adverse effects

Studies	AED	No of dogs treated	Prevalence	95 % CI affected cases	Doses of AEDs	Serum levels of AEDs	Treatment period	Body system affected and adverse effects	Most common adverse effects	Adverse effect type
Boothe et al. 2012	PHB	20	78.5 %	60.5 %–96.5 %	mean, 4.11+/−1.1; range, 3.9–4.9 mg/kg PO BID	mean, 27+/−6; range, 12.4–36 µg/mL	6 m	Neurological (ataxia, hyperactivity, sedation), GI (vomiting, diarrhea, PP), PU, PD, ClinPath (increased ALP, decreased albumin)	ataxia, sedation, increased serum ALP, decreased albumin	I
Heynold et al. 1997	PHB	37	35 %	19.6 %–50.4 %	mean, 2.5 mg/kg PO BID	range, 15–40 µg/ml	mean, 50; range, 8–108 m	Neurological (ataxia, sedation, aggression), GI (PP), Dermatological (itching)	sedation	I
Löscher et al. 2013	PHB	8	NA	NA	range, 10–40 mg/kg PO SID	14.7 µg/ml	2.5 m	Neurological (sedation, ataxia), PU, PD	sedation, ataxia, PU, PD	I
Gaskill et al. 2000	PHB	22	32 %	12.5 %–51.5 %	At 3 w: mean, 3.6+/−1.3; range, 1.3–6.0 mg/kg At 6 m: mean, 3.7+/−1.4; range, 1.3–8.3 mg/kg At 12 m: mean, 3.7+/−1.6; range, 1.3–8.3 mg/kg PO SID	At 3 w: mean, 58.6+/−15.0; range, 33–85 mmol/L At 6 m: 62.5+/−25.7; range, 8–120 mmol/L. At 12 m: mean, 62.2+/−23.51; range, 11–116 mmol/L	12 m	Endocrine (decreased total T4 levels, increased TSH levels, normal TSH stimulation test)	euthyroid sick syndrome	I
Steinberg 2004	PHB (monotherapy prior to the addition of other AEDs)	14	26.6 %	4.8 %–52.1 %	NA	PHB: mean, 32.1+/−14.4 µg/ml.	median, 17; range, 3.3–58.5 m	GI (chronic hepatotoxicity)	chronic hepatotoxicity	I
von Klopmann et al. 2006	PHB	34	68 %	52.3 %–83.7 %	NA	NA	NA	Endocrine (decreased total T4 levels, normal TSH levels, normal TSH stimulation test)	euthyroid sick syndrome	I
Chang et al. 2006	PHB	11	92.5 %	76.9 %–108.1 %	NA	NA	median, 18; range, 3–72 m	Neurological (ataxia, hyperactivity, sedation), GI (vomiting, diarrhea, PP), Dermatological (itching), PU, PD	PD, PU, PP, sedation, hyperactivity	I
Tipold et al. 2014	PHB	110	57.3 %	48.1 %–66.5 %	range, 2–6 mg/kg PO BID	<45 µg/mL	5 m	Neurological (sedation), GI (PP, diarrhea), PU, PD, ClinPath (increased ALP, γ-GT, ALT and GLDH)	sedation, PP, PU, PD	I
Fredso et al. 2015	PHB	6	93 %	70 %–114 %	median, 2.7; mean, 3; range 2.2–3 mg/kg PO BID	median, 77; mean, 77.3; range 55–111 µmol/L	2–12 m	Neurological (sedation, ataxia, hyperactivity, disobedience), GI (PP), PU, PD	PD, PP	I
Schwartz-Porsche et al. 1985	PHB	15	93 %	80.1 %–105.9 %	range, 5–17 mg/kg PO SID	range, 19–57 µg/ml	mean, 15; range, 7.3–32 m	Neurological (sedation, ataxia), GI (PP), PD, ClinPath (ALT, ALP, GLDH)	ataxia, sedation, PP, PD	I
Gaskill et al. 2005	PHB	12	NA	NA	median, 5; range, 2.1–12.9 mg/kg PO SID	mean, 22.8; range, 9.7–44.2 µg/ml	median, 20.4; range, 4–78 m	ClinPath (increased ALT, ALP)	increased ALT, ALP	I

Table 1 Details of number of dogs, 95 % CI affected cases, AED doses and serum levels, treatment period and adverse effects *(Continued)*

Farnbach et al. 1984	PHB	42	2.4 %	−2.2 %–7.2 %	range, 0.3–19.9 mg/kg PO SID	mean, 24.3; range, 6.5–81.3 μg/ml	NA	Neurological (hyperactivity)	hyperactivity	I
Gaskill and Kimber 2010	PHB	30	80 %	65.7 %–94.3 %	NA	NA	12 m	Neurological (ataxia, sedation, hyperactivity, aggression), GI (PP, anorexia, vomiting, diarrhoea), Dermatological (skin problems), ClinPath (increased ALP, ALT, lipase), PU, PD	PP, PU, PD, vomiting, skin problems, hyperactivity	I
Aitken et al. 2003	PHB	95	40 %	30.1 %–49.8 %	<2–> 10 mg/kg PO SID	<65–> 120 μmol/l	<3–> 12 m	ClinPath (increased ALT, ALP, γ-GT, GLDH, cholesterol, bile acids)	increased ALP, ALT, GLDH	I
Dayrell-Hart et al. 1991	PHB	18	NA	NA	median, 10.4; range, 3.1–27 mg/kg PO SID	mean, 49.7; range, 16–60 μg/ml (12 dogs had >40)	median, 39; range, 5–82 m	GI (hepatotoxicity) (also all dogs were ataxic and sedated)	NA	I
Andrik et al. 2010	PHB	30 (15 epileptic and 15 non-epileptic)	NA	NA	Epileptic dogs: 2 mg/kg PO BID (increased if necessary) Non-epileptic dogs: Initially at 2 mg/kg PO SID, then increased at 8 mg/kg PO SID	NA	Epileptic dogs: range, 12–60 m Non-epileptic dogs: 5 m	GI (chronic hepatotoxicity), ClinPath (increased ALP, ALT, AST, total bilirubin, decreased albumin and total protein)	increased ALT, ALP	I
Litchfield et al. 1972	PHB	4	NA	NA	range, 5–40 mg/kg IV SID	NA	0.5 m	ClinPath (increased ALP)	NA	I
Foster et al. 2000	PHB	Experimental dogs: 6 Epileptic dogs: 10	70 %	Experimental dogs: 0 % Epileptic dogs: 41.6 %–98.4 %	Experimental dogs: mean, 6 mg/kg; range, 5.9–6.4 mg/kg PO SID Epileptic dogs: range, 3.9–14.4 mg/kg PO SID	Experimental dogs: mean, 63+/−15, range, <65–194 μmol/L Epileptic dogs: mean, 110; range, 72–171 μmol/L	Experimental dogs: 3 m Epileptic dogs: range, 14–92 m	ClinPath (increased ALP, ALT, cholesterol)	increased ALP	I
Gaskil et al. 1999	PHB	78	40 %	28.8 %–50.6 %	median 4; range, 1–16.4 mg/kg PO SID	median, 17.6; range, 4–70 μg/ml	median, 12.5; range, 0.3–96	Endocrine (decreased total T4, free T4, increased TSH) Also, ClinPath abnormalities were reported, i.e. increased ALT, ALP, AST, γ-GT, fasting bile acids and cholesterol, but no further details are provided.	eythyroid sick syndrome	I
Muller et al. 2000	PHB	12	91.6 %	100 % or 50.5 %–99.5 %	mean, 5; range, 4.8–6.6 mg/kg PO BID	range, 20–40 μg/mL	7.1 m	Endocrine (decreased total T4, free T4, increased TSH, cholesterol and total T3), Neurological (sedation for the first 3 days) No significant PHB's effect on either of the adrenal function tests	euthyroid sick syndrome	I

Table 1 Details of number of dogs, 95 % CI affected cases, AED doses and serum levels, treatment period and adverse effects *(Continued)*

Muller et al. 2000	PHB	12	87.5 %	75.9 %–107.3 %	mean, 5; range, 4.8–6.6 mg/kg PO BID	range, 20–40 μg/ml	7.1 m	ClinPath (increased ALP, ALT, γ-GT, decreased albumin), Neurological (sedation for the first 3 days)	increased ALP, ALT, γ-GT	I
Kantrowitz et al. 1999	PHB	55	NA	NA	NA	median, 25.3; range, 8.0–74.3 μg/ml	median, 7 m; range, 1–120 m	Endocrine (decreased T4, increased TSH)	eythyroid sick syndrome	I
Chauvet et al. 1995	PHB	5	100 %	100 %	NA	range, 20–47 μg/ml	13 m	Endocrine (increased ACTH, altered ACTH stimulation and dexamethasone supression test), ClinPath (increased ALT, ALP, decreased albumin, cholesterol), PU, PD	increased ACTH, altered ACTH stimulation and dexamethasone supression test, increased ALT, ALP, decreased albumin, cholesterol	I
Balazs et al. 1978	PHB	4	100 %	100 %	40 mg/kg PO SID	NA	1.8 m	ClinPath (increased ALP)	increased ALP	I
Conning and Litchfield 1971	PHB	NA	NA	NA	NA	NA	NA	ClinPath (increased ALP)	increased ALP	I
Sturtevant et al. 1977	PHB	2	100 %	100 %	4.4 mg/kg PO TID	NA	1 m	ClinPath (Increased ALT, ALP)	increased ALT and ALP	I
Thrift et al. 2010	PHB	1	NA	NA	6.4 mg/kg PO BID	NA	2 m	ClinPath (anemia, increased ALT, ALP, AST)	idiosyncrasic anemia	I & II
Kube et al. 2006	PHB	1	NA	NA	Initially 5 mg/kg PO BID for 4 days, then 3 mg/kg PO BID	NA	2 m	Dyskinesia (twitching episodes)	NA	II
Steiner et al. 2008	PHB	118	14.4 %	8.1 %–20.7 %	NA	Unclear	NA	ClinPath (Increased cPLI)	NA	II
Gaskill et al. 2000	PHB	88	9 %	3.0 %–15.0 %	NA	range, 39–130 mol/L	16 m	GI (pancreatitis, increased amylase and/or lipase activities)	increased amylase and/or lipase activities	II
March et al. 2004	PHB	11	NA	NA	mean, 12.4+/−5.7; range, 3.8–19.8 mg/kg PO SID	mean, 43.5+/−15.1; range, 22.8–66 μg/ml	median, 6; range, 20.4–132 m	Dermatological (superficial necrolytic dermatitis)	NA	II
Weiss 2005	PHB	3	NA	NA	NA	NA	NA	Blood dyscrasias (bone marrow necrosis-myelofibrosis)	NA	II
Jacobs et al. 1998	PHB	2	NA	NA	Case 1: 2.2 mg/kg PO BID; Case 2: 4.4 mg/kg PO BID	NA	Case 1: 5 m; Case 2: 3 m	Blood dyscrasias (neutropenia, thrombocytopenia), ClinPath (increase ALP)	NA	II
Weiss et al. 2002	PHB	1	NA	NA	NA	NA	NA	Blood dyscrasias (myelofibrosis)	NA	II
Bevier et al. 2010	PHB	1	NA	NA	NA	NA	NA	Dermatological (superficial necrolytic dermatitis)	NA	II

Table 1 Details of number of dogs, 95 % CI affected cases, AED doses and serum levels, treatment period and adverse effects *(Continued)*

Bersan et al. 2014	PHB	16	NA	NA	median, 3; mean, 2.75+/−0.43; range, 1.60–7.25 mg/kg PO BID	median, 19; mean, 22.4+/−5.5; range, 13.2–30.5 µg/ml	median, 69.5; mean, 72.1+/−sd 45.8; range, 14–157 m	Blood dyscrasias (anemia and/or thrombocytopenia and/or neutropenia and/or pancytopenia)	anemia, pancytopenia	II
Volk et al. 2008 (case series)	PHB (monotherapy prior to the addition of other AEDs)	8	NA	NA	NA but was within normal reference values	NA	Approximately 2–3 m	Blood dyscrasias (bone marrow suppression)	NA	II
Habock and Pakozdy 2012	PHB	37	22 %	16.8 %–57.2 %	NA	NA	>1 m	Blood dyscrasias (anemia and/or thrombocytopenia and/or neutropenia and/or pancytopenia)	NA	II
Von Klopmann et al. 2006	PHB	1	NA	NA	2 mg/kg PO BID	NA		Blood dyscrasias (pancytopenia)	NA	II
Bizzeti et al. 2006	PHB	7	14.4 %	−11.6 %–40.2 %	NA	NA	NA	Pancreatitis, ClinPath (Increased amylase, lipase, cPLI)	NA	II
Mathis et al. 2014	PHB	1	NA	NA	2.1 mg/kg PO BID	27.5 µg/dL	6 m	Blood dyscrasias (bone marrow supression)	NA	II
Daminet et al. 1999	PHB	9	0 %	0 %	Initially 1.8–3 for one week, then 2.7–4.5 mg/kg PO BID	range, 65–150 pmol/L	0.8 m	No adverse effects	NA	NA
Dyer et al. 1994	PHB	6	0 %	0 %	5 mg/kg PO BID	range, 18–37 µg/ml	2 m	No PHB's effect on endogenous ACTH and ACTH stimulation test	NA	NA

Abbreviations: *AED(s)* anti-epileptic drug(s), *BID* bis in die (twice daily), *Chloraz* Chlorazepate, *CSF* cerebrospinal fluid, *CL* confidence level, *Gaba* Gabapentin, *IE* idiopathic epilepsy, *LEV* Levetiracetam, *m* month(s), *NA* Not Available, *PHB* phenobarbital, *PD* polydipsia, *PU* polyuria, *PP* polyphagia, *PBr* potassium bromide, *Prim* primidone, *PO* per os, *SID* semel in die (once daily), *TID* ter in die (three times daily), *TPM* topiramate, *w* week(s), *y* year(s)

Table 2 Details of number of dogs, 95 % CI affected cases, AED doses and serum levels, treatment period and adverse effects

Studies	AED	No of dogs treated	Prevalence	95 % CI affected cases	Doses of AEDs	Serum levels of AEDs	Treatment period	Body system affected and adverse effects	Most common adverse effects	Adverse effect type
Rundfeldt et sl. 2015	Imepitoin	127 Imepitoin high dose group: 66 Imepitoin low dose group: 61	Imepitoin high dose group: 86 % Imepitoin low dose group: 82 %	Imepitoin high dose group: 77.6 %–94.3 % Imepitoin low dose group: 72.3 %–91.6 %	Imepitoin high dose group: 30 mg/kg PO BID Imepitoin low dose group: 1 mg/kg PO BID	NA	1st phase: 3 m 2nd phase: 3 m	Neurological (hyperactivity, disorientation), musculoskeletal (unspecified), gastro-intestinal (unspecified), respiratory (unspecified), urogenital (unspecified), other systems (unspecified), general (unspecified)	Disorientation, hyperactivity	I
Tipold et al. 2014	Imepitoin	116	46.6 %	37.5 %–55.7 %	10–30 mg/kg PO BID	NA	5 m	Neurological (sedation, hyperactivity), GI (PP, diarrhoea), PU, PD, Renal/Urinary disorders, ClinPath (increased creatinine)	PP, PD, PU, sedation, hyperactivity	I
Tipold et al. 2014 (ELAS)	Imepitoin	32	NA	NA	30, 90 or 150 mg/kg PO BID (adverse effects occurred mainly in the higest doses, i.e. 3X and 5X the recommended dose)	NA	6 m	Neurological (loss of righting reflex, ataxia, intermittent tremors, decreased activity, nystagmus), GI (vomiting, hypersalivation, white material in the faeces), ClinPath (increased creatinine), Ophtalmological (lacrimation, eye dryness, eye discharges, relaxed nictitating membranes, eyelid closure)	NA (infrequent adverse effects)	I
Loscher et al. 2004, Rieck et al. 2006	Imepitoin as monotherapy (12 dogs) and imepitoin as an adjunct to PHB or Primidone (17 dogs)	29	58.6 %	40.7 %–76.5 %	Imepitoin: Initially 5 mg/kg PO BID for 1 week, then 10–30 mg/kg PO BID. PHB: 6–23 mg/kg PO SID. Primidone: 25–53 mg/kg PO SID	Imepitoin: mean, 4,000; range, 3400–7300 ng/ml (2 h after dosing) and mean, 650 ng/ml (12 h after dosing). PHB: range, 15–45 μg/ml (2 dogs with adverse effects had 56.6–58.9 lg/mL). Prim: NA	mean, 7.7 ± 0.7 m	Neurological (ataxia, sedation), GI (PP), ClinPath (increased ALT, ALP, GLDH)	PP	I
Löscher et al. 2004 (ELAS)	Imepitoin	1st experiment: 6 2nd experiment: 6	0 %	0 %	1st experiment: 5 mg/kg PO BID 2nd experiment: 40 mg/kg PO BID	1st experiment: range, 20–120 ng/ml 2nd experiment: range, 4800–7400 ng/ml	1st experiment: 1.2 m 2nd experiment: 1.2 m	1st experiment: none 2nd experiment: none but increase in body weight	NA	I
EMA report 2012 (US field trial)	Imepitoin	110	NA	NA	range, 10–30 mg/kg PO BID	NA	NA	Neurological (ataxia, hyperactivity, anxiety, disorientation), ClinPath (increased enzymes-unclear which) tachypnoea, PD	ataxia, hyperactivity, anxiety, PD, increased liver enzymes	I

Table 2 Details of number of dogs, 95 % CI affected cases, AED doses and serum levels, treatment period and adverse effects *(Continued)*

EMA report 2012 (unpublished clinical trials: Tipold 2006; Heit 2011; de Vries 2011)	Imepitoin	NA	NA	NA	30 mg/kg PO BID (Unclear if other doses were also used)	NA	NA	Neurological (ataxia, decreased motor activity, disorientation, hyperactivity, decreased sight, increased sensitivity to sound), GI (vomiting, diarrhoea, polyphagia), Renal (increase creatinine)	ataxia, decreased motor activity, disorientation, hyperactivity, decreased sight, increased sensitivity to sound, vomiting, diarrhoea	I
EMA report (GLP toxicity study 1)	Imepitoin	32	0 %	Doses of 0, 31.6 mg/kg: 0 % Other doses: NA	Doses of 0, 31.6, 100 and 316 mg/kg/day PO	NA	1 m	Neurological (decreased motor activity), GI (hypersalivation, vomiting), ECG modifications No adverse effects in the recommended doses; adverse effects occurred only in the highest doses	NA	I
EMA report (GLP toxicity study 2)	Imepitoin	NA	NA	NA	Doses of 0, 31.6, 82.5 and 215 mg/kg/day PO	NA	3.2 m (followed by a 1.2 m recovery period)	Only vomiting occurred in the 0 and 31.6 mg/kg/day doses; adverse effects occurred only in the highest doses	NA	I

Abbreviations: *AED(s)* anti-epileptic drug(s), *BID* bis in die (twice daily), *Chloraz* chlorazepate, *CSF* cerebrospinal fluid, *CL* confidence level, *Gaba* Gabapentin, *IE* idiopathic epilepsy, *LEV* Levetiracetam, *m* month(s), *NA* Not Available, *PHB* phenobarbital, *PD* polydipsia, *PU* polyuria, *PP* polyphagia, *PBr*, potassium bromide, *Prim* primidone, *PO* per os, *SID* semel in die (once daily), *TID* ter in die (three times daily), *TPM* topiramate, *w* week(s), *y* year(s)

Table 3 Details of number of dogs, 95 % CI affected cases, AED doses and serum levels, treatment period and adverse effects

Studies	AED	No of dogs treated	Prevalence	95 % CI affected cases	Doses of AEDs	Serum levels of AEDs	Treatment period	Body system affected and adverse effects	Most common adverse effects	Adverse effect type
Boothe et al. 2012	PBr	23	78.5 %	61.7 %–95.3 %	mean, 30.6; range, 26–35 mg/kg PO BID	mean, 1.9 +/− 0.6; range, 0.9–3.3 mg/ml	approximately 6 m	Neurological (ataxia, hyperactivity, sedation), GI (vomiting, diarrhoea, PP), PU, PD	sedation, hyperactivity, ataxia, PD, PU	I
Pearce 1990	PBr as an adjunct to PHB	10	40 %	9.6 %–70.4 %	PBr: 22 mg/kg PO SID (dose increases occurred) PHB: median, 3.3; mean, 3.8 mg/kg PO BID (dose was reduced by a mean of 50 % in 7/10 dogs during the PBr treatment)	PBr: mean, 810; range, 500–1625 mg/l PHB: mean, 29.7; range, 17–45 ug/ml	median, 7; mean, 7.8 m	Neurological (ataxia, sedation, hyperactivity), PU, PD	ataxia, letargy, PU, PD	I
March et al. 2002	PBr	6	20 %	−12.0 %–52.0 %	30 mg/kg PO BID	median, 245; range, 178–269 mg/dL	3.9 m (adverse effects occurred after this period when dose adjustments occurred (NA))	Neurological (ataxia, paraparesis, hyperactivity)	ataxia, paraparesis	I
Rossmeisl et al. 2009	PBr as an adjunct to PHB and/or other AEDs	1298	2 %	1.2 %–2.8 %	PBr: 44.9+/−1.7 mg/kg PO SID PHB: 6.3+/−0.4 mg/kg PO SID	PBr: 3.7+/−0.3 mg/ml PHB: 31.4+/−1.2 µg/dl	NA	Neurological (sedation, ataxia, paraparesis, tetraparesis)	sedation, ataxia, paraparesis, tetraparesis	I
Dayrell-Hart B et al. 1996	PBr	238	10.9 %	6.9 %–14.9 %	NA	21 affected dogs had >2.3 mg/ml and 5 affected dogs had <0.5 mg/ml	NA	Neurological (ataxia, sedation)	ataxia, sedation	I
Podell and Fenner 1993	PBr as an adjunct to PHB and/or other AEDs	23	78 %	61.1 %–94.9 %	PBr: mean, 20.75; range, 13–40 PO BID PHB: NA	PBr: 161 mg/dl PHB: 37.8 mcg/ml	mean, 15; range, 4–33 m	Neurological (ataxia, sedation), GI (PP), ClinPath (increased serum chloride), PU, PD	PU, PD, PP, sedation	I
Chang et al. 2006	PBr (monotherapy or as an adjunct to PHB)	Monotherapy: 4 Adjunctive Therapy: 10	Monotherapy: 62.5 % Adjunctive Therapy: 95 %	Monotherapy: 15.0–110.0 % Adjunctive therapy: 81 %–109 %	NA	NA	median, 18; range, 3–72 m	Neurological (ataxia, hyperactivity), Dermatological (pruritus), GI (PP), The adjunctive therapy group had also PU, PD and vomiting/diarhoea	Ataxia, hyperactivity, pruritus, PP	I
Yohn et al. 1992	PBr as an adjunct to PHB	1	NA	NA	NA	2.7 mg/ml	1 m	Neurological (sedation, ataxia, paraparesis, anisocoria)	NA	I

Table 3 Details of number of dogs, 95 % CI affected cases, AED doses and serum levels, treatment period and adverse effects *(Continued)*

Kantowitz et al. 1999	PBr (monotherapy or as an adjunct to PHB)	Monotherapry: 15 Adjunctive therapy: 8	NA	NA	NA	Monotherapy: median, 1985; range, 500–3419 mg/dL Adjunctive therapy: PBr: median, 1399; range, 584–2438 mg/dL. PHB: median, 22.4; range, 10.9–40 µg/ml	Monotherapy: median, 14.5; range, 3–37 m Adjunctive therapy: PBr: median, 5; range, 3–72 m. PHB: median, 22; range, 3–96 m	Monotherapy: Normal Adjunctive therapy: Endocrine (decreased total T4, free T4)	NA	I
Srivastava et al. 2013	PBr as an adjunct to PHB	6	100 %	100 %	PBr: 30 mg/kg PO SID PHB: Initially 2.5 mg/kg, then 5 mg/kg PO SID.	NA	mean, 11.50+/− 1.23; range, 8–15 m (on PHB). Then, PBr started and 3 m later a reduction of 50 % in the dose of PHB was performed. After 6 m, PHB was completely withdrawn.	Neurological (ataxia), GI (hepatoxicity, anorexia, PP), ClinPath (increased ALT, ALP, AST, bile acids), PU, PD (polyphagia, PU, PD appeared after 1–1.5 years of PBr therapy)	PU, PD, PP	I
Shaw et al. 1996	PBr as an adjunct to PHB	1	NA	NA	PBr: 20 mg/kg PO SID PHB: 3.75 mg/kg PO BID	PBr: 1100 mg/l. PHB: 20.4 µg/ml	Approximately 21 m	After PBr initiation: Neurological (sedation, ataxia)	NA	I
Paull et al. 2003	PBr	5	60 %	17.1 %–102.9 %	Initially 100 mg/kg PO BID for 2 days. Then, 30 mg/kg PO SID for 180 days.	range, 88–300 mg/dL (only one dog was >300 mg/dl)	6 m	Endocrine (Euthyroid sick syndrome with decreased TT4 and normal TSH) Placebo group had the same results	NA	I
Stabile et al. 2014	PBr as an adjunct to PHB	1	NA	NA	PBr: Initially, 400 mg/kg divided in six daily doses for four days. Then, 14 mg/kg PO BID PHB: Initially, 2.7 mg/kg, then 5 mg/kg and finally 6.4 mg/kg PO BID.	PBr: 15.9 mg/ml; PHB: 23.7 µg/ml	≥26 m	Neurological (sedation, ataxia, generalised appendicular repetitive myoclonus), ClinPath (pseudohyperchlormia, increased ALP)	NA	I & II
Gaskill and Kimber 2010	PBr	32	85.9 %	73.8 %–98.0 %	NA	NA	12 m	Neurological (ataxia, sedation, hyperactivity, aggression), GI (PP, anorexia, vomiting, diarrhoea, pancreatitis), Dermatological (skin problems), ClinPath (increased ALP, ALT, amylase, lipase), PU, PD	vomiting, sedation, PP, PU, PD	I & II

Table 3 Details of number of dogs, 95 % CI affected cases, AED doses and serum levels, treatment period and adverse effects *(Continued)*

Volk et al. 2008	PBr as an adjunct to PHB (prior to addition of other AEDs)	14	100 %	100 %	PBr and PHB: NA but were within normal reference values	PBr: 1.7+/−0.4 mg/ml PHB: 35.5+/−6.3 µg/ml	≥2–6 m	Neurological (ataxia, aggression), GI (PP, vomiting, pancreatitis), ClinPath (increased ALT, ALP) PU, PD	increased ALT, ALP, ataxia, aggression	I & II
Gaskill et al. 2000	PBr as an adjunct to PHB	Clinical trial: 6 Case series: 19	Clinical trial: 50 % Case series: 37 %	Clinical trial: 10.0 %–90.0 % Case series: 15.3 %–58.7 % (pancreatitis); 47.5 %–89.3 % (increased enzymes only)	Clinical trial: NA Case series: NA	Clinical trial: NA Case series: PBr: range, 12.5-37.5 mmol/L; PHB: range, 54–190 imol/L	Clinical trial: approximately 1 year Case series: NA	GI (pancreatitis, increased amylase and/or lipase activities)	pancreatitis, increased amylase and/ or lipase activities	II
Steinmetz et al. 2012	PBr as an adjunct to PHB	1	NA	NA	101.19 mg/kg SID PO (added at the beginning of the 4th year) PHB: 4.9 mg/kg BID PO	PBr: 45 mmol/l PHB: 168.52 µmol/l	48 m (adverse effect occurred after the 48 m)	Neurological (neuromyopathy with generalised low motor signs)	NA	II
Mackay and Mitchell 1998	PBr as an adjunct to PHB	1	NA	NA	PBr: Initially 200 mg/kg PO BID for 3 days, then 30 mg/kg PO SID PHB: 5 mg/kg PO BID.	PBr: NA. PHB: 126 umol/L	3 d (signs started 3 d after the loading dose of PBr was initiated)	ClinPath (artifactual hyperchloraemia and negative anion gap), Neurological (pacing, disorientation), GI (vomiting) The Neurological and GI signs were attributed to hypercloraemia	NA	II
Boynosky and Stokking 2014	PBr as an adjunct to PHB	2	NA	NA	Initially 40 mg/kg PO SID, then 60 mg/kg PO SID (case 1) or 86 mg/ kg PO SID (case 2)	Case 1: 2.9 mg/mL; Case 2: initially 0.8, then 3 mg/ml (after 7.5 months of treatment)	12 m [adverse effects occured 3 (case 1) and 8 (case 2) m after the dose increase]	Dermatological (panicculitis) accompanied by sedation and anorexia	NA	II
Steiner et al. 2008	PBr (monotherapy or as an adjunct to PHB)	Monotherapy: 98 Adjunctive therapy: 121	14 %	Monotherapy: 8.2 %–22.4 % Adjunctive: 5.9 %–17.3 %	NA	range, 0.5–4.2 mg/ml (majority of dogs; range, 1–2 mg/ml)	NA	ClinPath (increased cPLI)	NA	II
Bizzeti et al. 2006	PBr as an adjunct to PHB	7	43 %	6.1 %–79.4 %	NA	NA	NA	Pancreatitis, ClinPath (increased amylase, lipase,cPLI)	NA	II

Abbreviations: *AED(s)* anti-epileptic drug(s), *BID* bis in die (twice daily), *Chloraz* Chlorazepate, *CSF* cerebrospinal fluid, *CL* confidence level, *Gaba* Gabapentin, *IE* idiopathic epilepsy, *LEV* Levetiracetam, *m* month(s), *NA* Not Available, *PHB* phenobarbital, *PD* polydipsia, *PU* polyuria, *PP* polyphagia, *PBr* potassium bromide, *Prim* primidone, *PO* per os, *SID* semel in die (once daily), *TID* ter in die (three times daily); *TPM* Topiramate; *w* week(s), *y* year(s)

Table 4 Details of number of dogs, 95 % CI affected cases, AED doses and serum levels, treatment period and adverse effects

Studies	AED	No of Dogs	Prevalence	95 % CI affected case	Doses of AEDs	Serum levels of AEDs	Treatment period	Body system affected and adverse effects	Most common adverse effects	Adverse effect type
Volk et al. 2008	LEV as an adjunct to PHB and/or PBr	14	7.14 %	−6.3 %–20.6 %	LEV: 10 mg/kg for 2 m, 20 mg/kg for further 2 m, 10–20 mg/kg until 6 m and then 10–20 mg/kg long-term PO TID PHB and PBr: NA but were within normal reference values	PHB: 35.5+/−6.3 μg/ml, PBr:1.7+/−0.4 mg/ml, (prior LEV initiation and 2 m after initiation).	≥2–6 m	Neurological (sedation)	sedation	I
Volk et al. 2008 (case series)	LEV as an adjunct to PHB and/or PBr and/or gaba and/or TPM	8	25 %	−2.6 %–18.6 %	LEV: 30–32 mg/kg PO TID TID PHB and PBr: NA but were within normal reference values	NA	Approximately 2–3 m	Neurological (sedation)	sedation	I
Muñana et al. 2012	LEV as an adjunct to PHB and/or PBr and/or gaba and/or zonisamide	28	57 %	38.7 %–75.3 %	LEV: median, 20.6; range, 17–23.1 PO TID PHB: median, 7.2; range, 3.8–17.2 mg/kg PO SID. PBr: median, 34.0; range, 13.6–84.2 mg/kg PO SID	LEV: range, <2-50.8 μg/mL. PHB: mean, 28.13; range, 15.77–36.40 μg/mL PBr: mean, 186.20; range, 71.18–390 mg/dL	9 m (during the 5th m no AED was administered)	Neurological (ataxia, hyperactivity), GI: (anorexia, vomiting)	ataxia	I
Steinberg 2004	LEV as an adjunct to PHB and PBr	15	0 %	0 %	LEV: range, 7.1–23.8 mg/kg PO TID PB and PBr: NA	PHB: mean, 32.1+/−14.4 μg/ml. LEV: NA PBr: 2.2+/−0.7 mg/dl	median, 38; range, 13.8–95.5 m	No adverse effects attributed to LEV	NA	I
Packer et al. 2015	LEV as an adjunct to PHB and PBr	52	46 %	32.5 %–59.6 %	Maintenance group: mean, 19.5; range, 9–26 mg/kg PO TID. Pulse group: Initial dose at 60 mg/kg followed by 20 mg/kg PO TID	NA	Maintenance group: mean, 1.4; range, 0.3–7.5 y Pulse group: mean, 0.8; range, 0.3–3.4 y	Neurological (ataxia, sedation, aggression, hyperactivity), GI (PP, vomiting, diarrhoea), PD (Three times more often in the pulse group)	ataxia, sedation	I
Fredso et al. 2015	LEV	6	84 %	53.8 %–113.2 %	median, 31; mean, 30.4; range, 27.6–51.5 PO TID	median, 114; mean, 93; range, 18–137 μmol/L	2–12 m	Neurological (ataxia, sedation, hyperactivity, disobedience, attention seeking), GI (PP, anorexia, vomiting), PU, PD	PP	I
Moore et al. 2010	LEV	6	16.6 %	−13.2 %–46.4 %	At day one, a single dose was administered: mean, 21.7; range, 20.8–22.7 mg/kg PO. Then: range, 20.8–22.7 mg/kg PO TID for 6 d	289.31+/−51.68 μg/mL	0.25 m	GI (vomiting) (only one episode at the first d)	NA	I

Abbreviaions: *AED(s)* anti-epileptic drug(s), *BID* bis in die (twice daily), *Chloraz* Chlorazepate, *CSF* cerebrospinal fluid, *CL* confidence level, *Gaba* Gabapentin, *IE* idiopathic epilepsy, *LEV* Levetiracetam, *m* month(s), *NA* Not Available, *PHB* phenobarbital, *PD* polydipsia, *PU* polyuria, *PP* polyphagia, *PBr* potassium bromide, *Prim* primidone, *PO* per os, *SID* semel in die (once daily), *TID* ter in die (three times daily), *TPM* Topiramate, *w* week(s), *y* year(s)

Table 5 Details of number of dogs, 95 % CI affected cases, AED doses and serum levels, treatment period and adverse effects

Study	AED	No of dogs	Prevalence	95 % CI affected case	Doses of AEDs	Serum levels of AEDs	Treatment period	Body system affected and adverse effects	Most common adverse effects	Adverse effect type
von Klopmann et al. 2007	Zonisamide as an adjunct to PHB and/or PBr	11	72.7 %	46.4 %–99.0 %	Zonisamide: mean, 8.9; range, 5–11 mg/kg PO BID PHB and PBr: NA but continued unchanged or reduced if appropriate	Zonisamide: median, 19.2; range, 15.2–38.4 lg/ml. PHB: median, 121; range, 66–150 5 lmol/l. PBr: median 1.2; range, 0.7–1.7 g/l.	range, 4–17 m	Neurological (ataxia, sedation), ClinPath (increased ALP, ALT and GLDH)	ataxia, sedation, increased ALP	I
Chung et al. 2012	Zonisamide	10	10 %	−8.6 %–28.6 %	median 9.5; mean 8.65; range 2.5–12 mg/kg PO BID	range, 15.24–22.41 mg/mL	median, 12; mean, 11.2 m	Neurological (sedation), GI (vomiting, anorexia)	sedation, vomiting, anorexia	I
Dewey et al. 2004	Zonisamide as an adjunct to PHB and/or PBr and/or felbamate and/or gaba and/or cloraz	12	50 %	21.7 %–78.3 %	Zonisamide: mean, 8.9; range, 5–11 mg/kg PO BID. Other AEDs: NA but in 9/12 dogs concurrent AEDs doses were eliminated or reduced.	Zonisamide: median, 23.5; mean, 21.2 µg/mL.	mean, 8; median, 9; range, 2–18 m	Neurological (ataxia, sedation), GI (vomiting), ClinPath (ALP)	ataxia, increased ALP	I
Walker et al. 1988	Zonisamide	40	NA	NA	10, 30 or 75 mg/kg PO SID	range, 10–140 ug/ml	13 m	Neurological (aggression) GI (emaciation), ClinPath (increased ALP, decreased albumin)	aggression, increased ALP, decreased albumin	I
Boothe et al. 2008	Zonisamide	8	0 %	0 %	6.9 mg/kg IV SID or 10.3 mg/kg PO SID	range, 6–55 mcg/ml	2 m	Endocrine (Decreased total T4) (However, total T4 was only slightly decreased at the study end)	NA	I
Cook et al. 2011	Zonisamide	1	NA	NA	range, 7.9–8.4 mg/kg PO BID	38 µg/mL	18 m	ClinPath (mixed acid base disorder)	NA	II
Miller et al. 2011	Zonisamide	1	NA	NA	7.7 mg/kg PO BID	NA	0.3 m	GI (hepatoxicity)	NA	II

***Abbreviations*: *AED(s)* anti-epileptic drug(s), *BID* bis in die (twice daily), *Chloraz* Chlorazepate, *CSF* cerebrospinal fluid, *CL* confidence level, *Gaba* Gabapentin, *IE* idiopathic epilepsy, *LEV* Levetiracetam, *m* month(s), *NA* Not Available, *PHB* phenobarbital, *PD* polydipsia, *PU* polyuria, *PP* polyphagia, *PBr* potassium bromide, *Prim* primidone, *PO* per os, *SID* semel in die (once daily), *TID* ter in die (three times daily), *TPM* Topiramate, *w* week(s), *y* year(s)**

Table 6 Details of number of dogs, 95 % CI affected cases, AED doses and serum levels, treatment period and adverse effects

Studies	AED	No of dogs treated	Prevalence	95 % CI affected cases	Doses of AEDs	Serum levels of AEDs	Treatment period	Body system affected and adverse effects	Most common adverse effects	Adverse effect type
Schwartz-Porsche et al. 1982	Prim	30	NA	NA	range, 13–100 mg/kg PO SID	range, 6–37 μg/ml	range 6–96 m	Neurological (sedation, hind limb weakness), GI (PP), PU, PD, ClinPath (ALP, SGPT)	sedation, PU, PD	I
Schwartz-Porsche et al. 1985	Prim	20	NA	NA	range, 17–107 mg/kg PO SID	range, 0.5–58 μg/ml	mean, 14; range, 6.0–35 m	Neurological (sedation, hind limb weakness, ataxia), GI (PP), PD, ClinPath (ALT, ALP, GLDH)	sedation, PU, increased ALT, ALP and GLDH	I
Farnbach et al. 1984	Prim	23	4.3 %	−4.0 %–12.6 %	range, 15.2–82 mg/kg PO SID	range, 4.8–70.7 μg/ml	NA	Neurological (sedation, ataxia)	sedation, ataxia	I
Cunningham et al. 1983	Prim	15	NA	NA	10.6–39.4 mg/kg PO TID	mean, 2.4 μg/ml	9 m	Neurological (disorientation, ataxia, hyperactivity, pacing), GI (PP), PU, PD	PU, PD, PP, drowsiness, ataxia	I
Poffenbarger et al. 1985	Prim (monotherapy or as an adjunct to PHB)	3	NA	NA	Varied	NA	8–84 m	GI (chronic hepatopathy/ toxicity-hepatic chirosis)	chronic hepatopathy/toxicity	I
Bunch et al. 1987	Prim	1	NA	NA	13 mg/kg PO BID	NA	4 d	Neurological (hyperactivity)	NA	I
Bunch et al. 1984	Prim	22	93 %	82.3 %–103.6 %	Prim: 33+/−19 mg/kg PO SID Other AEDs: NA	NA	range, 6–120 m	GI (chronic hepatopathy/toxicity), ClinPath (increased ALP, ALT, AST, γ-GT, bile acids)	chronic hepatoxicity, increased ALP, ALT, AST, bile acids	I
Bunch et al. 1982	Prim	2	NA	NA	Case 1: 750 mg in total PO BID Case 2: 250 mg in total PO BID	NA	24 m	GI (chronic hepatopathy/toxicity)	chronic hepatoxicity	I
EPAR (US field trial)	Prim	110	NA	NA	NA	NA	NA	Neurological (ataxia, hyperactivity, anxiety, disorientation), ClinPath (increased enzymes-unclear which) tachypnoea, PD	ataxia, PD, increased liver enzymes	I
Raw and Gaskell 1985	Prim	52	35 %	22.0 %–48.0 %	NA	NA	48 m	Neurological (ataxia), GI (PP), PD	ataxia, PD, PP	
Meyer and Noonan 1981	Prim	6	100 %	100 %	30–40 mg/kg PO BID	NA	3 m	ClinPath (increased ALP, ALT)	increased ALT, ALP	I
Sturtevant et al. 1977	Prim	2	100 %	100 %	17.6 mg/kg POTID	NA	1 m	ClinPath (anemia, increased ALP)	increased ALP	I & II
Jacobs et al. 1998	Prim	1	NA	NA	25 mg/kg PO BID	NA	2 m	Blood dyscrasias (neutropenia, anemia, thrombocytopenia), ClinPath (decreased albumin, increased ALP)	NA	II
Henricks 1987	Prim	1	NA	NA	62 mg in total PO BID	NA	2 m	Dermatitis	NA	II
Balazs et al. 1978	Prim	4	0 %	0 %	40–80 mg/kg PO SID	NA	1.75 m	No adverse effects	NA	NA
Bunch et al. 1985	Prim	6	0 %	0 %	NA	NA	NA	No adverse effects	NA	NA

Abbreviations: *AED(s)* anti-epileptic drug(s), *BID* bis in die (twice daily), *Chloraz* Chlorazepate, *CSF* cerebrospinal fluid, *CL* confidence level, *Gaba* Gabapentin, *IE* idiopathic epilepsy, *LEV* Levetiracetam, *m* month(s), *NA* Not Available, *PHB* phenobarbital, *PD* polydipsia, *PU* polyuria, *PP* polyphagia, *PBr* potassium bromide, *Prim* primidone, *PO* per os, *SID* semel in die (once daily), *TID* ter in die (three times daily), *TPM* Topiramate, *w* week(s), *y* year(s)

Table 7 Details of number of dogs, 95 % CI affected cases, AED doses and serum levels, treatment period and adverse effects

Studies	AED	No of dogs	Prevalence	95 % CI affected cases	Doses of AEDs	Serum levels of AEDs	Treatment period	Body system affected and adverse effects	Most common adverse effects	Adverse effect type
Govendir et al. 2005	Gaba as an adjunct to PHB and/or PBr	17	76.5 %	56.3 %–96.6 %	Gaba: median, 35; range, 32–40 mg/kg PO SID. PHB: median, 8; range, 6–26 mg/kg PO SID. PBr: median, 24; range, 14–56 mg/kg PO SID.	Gabapentin: NA PHB and PBr: within normal reference values	4 m	Neurological (sedation, ataxia), GI (PP, pancreatitis, chronic hepatoxicity), ClinPath (increased ALP, triglycerides), PU, PD	ataxia, sedation	I
Platt et al. 2006	Gaba as an adjunct to PHB and PBr	11	54.5 %	25.1 %–83.9 %	mean, 10.9; range, 9.3–13.6 mg/kg PO TID	median, 6.8; mean, 8.4; range, 2.2–20.7 mg/l	3 m	Neurological (ataxia, sedation)	ataxia, sedation	I
Dewey et al. 2009	Pregabalin as an adjunct to PHB and PBr	11	91 %	74.1 %–107.9 %	Pregabalin: 2 mg/kg PO TID. The dose was increased by 1 mg/kg PO TID each w until 3 or 4 mg/kg PO TID. PHB and PBr: NA but were within normal reference values	Pregabalin: median, 7.3; mean, 6.4; range 2–11 µg/ml PHB: median, 27.1; mean, 27.7; range 19.8–40 µg/ml PBr: median, 1,6; mean, 1.9; range, 0.2–2.81 mg/ml	3 m	Neurological (ataxia, sedation), ClinPath (increased ALP, ALT) PU, PD, PP were also recorded but were associated to the combination therapy with PHB and PBr	ataxia, sedation	I
Ruehlmann et al. 2001	Felbamate as an adjunct to PHB	6	33.3 %	−4.4 %–71.0 %	Felbamate: median, 63 (initial dose) and 77 (final dose); range, 62–220 mg/kg PO SID. PHB: 3.75 mg/kg PO BID (discontinued 2 m after felbamate initiation)	median, 35; mean, 13–55 mg/l	median, 9 m	Haematological (leucopenia, lymphopenia, thrombocytopenia), keratoconjunctivitis sicca	leucopenia, lymphopenia, thrombocytopenia	I
McGee et al. 1998	Felbamate	NA	NA	NA	Sub-chronic group: 250, 500, and 1000 mg/kg PO SID Chronic group: 100 and 300 mg/kg PO SID	range, 16.5–79 µg/ml	Sub-chronic group: 3 m chronic group: 12 m	Sub-chronic group: Neurological (ataxia, sedation, tremors), GI (vomiting, salivation), ClinPath (increased ALT) Chronic group: Neurological (ataxia, limb rigidity, tremors), GI (vomiting, salivation), ClinPath (increased ALT, ALP)	Sub-chronic group: ataxia, sedation, tremors, vomiting, salivation, increased ALT. Chronic group: ataxia, limb rigidity, convulsions, vomiting, salivation, increased ALT, ALP.	I
Dayrell-Hart et al. 1996	Felbamate as an adjunct to PHB and PBr	16	25 %	3.8 %–46.2 %	NA	NA	NA	GI (chronic hepatotoxicity)	chronic hepatotoxicity	I

Table 7 Details of number of dogs, 95 % CI affected cases, AED doses and serum levels, treatment period and adverse effects *(Continued)*

Bunch et al. 1985	Phenytoin (monotherapy or as an adjunct to Prim)	Monotherapy: 8 Adjunctive therapy: 8	Monotherapy: 0 % Adjunctive therapy: 37 %	Monotherapy: 0 % Adjunct therapy: −1 %–16.7 %	NA	NA	NA	Monotherapy: None Adjunctive therapy: GI (anorexia, emaciation), ClinPath (increased ALP, ALT, bilirubin, bile acids, γ-GT, decreased albumin) These dogs were eventually euthanised.	Monotherapy: NA Adjunctive therapy: anorexia, increased ALP, ALT, bilirubin, bile acids, γ-GT, decreased albumin	I
Bunch et al. 1984	Phenytoin (monotherapy or as an adjunct to other AED(s))	Monotherapy: 7 Adjunctive therapy: 19	NA	NA	Phenytoin: mean, 21+/− 11 mg/kg PO SID Prim: mean, 33+/−19 mg/kg PO SID. Other AEDs: NA	NA	range, 6–120 m	GI (chronic hepatotoxicity), ClinPath (increased ALP, ALT, AST, bile acids)	Chronic hepatotoxicity, increased ALP, ALT, AST, bile acids	I
Meyer and Noonan 1981	Phenytoin	6	100 %	100 %	13–19 mg/kg PO TID	NA	3 m	ClinPath (increased ALP, ALT)	increased ALP and ALT	I
Sturtevant et al. 1977	Phenytoin	2	100 %	100 %	22 mg/kg PO TID	NA	1 m	ClinPath (increased ALP, ALT)	increased ALP and ALT	I
Bunch et al. 1982	Phenytoin as an adjunct to Prim	3	NA	NA	Case 1: Prim: 250 mg PO BID; Phenytoin: NA. Case 2: Prim: 750 mg PO BID Phenytoin: 100–233 mg PO TID Case 3: Prim: NA PHB: 150 mg PO SID Phenytoin: 750 mg PO SID 1000 mg PO SID	NA	Case 1: 48 m. Case 2: 30 m Case 3: 36 m	GI (chronic hepatotoxicity)	chronic hepatotoxicity	I
Weiss et al. 2002	Phenytoin	1	NA	NA	NA	NA	NA	Blood dyscrasias (myelofibrosis)	NA	II
Bunch et al. 1987	Phenytoin as an adjunct to PHB and/or Prim	3	NA	NA	Case 1: Phenytoin: 5 mg/kg PO BID, then increased up to 15 mg/kg PO TID. PHB: 0.8 mg/kg PO BID, then increased up to 13 mg/kg PO BID Case 2: Phenytoin: 7.5 mg/kg PO BID, then increased up to 15 mg/kg PO TID. PHB: 1.1 mg/kg PO BID, then increased up to 4.5 mg/kg PO TID. Prim: 18.5 mg/kg PO TID Case 3: Phenytoin: 5 mg/kg PO SID, then increased up to 21 mg/kg PO BID. PHB: 3 mg/kg PO BID. Prim: 13 mg/kg PO SID, then increased up to 26 mg/kg PO BID	Case 1: NA Case 2: NA Case 3: NA	Case 1: 27 months Case 2: 15 months Case 3: 8 months	GI (hepatotoxicity)	NA	II
Nash et al. 1977	Phenytoin	1	NA	NA	100 mg in total	NA	1 d	Idiosyncrasic hepatitis	NA	II
Bunch et al. 1990	Phenytoin	8	0 %	0 %	40 mg/kg PO TID	NA	13.5 m	No adverse effects	NA	NA

Table 7 Details of number of dogs, 95 % CI affected cases, AED doses and serum levels, treatment period and adverse effects *(Continued)*

Nafe 1981	Valproate (monotherapy or as an adjunct to PHB and/or Prim and/or phenytoin)	Monotherapy: NA Adjunctive therapy: 57	Monotherapy: NA Adjunctive therapy: 2 %	Monotherapy: NA Adjunctive therapy: −1.7 %–5.1 %	Sodium Valproate: Monotherapy: 200 mg/kg. Adjunctive therapy: range, 25–40 mg/kg PO SID. PHB, Prim and Phenytoin: NA.	NA	mean, 4.9; range, 1–8 m	Neurological (ataxia, sedation), dermatological (alopecia), GI (vomiting)	Sedation, alopecia	I
Kiviranta et al. 2013	TPM	10	NA	NA	TPM: Initially 2 mg/kg PO BID for 0.5 m, then 5 mg/kg PO BID for 2 m, and then 10 mg/kg PO BID for 2 m and then 10 PO TID for 2 m. PHB, PBr and LEV: NA but were within normal reference values	NA	2–6 m	Neurological (sedation, ataxia), ClinPath (increased ALP, ALT), weight lose	sedation, ataxia, increased ALP, ALT	I

Abbreviations: *AED(s)* anti-epileptic drug(s), *BID* bis in die (twice daily), *Chloraz* Chlorazepate, *CSF* cerebrospinal fluid, *CL* confidence level, *Gaba* Gabapentin, *IE* idiopathic epilepsy, *LEV* Levetiracetam, *m* month(s), *NA* Not Available, *PHB* phenobarbital, *PD* polydipsia, *PU* polyuria, *PP* polyphagia, *PBr* potassium bromide, *Prim* primidone, *PO* per os, *SID* semel in die (once daily), *TID* ter in die (three times daily), *TPM* Topiramate, *w* week(s), *y* year(s)

but no correlation could be found between serum levels and safety profile. In one study, however [90], there was a correlation between the administered dose and the safety profile; dogs treated with a higher initial dose (i.e. 60 mg/kg) experienced more adverse effects compared to dogs started on lower doses (20 mg/kg) (65 % (95 % CI: 43.6–86.5 %) vs. 34 % (95 % CI: 14.6–53.4 %), p = 0.03).

Zonisamide

There was an overall weak level of evidence provided for the zonisamide safety profile either as monotherapy or adjunctive therapy. Seven studies [30, 56, 57, 61, 68, 97, 99] presented data about the safety profile of oral zonisamide either as monotherapy (5 studies) [30, 61, 68, 97, 99] or as an adjunct to other AEDs (2 studies) [56, 57], giving a combined sample size of 83 dogs.

Five studies reported type I and type II adverse effects (Table 5). From these, 3/5 (60 %) and 2/5 (40 %) studies reported type I adverse effects for zonisamide monotherapy and adjunctive therapy (mainly to phenobarbital and/or potassium bromide) respectively. Specifically, in all of the studies, adverse effects most commonly included sedation, followed by ataxia, vomiting and decreased serum ALP activity. Less commonly, increased serum ALT and GLDH activity, aggression, anorexia, emaciation and decreased T4 and serum albumin were reported. In adjunctive therapy studies, adverse effects most commonly included sedation, ataxia and increased serum ALP activity, followed by vomiting, increased serum ALT and GLDH activity. In monotherapy studies all the adverse effects occurred at the same frequency; increased serum GLDH and ALT activity were not reported (Fig. 8). Two studies reported type II adverse effects including idiosyncratic hepatotoxicity and mixed acid–base disorder (Table 5).

Adequate data to allow calculations of the prevalence of adverse effects was reported in 4/7 (57 %) studies (Table 5). From these, only one showed >50 % prevalence of adverse effects for the specific period of treatment they conducted. Based on the 95 % CI, the majority of the population experienced at least one adverse effect in 25 % of the studies (Table 5).

Adequate information about the treatment period was reported in all of the studies (Table 5). From these, in 3/6 (50 %) the treatment period was relatively short (<6 months). Adequate information about the doses was provided in all studies (Table 5). The zonisamide maintenance doses exceeded the recommended dose margins in two studies. Adequate information about the zonisamide serum levels was reported in 6/7 (86 %) studies (Table 5), but no correlation could be found between serum levels and the safety profile.

Primidone

There was an overall weak level of evidence provided for the primidone safety profile either as monotherapy or adjunctive therapy. Sixteen studies [28, 32, 35, 52, 64, 65, 76, 82, 89, 91, 92, 95, 103–105, 113] presented data about the safety profile of primidone as an adjunct to phenobarbital [104] and as a monotherapy agent (remaining studies), giving a combined sample size of 298 dogs.

Twelve studies reported type I adverse effects including gastro-intestinal and neurological signs as the most common (Table 6). Specifically, adverse effects most commonly included increased serum ALP activity, ataxia and polydipsia followed by sedation, hyperactivity, chronic clinical hepatopathy/toxicity, polyphagia, disorientation and then increased serum ALT activity, hind limb weakness and polyuria. Less commonly reported effects included anxiety, tachypnea and increased serum AST, γ-GT, bile acids, SGPT and GLDH activity (Fig. 9). In two studies [32, 76] no adverse effects attributed to primidone were reported. Three studies reported type II adverse effects (Table 6). Specifically, blood dyscrasias (anemia, thrombocytopenia and/or neutropenia) and dermatitis were reported.

Adequate data to allow calculations of the prevalence of adverse effects was reported in 7/16 (44 %) of the studies (Table 6). From these, 3/7 (43 %) showed >50 % prevalence of adverse effects for the specific period of treatment over which it was conducted. Based on the 95 % CI, the majority of the population experienced at least one adverse effect in 3/7 (43 %) studies (Table 6).

Adequate information about the treatment period was reported in 13/16 (81 %) (Table 6). From these, in 6/13 the treatment period was relatively short (<6 months). Adequate information about the dose was provided in 14/16 (88 %) studies (Table 6). From these 11/14 (79 %) and 3/14 (21 %) reported doses for type I and type II adverse effects respectively. The primidone maintenance doses were higher than the recommended dose margins in type I and type II adverse effects in 5/11 (45 %) and 1/3 (33 %) studies, respectively. Adequate information about the primidone (phenobarbital) serum levels was reported in 5/16 (31 %) studies (Table 6). Of these, all reported type I adverse effects. The phenobarbital serum levels were higher than the recommended margins in 3/5 (60 %) studies.

Gabapentin

There was an overall weak level of evidence provided for the gabapentin safety profile. Two studies [58, 59] presented data about the safety profile of oral gabapentin as an adjunct to other AEDs, giving a combined sample size of 28 dogs.

Both studies reported only type I adverse effects, including neurological signs as the most common (Table 7). Specific adverse effects most commonly included sedation and ataxia. Less commonly reported adverse effects were polyphagia, pancreatitis, chronic clinical hepatopathy/toxicity, polydipsia, polyuria and increased ALP activity.

Both studies showed >50 % prevalence of adverse effects for the specific period of treatment during which they were conducted (Table 7). Based on the 95 % CI, the majority of the population experienced at least one adverse effect in one study (Table 7). In both studies the treatment period was relatively short (<6 months). The gabapentin maintenance doses were high but within the upper recommended dose margins in one study. Gabapentin serum levels were not measured and, thus, no analysis to detect associations between serum levels and adverse effects was performed.

Pregabalin

There was an overall insufficient level of evidence provided for the pregabalin safety profile. One study [55] presented data about the safety profile of oral pregabalin as an adjunct to phenobarbital and potassium bromide in 11 dogs.

The study reported only type I adverse effects including neurological signs as the main ones (Table 7). Specifically, sedation, ataxia and increased ALP activity and ALT activity were reported.

The study showed 91 % prevalence of adverse effects for the specific treatment period in which it was conducted. Based on the 95 % CI, the majority of the population experienced adverse effects (Table 7). The treatment period was relatively short (<6 months). No correlation was found between pregabalin dose/serum levels and adverse effects.

Valproate

There was an overall weak level of evidence provided for the valproate safety profile. One study [62] presented data about the safety profile of sodium valproate in different groups either as a monotherapy or as an adjunct to phenobarbital, primidone or a combination of phenobarbital and phenytoin in 57 dogs. The study reported only type I adverse effects including neurological, gastro-intestinal and dermatological ones (Table 7). Specifically, vomiting, sedation, ataxia and alopecia were reported.

The study did not show >50 % prevalence of adverse effects for the specific period of treatment during which it was conducted. Based on the 95 % CI, the majority of the population did not experience adverse effects (Table 7). The treatment period was unclear. No correlation was found between valproate dose and adverse effects. The serum levels were not measured.

Felbamate

There was an overall weak level of evidence provided for the felbamate safety profile either as monotherapy or adjunctive therapy. Three studies [47, 70, 78] presented data about the safety profile of felbamate as monotherapy [47] or as an adjunct to phenobarbital in particular and potassium bromide (remaining studies), giving a combined sample size of 22 dogs.

All studies reported type I adverse effects including gastro-intestinal and neurological signs as the most common (Table 7). Specifically, adverse effects most commonly included ataxia, tremors, vomiting, hypersalivation and increased ALP activity. Less commonly, clinical hepatopathy/toxicity, increased ALT activity, sedation, limb rigidity, leucopenia, lymphopenia, thrombocytopenia and keratoconjunctivitis sicca were reported (Fig. 10).

Two studies reported type II adverse effects (Table 7). Specifically, blood dyscrasias (anemia, thrombocytopenia and neutropenia) and dermatitis were reported.

Adequate data to allow calculations of the prevalence of adverse effects was reported in 2/3 (67 %) of the studies (Table 7) and none showed >50 % prevalence of adverse effects for the specific period of treatment during which they were conducted. Based on the 95 % CI, the majority of the population did not experience adverse effects (Table 7).

Adequate information about the treatment period was reported in 2/3 (67 %) (Table 7) and it was relatively short in one study (<6 months). Adequate information about the dose and serum levels was provided in 2/3 (67 %) studies (Table 7). In both of these the maintenance doses were higher than the recommended dose margins. No correlation was found between serum levels and adverse effects.

Topiramate

There was an overall weak level of evidence provided for the topiramate safety profile. One study [54] presented data about the safety profile of topiramate as an adjunct to phenobarbital, potassium bromide and levetiracetam in 10 dogs. The study reported type I adverse effects, including neurological and gastro-intestinal as the most common. Specific adverse effects most commonly reported were ataxia, sedation, weight loss and increased ALP and ALT activity. However, these adverse effects could be attributed in part to the co-administered AEDs such as phenobarbital and/or potassium bromide. The prevalence of adverse effects was approximately 50 %. The treatment period was relatively short (<6 months). The maintenance dose was within recommended dose margins (Table 7). Topiramate serum levels were not measured.

Phenytoin

There was an overall weak level of evidence provided for the phenytoin safety profile either as monotherapy or adjunctive therapy. Nine studies [32, 35, 52, 87, 89, 91, 92, 108] presented data about the safety profile of phenytoin as monotherapy (7 studies) [32, 34, 35, 52, 87, 91, 108] as an adjunct to primidone in particular and/or potassium bromide (4 studies) [32, 89, 91, 92], giving a combined sample of 66 dogs.

Five studies reported type I adverse effects including gastro-intestinal as the most common (Table 7). Specifically, increased serum ALP, ALT, bile acids and chronic clinical hepatopathy/toxicity were most commonly included. Less commonly, increased serum AST, γ-GT, bilirubin and bile acids activity, decreased albumin, anorexia and emaciation were reported (Fig. 11). In the monotherapy group, no adverse effects occurred in two studies [32, 34].

Three studies reported type II adverse effects (Table 7). Specifically, idiosyncratic hepatotoxicity in particular and blood dyscrasias (anemia, thrombocytopenia and/or neutropenia) occurred. Blood dyscrasias (pancytopenia) were reported by the monotherapy study [87].

Adequate data to allow calculations of the prevalence of adverse effects was reported in 4/9 (44 %) of the studies and all but two did not show >50 % prevalence of adverse effects for the specific period of treatment they were conducted. Based on the 95 % CI, the majority of the population experienced adverse effect in two studies (Table 7).

Adequate information about the treatment period was reported in 8/9 (89 %) (Table 7). From these, in 6/8 (75 %) the treatment period was relatively short (<6 months). Adequate information about the dose and/or serum levels was provided in 7/9 (77 %) (Table 7). No correlation could be found between dose and adverse effects. Phenytoin serum levels were not measured.

B) Safety profile comparisons between AEDs or between AEDs-placebo

Phenobarbital monotherapy vs placebo or untreated control

Total safety information was available in five studies [33, 36, 40, 43, 80]. Adequate information to calculate OR was provided in all the studies. Studies compared endocrinal factors and liver enzymes between phenobarbital and untreated or placebo-control groups. Four adverse effects were reported. The common estimated OR was 6.21 (95 % CI: 3.28–11.75), showing a statistically significant association ($P < 0.001$), with reduced odds of overall adverse effects in the untreated controls. Thus, treated dogs were over 6 times as likely to experience an adverse effect compared to controls. However, moderate heterogeneity was shown between studies ($chi^2 = 6.62$, $P = 0.09$). The OR for abnormal total T4, TSH and increased ALP and ALT activity showed a statistically significant association, with reduced odds of these adverse effects in the controls (Fig. 12).

Phenobarbital monotherapy vs potassium bromide monotherapy

Total safety information was available in five studies [3, 23, 29, 39, 75]. Adequate information to calculate OR was provided in all the studies. Twelve adverse effects were reported. The common estimated OR was 0.80 (95 % CI: 0.31-2.04), showing a statistically non-significant association ($P = 0.64$) between monotherapies. Low heterogeneity was shown between studies ($chi^2 = 1.07$, $P = 0.59$). The OR for increased serum ALP activity showed a statistical trend in favour of potassium bromide. The OR for pancreatitis, vomiting and increased serum amylase and lipase activity showed a statistically significant association, with reduced odds of these adverse effects in the phenobarbital group (Fig. 13).

Phenobarbital monotherapy vs levetiracetam monotherapy

Total safety information was available in one study [27]. Eleven main adverse effects were reported. The common estimated OR was 2.5 (95 % CI: 0.16–38.6), showing a statistically non-significant association ($P = 0.51$) between monotherapies. The OR for hypoactivity showed a statistically significant association, with reduced odds of this adverse effect in levetiracetam monotherapy (Fig. 14). Although the number of affected dogs did not significantly differ between the groups, the frequency of adverse effects (per dog) was higher in the phenobarbital group in this study.

Phenobarbital monotherapy vs imepitoin monotherapy

Total safety information was available in two studies [25, 42]. Adequate information to estimate OR was provided in one study [25] (Fig. 15). Four adverse effects were reported. The common estimated OR was 0.65 (95 % CI: 0.38–1.10), showing a statistically non-significant association ($P = 0.11$) between monotherapies. The OR for polydipsia and polyuria showed a statistical trend in favor of imepitoin. The OR for sedation and hyperactivity showed a statistically significant association, with reduced odds of these adverse effects in imepitoin and phenobarbital, respectively.

The same study [25] reported that liver enzymes (serum ALP, γ-GT, ALT and GLDH) were increased significantly ($P < 0.001$) in the phenobarbital group, along with a statistically significant ($P < 0.05$) association for dose dependence; neither such increase nor dose dependence trend was seen in the imepitoin group.

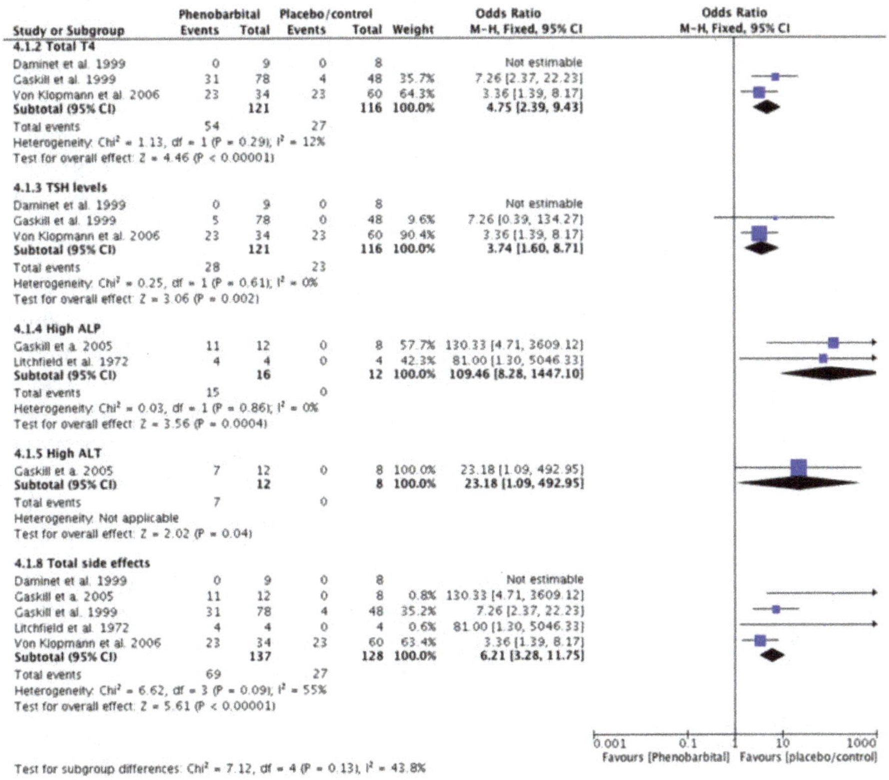

Fig. 12 Forest plot comparing phenobarbital vs placebo/control. Odd ratios (95 % CI) of specific and total adverse effects for phenobarbital and control groups

The second study [42], although the OR could not be estimated, reported sedation, ataxia, polydipsia and polyuria in phenobarbital group, whereas no adverse effects were observed in the imepitoin group.

Imepitoin monotherapy vs imepitoin adjunctive therapy

Total safety information was available in two studies [44, 48]. Imepitoin monotherapy was compared to imepitoin adjunctive therapy to phenobarbital and/or potassium bromide. Three adverse effects were reported. The common estimated OR was 0.58 (95 % CI: 0.19–1.75), showing a statistically non-significant association (P = 0.34) between the two therapies. No heterogeneity was shown between studies ($chi^2 = 0.00$, P = 1.00). The OR for increased serum ALP activity showed a statistically significant association, with reduced odds of this adverse effect in imepitoin monotherapy (Fig. 16).

Imepitoin monotherapy vs pseudo-placebo

Total safety information was available in one study [26]. Imepitoin monotherapy (high dose) was compared to imepitoin monotherapy (low dose; pseudo-placebo group). The study grouped the adverse effects into broad categories (e.g. neurological, gastro-intestinal, etc.). The adverse effects were reported on the grounds of these categories but they were not specified. The common estimated OR was 1.39 (95 % CI: 0.53–3.64), showing a statistically non-significant association (P = 0.5) between monotherapy and pseudo-placebo. The OR for neurological signs (ataxia and hyperactivity/restlessness) showed a statistically significant association, with reduced odds of this adverse effect in low-dose imepitoin monotherapy (Fig. 17).

The study reported that the findings from the hematology and biochemistry evaluation were unremarkable and remained within normal reference ranges. There was only a very low tendency for serum creatinine activity to increase in the high-dose imepitoin monotherapy compared to low-dose, but this change was also within normal ranges.

Levetiracetam adjunctive therapy vs placebo

Total safety information was available in one study [24]. The study compared adverse effects between levetiracetam (as an adjunct to phenobarbital, potassium bromide, gabapentin and/or zonisamide) and placebo-control (as an adjunct to phenobarbital, potassium bromide, gabapentin and/or zonisamide). Four adverse effects were reported. The common estimated OR was 1.82 (95 % CI: 0.62–5.35), showing a statistically non-significant association (P = 0.28) between treatment and placebo (Fig. 18). However, according to the study [24], a significant

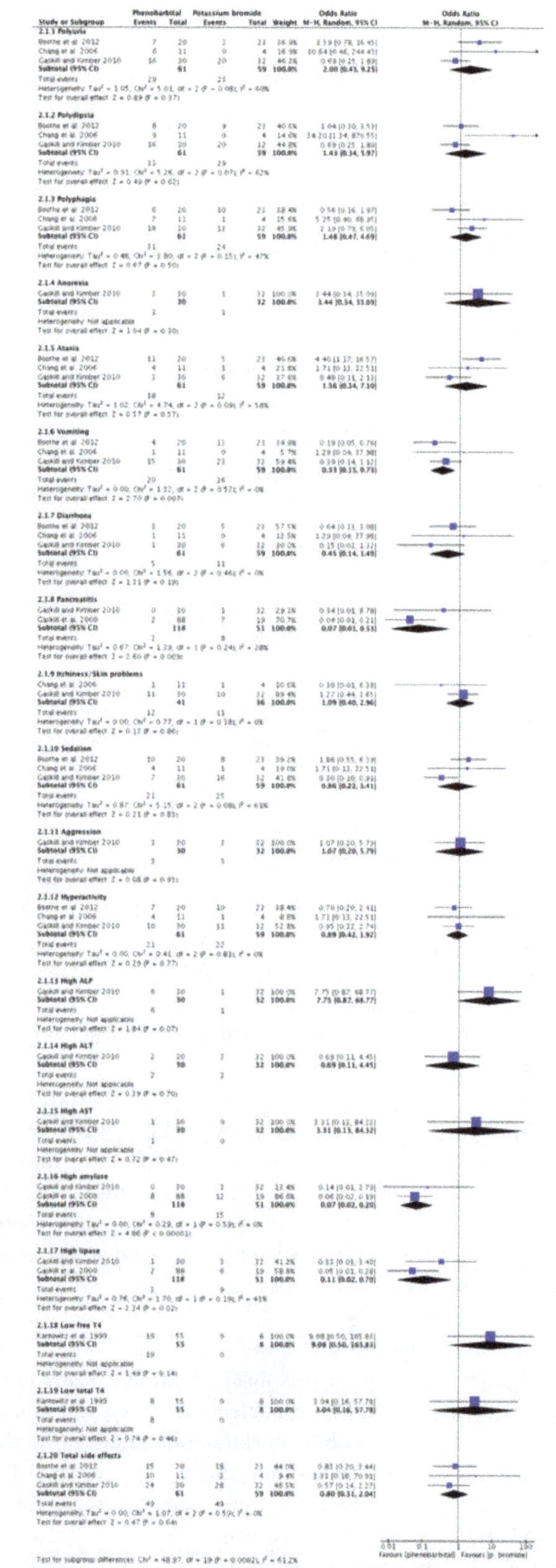

Fig. 13 Forest plot comparing phenobarbital vs potassium bromide. Odd ratios (95 % CI) of specific and total adverse effects for phenobarbital and potassium bromide groups

increase in the prevalence of any of the reported adverse effects (P = 0.013) and ataxia in particular (p = 0.002) was noted in dogs receiving levetiracetam compared to baseline.

Further comparisons between AEDs were not possible due to the lack of comparison studies and/or insufficient report of power analysis and data to allow additional statistical analysis.

Discussion

To the authors' knowledge, this is the first systematic review, including a meta-analytic approach, of AEDs' adverse effects in dogs. The authors followed the PRISMA statement to report this systematic review [120]. The potential for development of AEDs' adverse effects in dogs are well accepted. Our systematic review found, however, that the strength of evidence as well as the prevalence and occurrence of adverse effects were variable among different AEDs and even among studies evaluating the same AED.

Main categories of adverse effects are type I (pharmacology-related) and type II (idiosyncratic). While type I effects are dose-dependent, occur predictably and are usually caused by a known pharmacological property of the drug, idiosyncratic reactions cannot be explained on the grounds of the drug's known mechanisms of action and usually occur unpredictably and irrespective of dosage [121]. In our study, type II adverse effects occurred mainly in dogs receiving doses within the recommended margins; however, these adverse effects occurred at any dose. Type II adverse effects occurred in primidone, phenobarbital, potassium bromide and zonisamide. Idiosyncratic reactions were usually caused either by immune-mediated hypersensitivity reactions or by cytotoxic effects of the drug or one of its metabolites [121]. Due to the liver's central role in drug metabolism it is one of the major sites where idiosyncratic drug reactions manifest. Individual differences in rate of formation and detoxification of reactive metabolites may explain why only certain patients develop idiosyncratic reactions [121]. These unpredictable adverse reactions occur rarely and therefore frequently remain undetected during clinical trials until approval and marketing of drugs. Once a large number of patients is exposed to new or more AEDs, these adverse effects may increase in frequency [122].

This systematic review identified and evaluated ninety studies, the vast majority of which were UCTs, retrospective case series, and reports derived from second and third groups. In total, the data of 4102 dogs were included. Direct and indirect comparisons among drugs based on the frequency, proportion and prevalence of adverse effects in each AED and study showed that levetiracetam and secondary imepitoin might be amongst

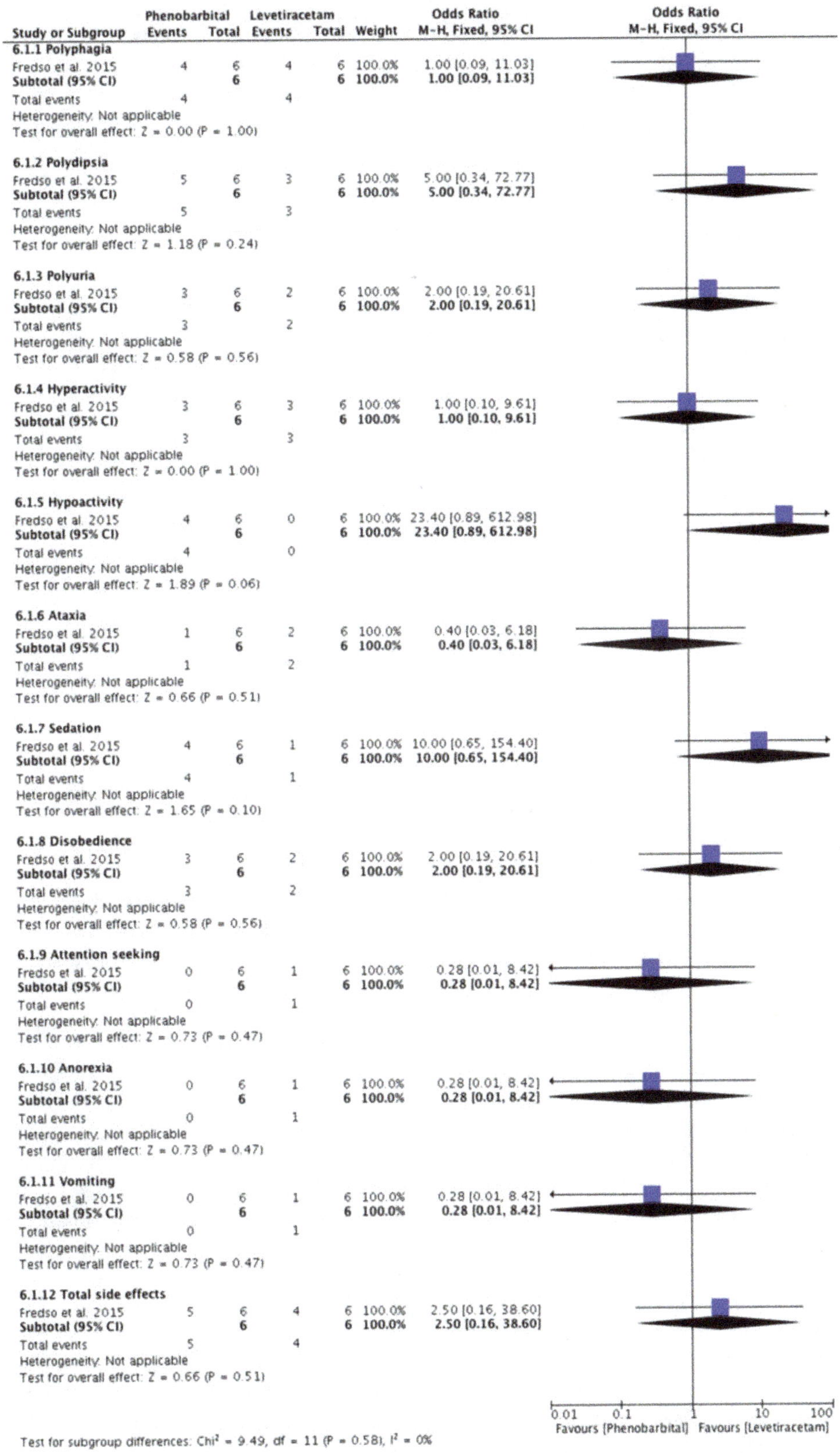

Fig. 14 Forest plot comparing phenobarbital vs levetiracetam. Odd ratios (95 % CI) of specific and total adverse effects for phenobarbital and levetiracetam groups

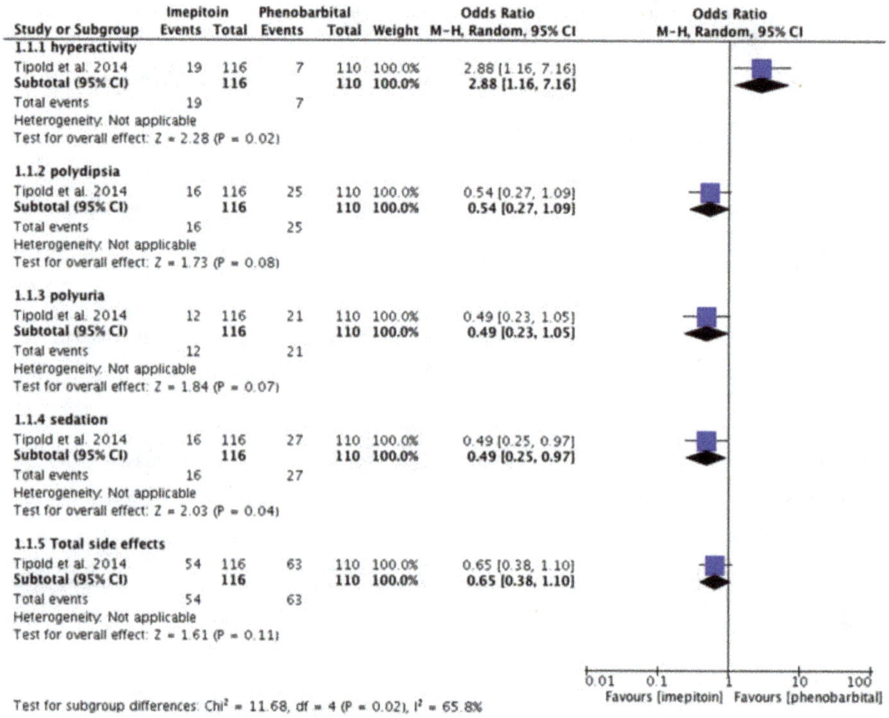

Fig. 15 Forest plot comparing phenobarbital vs imepitoin. Odd ratios (95 % CI) of specific and total adverse effects for phenobarbital and imepitoin groups

the safest AEDs, followed by phenobarbital and potassium bromide; a strong level of evidence was identified supporting their safety profile. The remaining AEDs showed a variety of adverse effects, but there was weak evidence to support their safety profile. Direct comparisons could be made only between specific AEDs based on the results of comparison group studies. It was found that imepitoin tended to have a better safety profile than phenobarbital. Levetiracetam appeared to have a better safety profile than phenobarbital, and phenobarbital appeared to have a better safety profile than potassium bromide. However, neither association was statistically significant. The trend for phenobarbital to have a safer profile than potassium bromide supports a former high-quality study which showed that phenobarbital had a better safety profile than potassium bromide [23]. It is interesting that this association was not statistically different in our meta-analysis. It could be that our statistical methods applied were too stringent or that data in our study were more heterogenous, due to the data deriving from various studies, making it less likely in this systematic review to detect a statistical difference. Equally though, it is acknowledged there may be no major underlying biological difference in adverse event rates between these therapies.

Similar to a previous systematic review of AED efficacy [13], the majority of the studies included in this review did not offer high quality of evidence. Studies in the first group, which were considered to offer lower overall risk of bias, were too few compared to other groups (study group 1st:2nd:3rd proportion was 1:4:3). In addition, only 16 and 33 % of studies included well-characterised groups of IE and healthy non-epileptic dogs respectively. Only 13 % of studies included good study population size. Many studies had only a very limited follow-up time to assess efficacy and tolerability (<6 months). Therefore, the results should always be interpreted with caution.

In contrast to AEDs' efficacy evaluation, case reports do have an important role in forming a safety profile of an individual AED. Specifically, type II or other rare adverse events are unlikely to be recognized by standard clinical trials [123]. Searching the whole range of publications and including NRCTs, UCTs, observational and descriptive studies might avoid missing important information about rare adverse effects and removes potential biases that could occur in systematic reviews which use stricter exclusion criteria and do not include studies other than RCTs [124]. A number of reviews of human drugs have found that case reports and spontaneous reporting systems provide better information about adverse effects than clinical trials do [115, 125]. Indeed, in our review, we found that case reports provided valuable specifics for several kinds of adverse effects not reported in other study designs. Therefore, although small case series and in particular case reports are considered to

Study or Subgroup	Imepitoin mono Events	Imepitoin mono Total	Imepitoin add-on Events	Imepitoin add-on Total	Weight	Odds Ratio M-H, Fixed, 95% CI
3.1.1 polyphagia						
Loscher et al. 2004	7	12	10	17	50.0%	0.98 [0.22, 4.39]
Rieck et al. 2006	7	12	10	17	50.0%	0.98 [0.22, 4.39]
Subtotal (95% CI)		**24**		**34**	**100.0%**	**0.98 [0.34, 2.83]**
Total events	14		20			
Heterogeneity: Chi² = 0.00, df = 1 (P = 1.00); I² = 0%						
Test for overall effect: Z = 0.04 (P = 0.97)						
3.1.2 ataxia						
Loscher et al. 2004	0	12	2	17	50.0%	0.25 [0.01, 5.65]
Rieck et al. 2006	0	12	2	17	50.0%	0.25 [0.01, 5.65]
Subtotal (95% CI)		**24**		**34**	**100.0%**	**0.25 [0.03, 2.26]**
Total events	0		4			
Heterogeneity: Chi² = 0.00, df = 1 (P = 1.00); I² = 0%						
Test for overall effect: Z = 1.24 (P = 0.22)						
3.1.3 sedation						
Loscher et al. 2004	0	12	2	17	50.0%	0.25 [0.01, 5.65]
Rieck et al. 2006	0	12	2	17	50.0%	0.25 [0.01, 5.65]
Subtotal (95% CI)		**24**		**34**	**100.0%**	**0.25 [0.03, 2.26]**
Total events	0		4			
Heterogeneity: Chi² = 0.00, df = 1 (P = 1.00); I² = 0%						
Test for overall effect: Z = 1.24 (P = 0.22)						
3.1.4 High ALP						
Loscher et al. 2004	0	12	6	17	50.0%	0.07 [0.00, 1.40]
Rieck et al. 2006	0	12	6	17	50.0%	0.07 [0.00, 1.40]
Subtotal (95% CI)		**24**		**34**	**100.0%**	**0.07 [0.01, 0.58]**
Total events	0		12			
Heterogeneity: Chi² = 0.00, df = 1 (P = 1.00); I² = 0%						
Test for overall effect: Z = 2.46 (P = 0.01)						
3.1.5 High ALT						
Loscher et al. 2004	0	12	1	17	50.0%	0.44 [0.02, 11.74]
Rieck et al. 2006	0	12	1	17	50.0%	0.44 [0.02, 11.74]
Subtotal (95% CI)		**24**		**34**	**100.0%**	**0.44 [0.04, 4.49]**
Total events	0		2			
Heterogeneity: Chi² = 0.00, df = 1 (P = 1.00); I² = 0%						
Test for overall effect: Z = 0.69 (P = 0.49)						
3.1.6 High GLDH						
Loscher et al. 2004	0	12	3	17	50.0%	0.17 [0.01, 3.53]
Rieck et al. 2006	0	12	3	17	50.0%	0.17 [0.01, 3.53]
Subtotal (95% CI)		**24**		**34**	**100.0%**	**0.17 [0.02, 1.44]**
Total events	0		6			
Heterogeneity: Chi² = 0.00, df = 1 (P = 1.00); I² = 0%						
Test for overall effect: Z = 1.63 (P = 0.10)						
3.1.7 Total side effects						
Loscher et al. 2004	7	12	12	17	50.0%	0.58 [0.12, 2.75]
Rieck et al. 2006	7	12	12	17	50.0%	0.58 [0.12, 2.75]
Subtotal (95% CI)		**24**		**34**	**100.0%**	**0.58 [0.19, 1.75]**
Total events	14		24			
Heterogeneity: Chi² = 0.00, df = 1 (P = 1.00); I² = 0%						
Test for overall effect: Z = 0.96 (P = 0.34)						

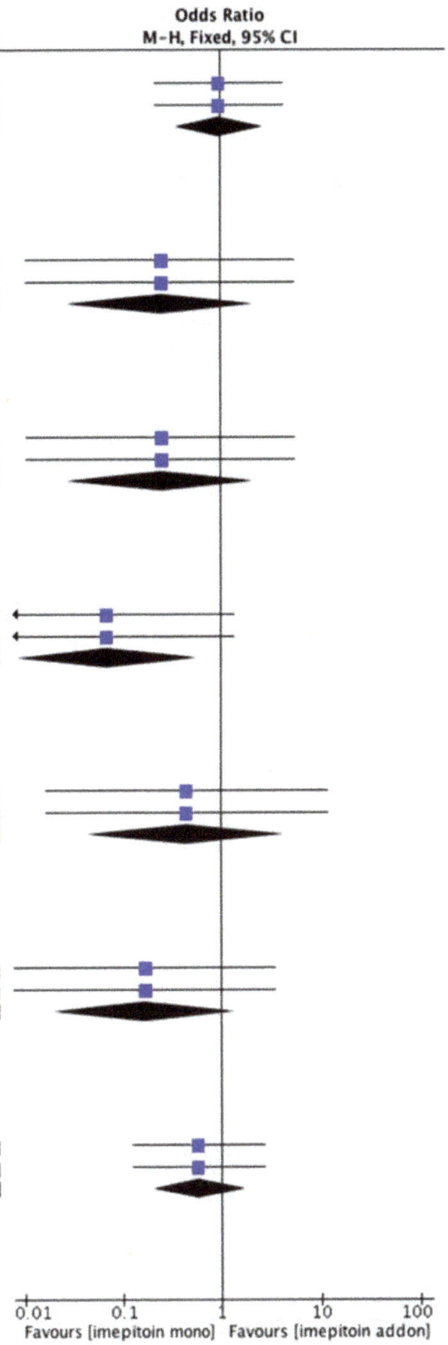

Test for subgroup differences: Chi² = 6.61, df = 6 (P = 0.36), I² = 9.2%

Fig. 16 Forest plot comparing imepitoin monotherapy vs imepitoin adjunctive therapy. Odd ratios (95 % CI) of specific and total adverse effects for imepitoin monotherapy and adjunctive therapy groups

provide overall low quality evidence for many measurement outcomes (e.g. AEDs' efficacy), they can reveal valuable information as far as the safety profile is concerned and were included in the current systematic review.

Difficulties in describing adverse effects among studies

It has been suggested that reporting of AEDs' adverse events in clinical trials is poor and has not improved over the years [126]. Searching for information about adverse effects can be quite complicated [127–129]. Little evidence exists on the most appropriate searching methods, and a study has assessed different methods in retrieving studies of adverse effects [4]. This study found that a combination of different search methods is required to retrieve as many studies as possible. The same study, however, has also concluded that the most

Study or Subgroup	Imepitoin Events	Imepitoin Total	Pseudo-placebo Events	Pseudo-placebo Total	Weight	Odds Ratio M-H, Fixed, 95% CI
7.1.1 Neurological						
Rundfeldt et al. 2015	48	66	32	61	100.0%	2.42 [1.15, 5.06]
Subtotal (95% CI)		**66**		**61**	**100.0%**	**2.42 [1.15, 5.06]**
Total events	48		32			
Heterogeneity: Not applicable						
Test for overall effect: Z = 2.34 (P = 0.02)						
7.1.2 Gastro-intestinal						
Rundfeldt et al. 2015	32	66	25	61	100.0%	1.36 [0.67, 2.74]
Subtotal (95% CI)		**66**		**61**	**100.0%**	**1.36 [0.67, 2.74]**
Total events	32		25			
Heterogeneity: Not applicable						
Test for overall effect: Z = 0.85 (P = 0.40)						
7.1.3 Musculoskeletal						
Rundfeldt et al. 2015	12	66	8	61	100.0%	1.47 [0.56, 3.89]
Subtotal (95% CI)		**66**		**61**	**100.0%**	**1.47 [0.56, 3.89]**
Total events	12		8			
Heterogeneity: Not applicable						
Test for overall effect: Z = 0.78 (P = 0.44)						
7.1.4 Respiratory						
Rundfeldt et al. 2015	7	66	8	61	100.0%	0.79 [0.27, 2.31]
Subtotal (95% CI)		**66**		**61**	**100.0%**	**0.79 [0.27, 2.31]**
Total events	7		8			
Heterogeneity: Not applicable						
Test for overall effect: Z = 0.44 (P = 0.66)						
7.1.5 Urogenital						
Rundfeldt et al. 2015	4	66	5	61	100.0%	0.72 [0.18, 2.83]
Subtotal (95% CI)		**66**		**61**	**100.0%**	**0.72 [0.18, 2.83]**
Total events	4		5			
Heterogeneity: Not applicable						
Test for overall effect: Z = 0.47 (P = 0.64)						
7.1.6 Other systems						
Rundfeldt et al. 2015	14	66	15	61	100.0%	0.83 [0.36, 1.89]
Subtotal (95% CI)		**66**		**61**	**100.0%**	**0.83 [0.36, 1.89]**
Total events	14		15			
Heterogeneity: Not applicable						
Test for overall effect: Z = 0.45 (P = 0.65)						
7.1.7 General						
Rundfeldt et al. 2015	5	66	5	61	100.0%	0.92 [0.25, 3.34]
Subtotal (95% CI)		**66**		**61**	**100.0%**	**0.92 [0.25, 3.34]**
Total events	5		5			
Heterogeneity: Not applicable						
Test for overall effect: Z = 0.13 (P = 0.90)						
7.1.8 Total adverse effects						
Rundfeldt et al. 2015	57	66	50	61	100.0%	1.39 [0.53, 3.64]
Subtotal (95% CI)		**66**		**61**	**100.0%**	**1.39 [0.53, 3.64]**
Total events	57		50			
Heterogeneity: Not applicable						
Test for overall effect: Z = 0.68 (P = 0.50)						

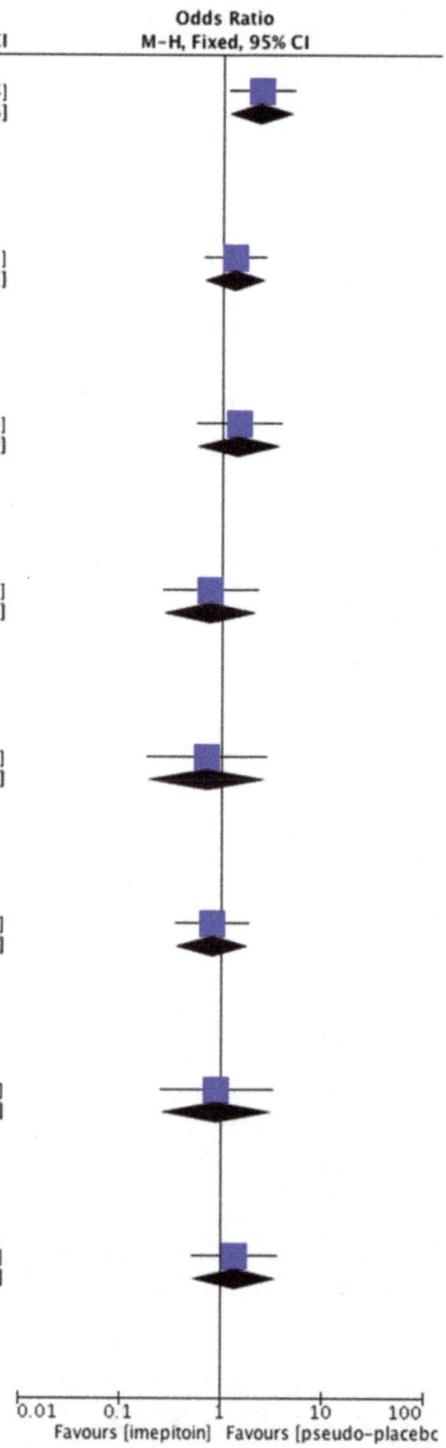

Test for subgroup differences: $Chi^2 = 5.76$, $df = 7$ ($P = 0.57$), $I^2 = 0\%$

Fig. 17 Forest plot comparing imepiton vs pseudo-placebo. Odd ratios (95 % CI) of specific and total adverse effects for imepitoin and control groups

effective search methods might not be possible until there is better reporting and indexing of records concerning the adverse effects. Another recent study has indicated that database searching using adverse effects terms can retrieve the majority of articles (around 92 %) on drugs' adverse effects [130]. Our review used all the possible searching methods and combinations of these methods and terms in order to retrieve all or the vast

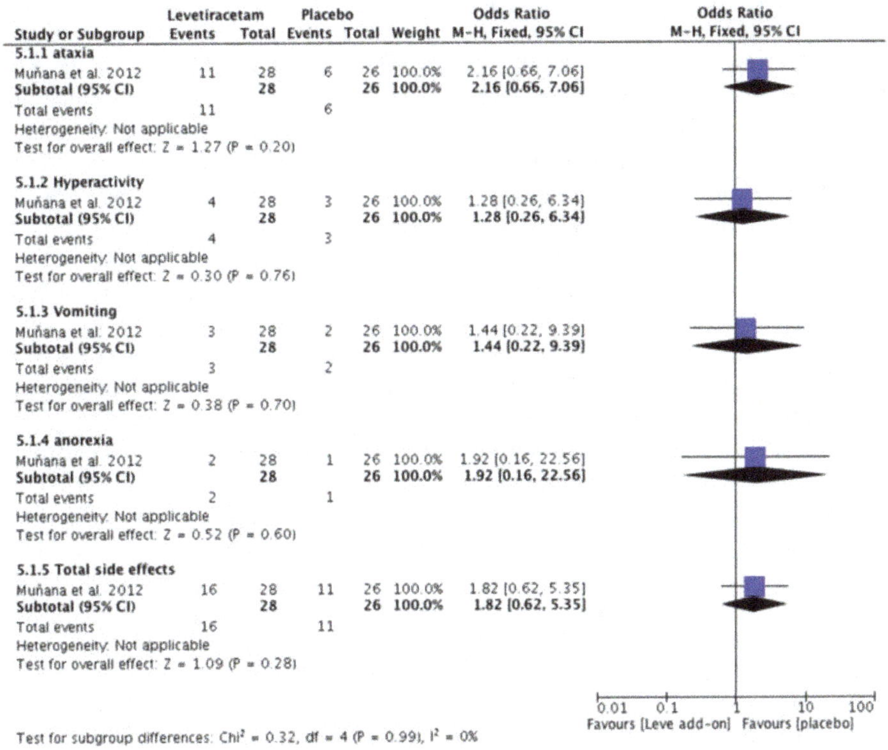

Fig. 18 Forest plot comparing levetiracetam vs placebo. Odd ratios (95 % CI) of specific and total adverse effects for levetiracetam and control groups

majority of the available studies reporting or assessing AEDs' adverse effects.

The majority of the studies for many AEDs, apart from phenobarbital, primidone, imepitoin and secondary potassium bromide and zonisamide, evaluated the drugs when administered in combination with other AEDs, making it sometimes difficult to determine whether clinical signs could always be attributed to AEDs' administration. Therefore, should these AEDs be used and investigated more frequently as monotherapy, future analyses (i.e. randomised controlled clinical trials) may allow even clearer conclusions on the safety questions raised in the present systematic review.

In newer standardized trials every sign that occurs during the study will be recorded as an adverse effect even if it is not always associated with the treatment. In addition, newer trials tend to include toxicology studies in which the doses that are administered are sometimes beyond the recommended treatment doses. Therefore, newer trials will report more adverse reactions than others. As imepitoin is a newly developed antiepileptic drug it is possible that the adverse effects have been more adequately captured than for older AEDs and that certain reported adverse effects might have been over-reported or drug unrelated. Furthermore, a few infrequent adverse effects were recorded and mainly occurred in doses higher than the recommended therapeutic ones. The longer a drug is on the market, the likelihood of reports of adverse effects increases. This should be considered when evaluating older AEDs.

The prevalence is a good indicator for evaluating the safety profile of an AED in a study. However, a few limitations originating from the evaluated studies were detected in this review. For instance, in three studies [31, 33, 76], the prevalence was 0 %, but the duration was quite short and only a very small population was included. In another study [75], although a very large population was included, the prevalence was 1 %, possibly because the authors focused on reporting the prevalence of pancreatitis only and the cases were reviewed retrospectively. Similarly, in 23 studies [31, 34–36, 38–40, 43, 45, 46, 49–52, 69, 76, 81, 83–85, 87, 93, 103], the authors focused on reporting only specific adverse effects and, therefore, other adverse effects may have been under- or misreported. In seven studies [36, 81, 83, 85, 87, 89, 104], prevalence was not calculated because only dogs with adverse effects were included. In 16 studies [28, 30, 37, 39, 42, 47, 49, 54, 64, 65, 84, 85, 87, 91, 112, 113], the total number of affected dogs was not very clear and therefore prevalence could not be calculated (risk of prevalence data loses). Lastly, prevalence is difficult to derive from case reports.

There have been some characteristics in the included studies that might have influenced AEDs' safety profile

[1]. First of all, the dose range of a particular AED significantly varied among studies. Another characteristic could be the differences in AEDs' titration. The safety of some drugs can be influenced by the method and speed of titration [1]. For instance, imepitoin allows quick titration and dose adjustments in dogs with poor response to the drug. However, this was not followed in one study [25] due to the comparison with phenobarbital which demands slow titration. Therefore, this could have negatively affected imepitoin's safety profile. In addition, the number or frequency of AEDs' administration could influence safety profiles. Specifically for the AEDs with a short half-life, the number of daily administrations might affect the probability of the occurrence of adverse-effects that correlate to fluctuations of blood levels. However, it has been suggested that this characteristic is not as important as the titration speed [1].

The duration of the study should be sufficient to allow the most frequent adverse effects to occur. In many studies, the relatively small treatment period provided limited time for some adverse effects to occur. Durations of the studies were very heterogeneous and thus the spectrum of the observed adverse effects might have been affected by it. However, one human study [1], which evaluated the AEDs' central nervous system adverse effects, found that most of them occurred soon after the beginning of treatment or shortly after a dose increase. In our review, adverse effects occurred throughout the treatment duration of the studies.

As was found in the previous systematic review of AEDs' efficacy [13], several aspects may have also adversely affected the assessment of the reviewed studies. Similarly, the main aspects in the current systematic review were the difference of baseline signalment characteristics, heterogeneity in treatment initiation and protocols between studies, range of study publication dates, publication bias, the several sources of biases related to the studies, the lack of high quality evidence studies (i.e. bRCTs and bRELAS), lack of studies designed with primary aim to investigate AEDs' safety profile and enrolment of relatively small numbers of animals.

In our study, although the safety profile for each individual AED could be reported and assessed, there were factors that limit definite conclusions on safety profile among AEDs. In a few of the human systematic reviews and/or meta-analysis on AEDs' safety profile, statistical methods (e.g. comparisons of odds ratio based on study's evaluated AED and the control group, difference risk ratio, etc.) were conducted for contrasting and combining results from different groups and studies with the aim to identify similar patterns and sources of disagreement among study results or other interesting relationships that may have come to light in the context of multiple studies. In veterinary medicine, though, due to the small number of comparison (i.e. control AED or placebo) clinical trials or ELAS, lack of standardized descriptions of adverse events, variation in methods for data collecting, significant differences among study designs, several potential sources of bias and the fact that objective quantifiable measures and severity of most complaints were not considered in reports, a rigorous statistical method analysis cannot widely be used and, therefore, a meta-analytic approach is very difficult or even impossible. However, in our study, we were able to perform a statistical analysis and meta-analytic exploration for comparison groups within individual studies as well as among a few studies retrieved, which allowed us to evaluate and compare the safety profile between specific AEDs. Only a few more reliable comparisons about the safety profiles could be made, mainly, among phenobarbital, imepitoin and potassium bromide.

Implications for research

The report and assessment of the safety profile of individual AEDs on systematic reviews is very important, but it is the authors' opinion that the assessment and comparison of the safety profile among AEDs through a meta-analytic approach could offer even more valuable information and facilitate the clinician's decision on which AED to choose in respect to its safety profile. Although the prevalence of adverse effects in each study provides a general indicator of each AED's safety profile and allows limited and indirect comparisons between AEDs, the statistical analysis of comparison group studies is the essential factor that allows direct and more established comparisons. Therefore, further comparison studies are widely needed in order to perform a larger scale meta-analytic study that would offer stronger conclusions and valuable information on which AED can be considered the most or least safe. Towards this goal further conduction of high quality controlled studies (bRCTs and bRELAS) for type I adverse effects and official report of type II adverse effects are vital.

Last, but not least, a further problem that was detected by the evaluation of the studies in this review was the lack of detailed or clear information. This resulted in difficulties when performing statistics for AEDs' safety profile comparisons. Therefore, it is essential that future studies include as much accurate information as possible and that scientists have wide access to results of clinical trials and experimental studies.

Implications for clinical practice

It was found that levetiracetam might be one of the safest AEDs based on individual drug assessments, which was also supported by a strong level of evidence. Although phenobarbital is believed to be more commonly associated with a higher adverse effects rate compared to other AEDs such as levetiracetam or imepitoin, it could be argued that it has been longer on the market and a greater number of studies have involved phenobarbital; therefore the number of adverse event reports is likely to be higher. The current evidence based on this systematic review and the previous one [13] shows that there is good level of evidence supporting phenobarbital as one of the most effective AED, but it might have a lower safety profile than other AEDs (i.e. levetiracetam and imepitoin). There was, however, no statistically significant association between the overall safety profile of phenobarbital and imepitoin or levetiracetam. Only for sedation, hypoactivity and hyperactivity, a statistically significant difference was detected in favour of imepitoin, levetiracetam and phenobarbital respectively. Phenobarbital was not compared to further AEDs because of the lack of data (i.e. comparison studies). The remaining AEDs showed a variable safety profile that, potentially, could be high or low; no evidence neither was identified to support any of these statements, nor to compare their safety to other AEDs.

In general, most of the adverse effects reported in all AEDs, apart from the idiosyncratic ones, were not usually life threatening and subsided once doses and serum levels were reduced or following complete AED withdrawal. It is important for clinicians to be able to evaluate the benefits (i.e. the efficacy, cost and frequency of administration, pharmacokinetic properties, need for blood monitoring and lack of possible drug interactions) and risks (i.e. the potential prevalence and severity of adverse effects, long-term impact of adverse effects on patient and owner's quality of life, drug interactions) before initiating treatment with a specific AED.

Conclusion

This systematic review provides an evidence-based evaluation of the data on the AEDs' adverse effects most common usage for canine IE. Case reports were included to ensure that this review would capture idiosyncratic or other rare adverse effects. Only very few studies were designed in a randomised, controlled, and blinded manner and many of the studies included only a small study population with unclear inclusion or exclusion criteria and short term follow-up. Direct comparisons suggested that imepitoin and levetiracetam might have a better safety profile than phenobarbital, whilst the latter might have a better safety profile than potassium bromide. None of the comparisons showed a statistically significant difference. Further comparisons for all the AEDs were not possible as a considerable amount of studies did not report power calculations or clear and adequate data to allow further statistical analysis. Individual AED assessments showed that levetiracetam might be one of the safest AEDs followed by imepitoin and then phenobarbital and potassium bromide; all supported by strong level of evidence. The safety profile in other AEDs was variable but insufficient level of evidence was found to permit firm conclusions.

Consent for publication

Not applicable.

Abbreviations

AED(s): anti-epileptic drug(s); bELAS: blinded experimental laboratory animal studies; BID: bis in die (twice daily); bRCTs: blinded randomised clinical trials; Chloraz: Chlorazepate; CL: confidence level; CSF: cerebrospinal fluid; CT: computer tomography; CTs: clinical trials; Gaba: Gabapentin; IE: idiopathic epilepsy; Leve: Levetiracetam; m: month(s); MRI: magnetic resonance imaging; NA: Not Available; nbELAS: non-blinded experimental laboratory animal studies; nbRCTs: non-blinded randomised clinical trials; NRCTs: non-randomised clinical trials; NRELAS: non-randomised experimental laboratory studies; OR: odds ratio; PB: phenobarbital; PBr: potassium bromide; PD: polydipsia; PO: per os; PP: polyphagia; PU: polyuria; SF: seizure frequency; SID: semel in die (once daily); TID: ter in die (three times daily); UCTs: uncontrolled clinical trials; UELAS: uncontrolled experimental laboratory studies; w: week(s).

Competing interests

The authors declare that they have no competing interests.

Authors' contributions

All authors helped to draft the manuscript and participated in its design. MC and SS collected the data for the study. MC assessed the data. All authors read and approved the final manuscript.

Acknowledgements

The authors would like to thank Dr Cynthia Gaskill (University of Kentucky) for assisting with our inquiries.

Funding

Not applicable.

Author details

[1]Faculty of Brain Sciences, UCL Institute of Neurology, University College London, London WC1E 6BT, UK. [2]College of Veterinary Medicine, Iowa State University, Ames, Iowa 50011, USA. [3]Department of Production and Population Health, Royal Veterinary College, Hawkshead Lane, Hatfield, Herts AL9 7TA, UK. [4]Department of Clinical Science and Services, Royal Veterinary College, Hawkshead Lane, Hatfield, Herts AL9 7TA, UK.

References

1. Zaccara G, Gangemi PF, Cincotta M. Central nervous system adverse effects of new antiepileptic drugs. A meta-analysis of placebo-controlled studies. Seizure. 2008;17(5):405–21.
2. Baulac M: Approach of the European Medicines Agency in Development of Antiepileptic Drugs. In: *Atlas of Epilepsies*. edn.: Springer; 2010: 1615–1619. http://link.springer.com/referenceworkentry/10.1007/978-1-84882-128-6_243.
3. Chang Y, Mellor DJ, Anderson TJ. Idiopathic epilepsy in dogs: owners' perspectives on management with phenobarbitone and/or potassium bromide. J Small Anim Pract. 2006;47(10):574–81.

4. Golder S, McIntosh HM, Duffy S, Glanville J, Centre for R, Dissemination, et al. Developing efficient search strategies to identify reports of adverse effects in MEDLINE and EMBASE. Health Info Libr J. 2006;23(1):3–12.
5. Loke YK. Assessing the benefit-harm balance at the bedside. BMJ. 2004; 329(7456):7–8.
6. Bracchi R. Drug companies should report side effects in terms of frequency. BMJ. 1996;312(7028):442.
7. Cuervo LG, Clarke M. Balancing benefits and harms in health care. BMJ. 2003;327(7406):65–6.
8. Ernst E, Pittler MH. Assessment of therapeutic safety in systematic reviews: literature review. BMJ. 2001;323(7312):546.
9. Papanikolaou PN, Ioannidis JP. Availability of large-scale evidence on specific harms from systematic reviews of randomized trials. Am J Med. 2004;117(8):582–9.
10. Ross SD. Drug-related adverse events: a readers' guide to assessing literature reviews and meta-analyses. Arch Intern Med. 2001;161(8):1041–6.
11. Chou R, Helfand M. Challenges in systematic reviews that assess treatment harms. Ann Intern Med. 2005;142(12 Pt 2):1090–9.
12. Berlin JA, Colditz GA. The role of meta-analysis in the regulatory process for foods, drugs, and devices. JAMA. 1999;281(9):830–4.
13. Charalambous M, Brodbelt D, Volk HA. Treatment in canine epilepsy–a systematic review. BMC Vet Res. 2014;10:257.
14. Perucca E. Clinical pharmacology and therapeutic use of the new antiepileptic drugs. Fundam Clin Pharmacol. 2001;15(6):405–17.
15. Baird-Heinz HE, Van Schoick AL, Pelsor FR, Ranivand L, Hungerford LL. A systematic review of the safety of potassium bromide in dogs. J Am Vet Med Assoc. 2012;240(6):705–15.
16. Guyatt GH, Oxman AD, Kunz R, Vist GE, Falck-Ytter Y, Schunemann HJ, Group GW. What is "quality of evidence" and why is it important to clinicians? BMJ. 2008;336(7651):995–8.
17. Straus E.S. RWS, Glasziou P., Haynes R.B.: Evidence-Based Medicine: How to Practice and Teach It, 4 edn: Churchill livingstone elsevier; 2010.
18. Holmes MA. Philosophical foundations of evidence-based medicine for veterinary clinicians. J Am Vet Med Assoc. 2009;235(9):1035–9.
19. Summers JF, Brodbelt DC, Forsythe PJ, Loeffler A, Hendricks A. The effectiveness of systemic antimicrobial treatment in canine superficial and deep pyoderma: a systematic review. Vet Dermatol. 2012;23(4):305–29. e361.
20. Higgins JPT AD, Sterne JAC et al.: In: Higgins JPT, Green S, eds. Cochrane Handbook for Systematic Reviews of Interventions Version 5.1.0. Part 2: General methods for Cochrane reviews, Chapter 8: Assessing risk of bias in included studies, Table 8.5.d: Criteria for judging risk of bias in the 'Risk of bias' assessment tool. In.: The Cochrane Collaboration; 2011. http://www.ncbi.nlm.nih.gov/pubmed/24667063.
21. Hooijmans CR, Rovers MM, de Vries RB, Leenaars M, Ritskes-Hoitinga M, Langendam MW. SYRCLE's risk of bias tool for animal studies. BMC Med Res Methodol. 2014;14:43.
22. Kirkwood B. SJ: Essential Medical Statistics, Second edn: Wiley; 2003.
23. Boothe DM, Dewey C, Carpenter DM. Comparison of Phenobarbital with bromide as a first-choice antiepileptic drug for treatment of epilepsy in dogs. J Am Vet Med Assoc. 2012;240(9):1073–83.
24. Munana KR, Thomas WB, Inzana KD, Nettifee-Osborne JA, McLucas KJ, Olby NJ, Mariani CJ, Early PJ. Evaluation of levetiracetam as adjunctive treatment for refractory canine epilepsy: a randomized, placebo-controlled, crossover trial. J vet intern med / Am Coll Vet Inter Med. 2012;26(2):341–8.
25. Tipold A, Keefe TJ, Loscher W, Rundfeldt C, de Vries F: Clinical efficacy and safety of imepitoin in comparison with phenobarbital for the control of idiopathic epilepsy in dogs. J. Vet. Pharmacol. Ther. 2014;38(2):160–8.
26. Rundfeldt C, Tipold A, Loscher W. Efficacy, safety, and tolerability of imepitoin in dogs with newly diagnosed epilepsy in a randomized controlled clinical study with long-term follow up. BMC Vet Res. 2015;11:228.
27. Fredso N, Sabers A, Toft N, Moller A, Berendt M: A single-blinded phenobarbital-controlled trial of levetiracetam as mono-therapy in dogs with newly diagnosed epilepsy. Vet. J. 2015;208:44–9.
28. Schwartz-Porsche D, Loscher W, Frey HH. Therapeutic efficacy of Phenobarbital and primidone in canine epilepsy: a comparison. J Vet Pharmacol Ther. 1985;8(2):113–9.
29. Gaskill CL, Kimber WJ. Comparison of Phenobarbital and potassium bromide monotherapies in the treatment of canine epilepsy. In: *ACVIM*. JVIM. 2010;24:696.
30. Walker RM, DiFonzo CJ, Barsoum NJ, Smith GS, Macallum GE. Chronic toxicity of the anticonvulsant zonisamide in beagle dogs. Fundam Appl Toxicol : off j Soc Toxicol. 1988;11(2):333–42.
31. Dyer KR, Monroe WE, Forrester SD. Effects of short- and long-term administration of Phenobarbital on endogenous ACTH concentration and results of ACTH stimulation tests in dogs. J Am Vet Med Assoc. 1994;205(2): 315–8.
32. Bunch SE, Castleman WL, Baldwin BH, Hornbuckle WE, Tennant BC. Effects of long-term primidone and phenytoin administration on canine hepatic function and morphology. Am J Vet Res. 1985;46(1):105–15.
33. Daminet S, Paradis M, Refsal KR, Price C. Short-term influence of prednisone and Phenobarbital on thyroid function in euthyroid dogs. Can vet j La revue veterinaire canadienne. 1999;40(6):411–5.
34. Bunch SE, Easley JR, Cullen JM. Hematologic values and plasma and tissue folate concentrations in dogs given phenytoin on a long-term basis. Am J Vet Res. 1990;51(11):1865–8.
35. Meyer DJ, Noonan NE. Liver tests in dogs receiving anticonvulsant drugs (diphenylhydantoin and primidone). J Am Anim Hosp Assoc. 1981;17:261–4.
36. Gaskill CL, Miller LM, Mattoon JS, Hoffmann WE, Burton SA, Gelens HC, Ihle SL, Miller JB, Shaw DH, Cribb AE. Liver histopathology and liver and serum alanine aminotransferase and alkaline phosphatase activities in epileptic dogs receiving Phenobarbital. Vet Pathol. 2005; 42(2):147–60.
37. Andric N, Popovic N, Stepanovic P, Francuski J, Durdevic D. Biochemical changes in the blood serum of dogs treated with Phenobarbital. Acta Vet (Beograd). 2010;60:573–84.
38. Foster SF, Church DB, Watson AD. Effects of phenobarbitone on serum biochemical tests in dogs. Aust Vet J. 2000;78(1):23–6.
39. Kantrowitz LB, Peterson ME, Trepanier LA, Melian C, Nichols R. Serum total thyroxine, total triiodothyronine, free thyroxine, and thyrotropin concetrations in epileptic dogs treated with anticonvulsants. JAVMA. 1999; 214(12):1804–8.
40. Gaskill CL, Burton SA, Gelens HC, Ihle SL, Miller JB, Shaw DH, Brimacombe MB, Cribb AE. Effects of Phenobarbital treatment on serum thyroxine and thyroid-stimulating hormone concentrations in epileptic dogs. J Am Vet Med Assoc. 1999;215(4):489–96.
41. Jambroszyk M, Tipold A, Potschka H. Add-on treatment with verapamil in pharmacoresistant canine epilepsy. Epilepsia. 2011;52(2):284–91.
42. Loscher W, Hoffmann K, Twele F, Potschka H, Tollner K. The novel antiepileptic drug imepitoin compares favourably to other GABA-mimetic drugs in a seizure threshold model in mice and dogs. Pharmacol res : off j Italian Pharmacol Soc. 2013;77:39–46.
43. Litchfield MH, Conning DM. Effect of phenobarbitone on plasma and hepatic alkaline phosphatase activity in the dog. Naunyn Schmiedebergs Arch Pharmacol. 1972;272(3):358–62.
44. Loscher W, Potschka H, Rieck S, Tipold A, Rundfeldt C. Anticonvulsant efficacy of the low-affinity partial benzodiazepine receptor agonist ELB 138 in a dog seizure model and in epileptic dogs with spontaneously recurrent seizures. Epilepsia. 2004;45(10):1228–39.
45. Muller PB, Taboada J, Hosgood G, Partington BP, VanSteenhouse JL, Taylor HW, Wolfsheimer KJ. Effects of long-term Phenobarbital treatment on the liver in dogs. J vet intern med / Am Coll Vet Inter Med. 2000;14(2):165–71.
46. Muller PB, Wolfsheimer KJ, Taboada J, Hosgood G, Partington BP, Gaschen FP. Effects of long-term phenobarbital treatment on the thyroid and adrenal axis and adrenal function tests in dogs. J vet intern med / Am Coll Vet Inter Med. 2000;14(2):157–64.
47. McGee JH, Erikson DJ, Galbreath C, Willigan DA, Sofia RD. Acute, subchronic, and chronic toxicity studies with felbamate, 2-phenyl-1,3-propanediol dicarbamate. Toxicol Sci : off j Soc Toxicol. 1998;45(2):225–32.
48. Rieck S, Rundfeldt C, Tipold A. Anticonvulsant activity and tolerance of ELB138 in dogs with epilepsy: a clinical pilot study. Vet J. 2006;172(1):86–95.
49. Conning DM, Litchfield MH. Increase of serum alkaline phosphatase activity due to enzyme "induction" in the liver of beagle dogs. J pathol. 1971;103(2):Pxii.
50. Steiner JM, Xenoulis PG, Anderson JA, Barr AC, Williams DA. Serum pancreatic lipase immunoreactivity concentrations in dogs treated with potassium bromide and/or phenobarbital. Vet Ther : res appl vet med. 2008;9(1):37–44.
51. Paull LC, Scott-Moncrieff JC, DeNicola DB, Glickman N, Refsal KR, Glickman LT. Effect of anticonvulsant dosages of potassium bromide on thyroid function and morphology in dogs. J Am Anim Hosp Assoc. 2003;39(2):193–202.
52. Sturtevant F, Hoffmann WE, Dorner JL. The effect of three anticonvulsant drugs and ACTH on canine serum alkaline phosphatase. J Am Anim Hosp Assoc. 1977;13:754–7.

53. Volk HA, Matiasek LA, Lujan Feliu-Pascual A, Platt SR, Chandler KE. The efficacy and tolerability of levetiracetam in pharmacoresistant epileptic dogs. Vet J. 2008;176(3):310–9.
54. Kiviranta A-MOL-V, Hielm-Björkman A, Jokinen T. Topiramate as an add-on antiepileptic drug in treating refractory canine idiopathic epilepsy. J Small Anim Pract. 2013;12130:1–9.
55. Dewey CW, Cerda-Gonzalez S, Levine JM, Badgley BL, Ducote JM, Silver GM, Cooper JJ, Packer RA, Lavely JA. Pregabalin as an adjunct to phenobarbital, potassium bromide, or a combination of phenobarbital and potassium bromide for treatment of dogs with suspected idiopathic epilepsy. J Am Vet Med Assoc. 2009;235(12):1442–9.
56. Dewey CW, Guiliano R, Boothe DM, Berg JM, Kortz GD, Joseph RJ, Budsberg SC. Zonisamide therapy for refractory idiopathic epilepsy in dogs. J Am Anim Hosp Assoc. 2004;40(4):285–91.
57. von Klopmann T, Rambeck B, Tipold A. Prospective study of zonisamide therapy for refractory idiopathic epilepsy in dogs. J Small Anim Pract. 2007; 48(3):134–8.
58. Govendir M, Perkins M, Malik R. Improving seizure control in dogs with refractory epilepsy using gabapentin as an adjunctive agent. Aust Vet J. 2005;83(10):602–8.
59. Platt SR, Adams V, Garosi LS, Abramson CJ, Penderis J, De Stefani A, Matiasek L. Treatment with gabapentin of 11 dogs with refractory idiopathic epilepsy. Vet Rec. 2006;159(26):881–4.
60. Steinberg MFD. Levetiracetam therapy for long-term idiopathic epileptic dogs. J vet intern med / Am Coll Vet Inter Med. 2004;18:410.
61. Chung JY, Hwang CY, Chae JS, Ahn JO, Kim TH, Seo KW, Lee SY, Youn HY. Zonisamide monotherapy for idiopathic epilepsy in dogs. N Z Vet J. 2012; 60(6):357–9.
62. Nafe LAPA, Kay WJ. Sodium valproate: a preliminary clinical trial in epileptic dogs. J Am Anim Hosp Assoc. 1981;17(1):131–3.
63. Schwartz-Porsche DJU. Wirksamkeit von Bromid bei den therapieresistenten Epilepsien des Hundes. Tierarztl Prax. 1991;19(4):395–401.
64. Cunningham JG, Haidukewych D, Jensen HA. Therapeutic serum concentrations of primidone and its metabolites, phenobarbital and phenylethylmalonamide in epileptic dogs. J Am Vet Med Assoc. 1983; 182(10):1091–4.
65. Schwartz-Porsche D, Loscher W, Frey HH. Treatment of canine epilepsy with primidone. J Am Vet Med Assoc. 1982;181(6):592–5.
66. Pearce LK. Potassium bromide as an adjunct to Phenobarbital for the management of uncontrolled seizures in dogs. Prog Vet Neurol. 1990;1:95–101.
67. Srivastava M, Singh N, Srivastava A. Management of Phenobarbital Refractory Idiopathic Epilepsy by Potassium Bromide in Dogs. Adv Anim Vet Sci. 2013;1(1):25–7.
68. Boothe DM, Perkins J. Disposition and safety of zonisamide after intravenous and oral single dose and oral multiple dosing in normal hound dogs. J Vet Pharmacol Ther. 2008;31(6):544–53.
69. Aitken MM, Hall E, Scott L, Davot JL, Allen WM. Liver-related biochemical changes in the serum of dogs being treated with phenobarbitone. Vet Rec. 2003;153(1):13–6.
70. Dayrell-Hart B, Tiches D, Vite C, Steinberg S: Efficacy and safety of felbamate as an anticonvulsant in dogs with refractory seizures. In: ACVIM Forum: J. Vet. Inter. Med. 1996;10:174.
71. Chauvet AE, Feldman EC, Kass PH. Effects of phenobarbital administration on results of serum biochemical analyses and adrenocortical function tests in epileptic dogs. J Am Vet Med Assoc. 1995;207(10):1305–7.
72. Moore SA, Munana KR, Papich MG, Nettifee-Osborne J. Levetiracetam pharmacokinetics in healthy dogs following oral administration of single and multiple doses. Am J Vet Res. 2010;71(3):337–41.
73. March PA, Podell M, Sams RA. Pharmacokinetics and toxicity of bromide following high-dose oral potassium bromide administration in healthy Beagles. J Vet Pharmacol Ther. 2002;25(6):425–32.
74. Gaskill CL, Burton SA, Gelens HC, Ihle SL, Miller JB, Shaw DH, Brimacombe MB, Cribb AE. Changes in serum thyroxine and thyroid-stimulating hormone concentrations in epileptic dogs receiving phenobarbital for one year. J Vet Pharmacol Ther. 2000;23(4):243–9.
75. Gaskill CL, Cribb AE. Pancreatitis associated with potassium bromide/ phenobarbital combination therapy in epileptic dogs. Can vet j La revue veterinaire canadienne. 2000;41(7):555–8.
76. Balazs T, Farber TM, Feuer G. Drug-induced changes in serum alkaline phosphatase and alanine aminotransferase activities not related to hepatic injuries. Archives of toxicology Supplement = Archiv fur Toxikologie Supplement. 1978;Suppl 1:159–163.
77. Podell M, Fenner WR. Bromide therapy in refractory canine idiopathic epilepsy. J vet intern med / Am Coll Vet Inter Med. 1993;7(5):318–27.
78. Ruehlmann D, Podell M, March P. Treatment of partial seizures and seizure-like activity with felbamate in six dogs. J Small Anim Pract. 2001;42(8):403–8.
79. Heynold Y, Faissler D, Steffen F, Jaggy A. Clinical, epidemiological and treatment results of idiopathic epilepsy in 54 labrador retrievers: a long-term study. J Small Anim Pract. 1997;38(1):7–14.
80. von Klopmann T, Boettcher IC, Rotermund A, Rohn K, Tipold A. Euthyroid sick syndrome in dogs with idiopathic epilepsy before treatment with anticonvulsant drugs. J vet intern med / Am Coll Vet Inter Med. 2006;20(3):516–22.
81. Bersan E, Volk HA, Ros C, De Risio L. Phenobarbitone-induced haematological abnormalities in idiopathic epileptic dogs: prevalence, risk factors, clinical presentation and outcome. Vet Rec. 2014;175(10):247.
82. Raw M, Gaskell C. A review of one hundred cases of presumed canine epilepsy. J Small Anim Pract. 1985;26:645–52.
83. March PA, Hillier A, Weisbrode SE, Mattoon JS, Johnson SE, DiBartola SP, Brofman PJ. Superficial necrolytic dermatitis in 11 dogs with a history of phenobarbital administration (1995–2002). J vet intern med / Am Coll Vet Inter Med. 2004;18(1):65–74.
84. Dayrell-Hart B, Steinberg SA, VanWinkle TJ, Farnbach GC. Hepatotoxicity of phenobarbital in dogs: 18 cases (1985–1989). J Am Vet Med Assoc. 1991; 199(8):1060–6.
85. Weiss DJ. Bone marrow necrosis in dogs: 34 cases (1996–2004). J Am Vet Med Assoc. 2005;227(2):263–7.
86. Dayrell-Hart B, Vite C, Tiches D, Aleman D, Steinberg SA: Serum bromide concentrations and seizure control in dogs with epilepsy. In: *ACVIM forum: 1996*: Journal of Veterinary Internal Medicine; 1996: 174.
87. Weiss DJ, Smith SA. A retrospective study of 19 cases of canine myelofibrosis. J vet intern med / Am Coll Vet Inter Med. 2002;16(2):174–8.
88. Rossmeisl JH, Inzana KD. Clinical signs, risk factors, and outcomes associated with bromide toxicosis (bromism) in dogs with idiopathic epilepsy. J Am Vet Med Assoc. 2009;234(11):1425–31.
89. Bunch SE, Castleman WL, Hornbuckle WE, Tennant BC. Hepatic cirrhosis associated with long-term anticonvulsant drug therapy in dogs. J Am Vet Med Assoc. 1982;181(4):357–62.
90. Packer RA, Nye G, Porter ES, Volk HA: Assessment into the usage of levetiracetam in a canine epilepsy clinic. BMC Vet. Res. 2015;11(25)1–8.
91. Bunch SE, Baldwin BH, Hornbuckle WE, Tennant BC. Compromised hepatic function in dogs treated with anticonvulsant drugs. J Am Vet Med Assoc. 1984;184(4):444–8.
92. Bunch SE, Conway MB, Center SA, Castleman WL, Baldwin BH, Hornbuckle WE, Tennant BC. Toxic hepatopathy and intrahepatic cholestasis associated with phenytoin administration in combination with other anticonvulsant drugs in three dogs. J Am Vet Med Assoc. 1987;190(2):194–8.
93. Bizzeti M, Croce I, Sgorbini M: Acute pancreatitis in the dog secondary to anti-convulsivant therapy with phenobarbital or with phenobarbital in association with potassium bromide. Annali Fac Med Vet. 2006;59:165–170.
94. Habock G, Pakozdy A. Hamatologische abweichungen wahrend der phenobarbital-therapie beim hund. Wien Tierarztl Monatsschr. 2012;99:242–9.
95. Farnbach GC. Serum concentrations and efficacy of phenytoin, phenobarbital, and primidone in canine epilepsy. J Am Vet Med Assoc. 1984;184(9):1117–20.
96. Stabile A, De Stefani A, De Risio L. Unusual manifestation of bromide toxicity (bromism) in an idiopathic epileptic dog already treated with phenobarbital. Vet Rec Case Rep. 2014;2:1–3.
97. Miller ML, Center SA, Randolph JF, Lepherd ML, Cautela MA, Dewey CW. Apparent acute idiosyncratic hepatic necrosis associated with zonisamide administration in a dog. J vet intern med / Am Coll Vet Inter Med. 2011; 25(5):1156–60.
98. Bevier DE, Miller MA, Rohleder JJ, Wozniak AD. Pathology in practice. Superficial necrolytic dermatitis. J Am Vet Med Assoc. 2010;237(4):365–7.
99. Cook AK, Allen AK, Espinosa D, Barr J. Renal tubular acidosis associated with zonisamide therapy in a dog. J vet intern med / Am Coll Vet Inter Med. 2011;25(6):1454–7.
100. Kube SA, Vernau KM, LeCouteur RA. Dyskinesia associated with oral phenobarbital administration in a dog. J vet intern med / Am Coll Vet Inter Med. 2006;20(5):1238–40.

101. Steinmetz S, Tipold A, Bilzer T, Schenk HC. Transient neuromyopathy after bromide intoxication in a dog with idiopathic epilepsy. Irish vet j. 2012;65(1):19.
102. Boynosky NA, Stokking LB. Potassium bromide-associated panniculitis. J Small Anim Pract. 2014;55(12):640–2.
103. Jacobs G, Calvert C, Kaufman A. Neutropenia and thrombocytopenia in three dogs treated with anticonvulsants. J Am Vet Med Assoc. 1998;212(5):681–4.
104. Poffenbarger EM, Hardy RM. Hepatic cirrhosis associated with long-term primidone therapy in a dog. J Am Vet Med Assoc. 1985;186(9):978–80.
105. Henricks PM. Dermatitis associated with the use of primidone in a dog. J Am Vet Med Assoc. 1987;191(2):237–8.
106. Yohn SE, Morrison WB, Sharp PE. Bromide toxicosis (bromism) in a dog treated with potassium bromide for refractory seizures. J Am Vet Med Assoc. 1992;201(3):468–70.
107. Thrift E, Wimpole JA, Malik R. Life-thratening anemia due to possible phenobarbitone idiosyncrasy in a dog. Aust Vet Practit. 2010;40(4):130–3.
108. Nash AS, Thompson H, Bogan JA. Phenytoin toxicity: a fatal case in a dog with hepatitis and jaundice. Vet Rec. 1977;100(14):280–1.
109. Mathis JC, Yoo SH, Sullivan LA. Diagnosis of secondary dysmyelopoiesis via costochondral rib aspirate in a dog. J Vet Emerg Crit Care. 2014;24(6):739–44.
110. Mackay B, Mitchell G. Spurious hyperchloraemia and negative anion gap in a dog with bromide toxicity. Aust Vet Practit. 1998;28(2):50–2.
111. von Klopmann T, Papenhagen H, Tipold A. Phenobarbitalinduzierte blutbildveranderungen bei einem Shi-Tzu. Tierarztl Prax. 2006;34:40–4.
112. EPAR: CVPM assesment report for pexion. European Medicines agency 2012; 1–23. http://www.ema.europa.eu/docs/en_GB/document_library/EPAR_-_Public_assessment_report/veterinary/002543/WC500140842.pdf.
113. EPAR US: CVPM assesment report for pexion. European Medicines agency. 2012;1–23. http://www.ema.europa.eu/docs/en_GB/document_library/EPAR_-_Public_assessment_report/veterinary/002543/WC500140842.pdf.
114. Speciale J, Dayrell-Hart B, Steinberg SA. Clinical evaluation of gamma-vinyl-gamma-aminobutyric acid for control of epilepsy in dogs. J Am Vet Med Assoc. 1991;198(6):995–1000.
115. Loke YK, Derry S, Aronson JK. A comparison of three different sources of data in assessing the frequencies of adverse reactions to amiodarone. Br J Clin Pharmacol. 2004;57(5):616–21.
116. Shaw N, Trepanier LA, Center SA, Garland S. High dietary chloride content associated with loss of therapeutic serum bromide concentrations in an epileptic dog. J Am Vet Med Assoc. 1996;208(2):234–6.
117. Tipold A: Efficacy, safety and tolerability of ELB 138 in dogs with newly diagnosed epilepsy. In EPAR. 2006.
118. Heit: A clinical field study evaluating the safety and efficacy of ELB 138 in dogs with idiopathic epilepsy. In EPAR. 2011.
119. de Vries F: Efficacy of imepitoin (ELB 138) in dogs suffering from newly diagnosed idiopathic epilepsy. In EPAR. 2011.
120. Moher D, Liberati A, Tetzlaff J, Altman DG, P Group. Preferred reporting items for systematic reviews and meta-analyses: the PRISMA statement. BMJ. 2009;339:b2535.
121. Zaccara G, Franciotta D, Perucca E. Idiosyncratic adverse reactions to antiepileptic drugs. Epilepsia. 2007;48(7):1223–44.
122. Navarro VJ, Senior JR. Drug-related hepatotoxicity. N Engl J Med. 2006; 354(7):731–9.
123. Papanikolaou PN, Christidi GD, Ioannidis JP. Comparison of evidence on harms of medical interventions in randomized and nonrandomized studies. CMAJ : Can Mil Assoc j = j de l'Assoc med can. 2006;174(5):635–41.
124. Turner RM, Spiegelhalter DJ, Smith GC, Thompson SG. Bias modelling in evidence synthesis. J R Stat Soc Ser A. 2009;172(1):21–47.
125. Aagaard L, Hansen EH. Information about ADRs explored by pharmacovigilance approaches: a qualitative review of studies on antibiotics. SSRIs and NSAIDs BMC clin pharmacol. 2009;9:4.
126. Shukralla AA, Tudur-Smith C, Powell GA, Williamson PR, Marson AG. Reporting of adverse events in randomised controlled trials of antiepileptic drugs using the CONSORT criteria for reporting harms. Epilepsy Res. 2011; 97(1–2):20–9.
127. Aronson JK, Derry S, Loke YK. Adverse drug reactions: keeping up to date. Fundam Clin Pharmacol. 2002;16(1):49–56.
128. Derry S, Loke YK, Aronson JK. Incomplete evidence: the inadequacy of databases in tracing published adverse drug reactions in clinical trials. BMC Med Res Methodol. 2001;1:7.
129. Wieland S, Dickersin K. Selective exposure reporting and Medline indexing limited the search sensitivity for observational studies of the adverse effects of oral contraceptives. J Clin Epidemiol. 2005;58(6):560–7.
130. Golder S, Loke YK. Failure or success of electronic search strategies to identify adverse effects data. J Mil Libr Assoc : JMLA. 2012;100(2):130–4.

12

Assessment of static posturography and pedobarography for the detection of unilateral forelimb lameness in ponies

Lidia Pitti[1], Maarten Oosterlinck[2], Maria L. Díaz-Bertrana[1], José M. Carrillo[3], Mónica Rubio[3], Joaquin Sopena[3], Angelo Santana[4] and José M. Vilar[5*]

Abstract

Background: Static posturography and pedobarography are based on the detection of postural imbalance and, consequently, the pressure redistribution between limbs in lame subjects. These techniques have proven to be useful for the detection of lameness in humans and dogs. The main objective of this study was to test the suitability of static posturography and pedobarography in diagnosing lameness in ponies.
A pressure platform was used to obtain postural data (statokinesiograms, mean X and Y, length, LFS ratio, and mean velocity) from 10 sound ponies and 7 ponies with unilateral forelimb lameness. Static pedobarographic data (pressure distribution, mean pressure, and peak pressure) were also collected and compared with force plate data (peak vertical force and vertical impulse) obtained from the same animals at the walk.

Results: Significant differences were seen between lame and sound ponies for almost all evaluated parameters. With this sample size, differences between lame and sound limbs/groups were detected with a statistical power of 90%, except for mean X and Y.

Conclusions: Static posturography and pedobarography provide a complementary approach for lameness detection in equids.

Keywords: Balance, Center of pressure, Postural sway, Stabilography, Posturography, Pedobarography, Pony

Background

To overcome the inherent limitations of a subjective visual evaluation of lameness, kinetic [1, 2] and kinematic [3, 4] analyses have been introduced in equine veterinary medicine. Force platforms are considered the "gold standard" in the evaluation of lameness, and inertial sensor and optical motion capture systems have recently become commercially available [5]. However, the installation of a force platform or an optical motion capture system is technically and financially demanding, precluding widespread use outside of highly specialized laboratories or hospitals [6].

Alternatively, pressure platforms may provide a more practical alternative to force plate analysis. This equipment is portable, rather inexpensive, and provides not only information on ground reaction forces (GRF) (e.g. peak vertical force (PVF) and vertical impulses (VI)) , but also pressure-related (i.e., pedobarographic (PB)) parameters as mean or peak pressures (MP, PP, respectively) [7–10].

In equine veterinary medicine, pressure plates have been used for studying hoof landing patterns and unrollment [11], effects of trimming [12], and symmetry and hoof balance in sound horses and ponies [13, 14].

A new approach to lameness detection in the veterinary medicine is based in the detection of postural (i.e., posturographic (PT)) characteristics determined by a number of body center of pressure (COP) path parameters as area, length, velocity, etc. Changes in these characteristics obtained from force plate analysis have been used to assess the development of postural balance in foals [15], the postural effects of administering

* Correspondence: jose.vilar@ulpgc.es
[5]Departamento de Patología Animal, Instituto Universitario de Investigaciones Biomédicas Y Sanitarias, Universidad de Las Palmas de Gran Canaria, Arucas, Spain
Full list of author information is available at the end of the article

detomidine® [16] and blindfolding in healthy horses [17]. Moreover, it has been suggested that COP analysis could have diagnostic value in differentiating lame from ataxic horses [18]. Regarding lameness, it has been shown in lame subjects that a load transfer towards the sound limbs occurs [19, 20], although this redistribution pattern could vary depending on a horse's gait [21]. Consequently, lameness would also affect static COP path characteristics and pressure values (MP, PP, etc.). This has been proven in dogs in which this technique was effective for diagnosing lameness and assessing the effect of treatments for osteoarthritis [22].

A unique advantage of this new technique for assessing lameness is that measurements are taken with the animal standing still; thus, data can be collected in relatively small spaces [23].

Based on widespread application in humans, the most frequently used PT parameters for the diagnosis of postural alterations are as follows: (1) statokinesiograms, defined as the area determined by an ellipse that contains 90% of the recorded points of the COP trajectory [24], measured in mm^2, and a smaller area is associated with superior stability [22, 25]; (2) mean COP X and Y (mm), which quantifies the mediolateral and craniocaudal COP displacements independently, and, similar to statokinesiograms, smaller displacement is associated with better stability [25, 26]; (3) COP length (m), which is also called total path length [24], is the length of the line that joins the recorded points of the COP trajectory, where a higher value means more instability [27]; (4) LFS (length in function of surface), which is defined as the correlation coefficient between the COP length and its surface. This parameter provides information about the accuracy of postural control and the effort made by the subject [28], which increases its value [29]; (5) mean velocity (mm/s) of COP sway increases with instability, and this parameter may be one of the most accurate variables for the assessment of postural stability [30, 31].

Secondly, main PB data have (1) static pressure distribution expressed as a percentage (%) of total pressure exerted by each limb [22] and (2) mean pressure (MP) and peak pressure (PP) of limbs detected by the activated platform sensors [32] measured in kilopascals.

We hypothesized that static PT and PB parameters may be valid to detect lameness in equids. Therefore, the aim of this study was to test the appropriateness of a set of static PT and PB parameters in lameness detection in ponies.

Methods

Animals

The study sample consisted of 17 unshod ponies of similar conformation used for pleasure riding by children. The animals' hooves were trimmed 1 week before the study. All ponies were examined and judged by an experienced veterinary clinician (LP) under AAEP criteria, i. e., absence of lameness in the medical history of the pony, visual and hands-on exams, application of hoof testers to the hooves, joint flexion tests and evaluation of ponies in motion (walk and trot). Lameness was graded according to the AAEP scoring system (0–5). In the case of lameness, further examination included diagnostic anesthesia and dedicated imaging in order to identify the cause of lameness.

Ten of the 17 ponies were judged to be clinically sound (AAEP score 0) and, consequently, were considered part of the control group. Age ranged from 5 to 13 years; body mass from 174 to 180 kg.. On the other hand, 7 ponies presented forelimb lameness (grade 2–3/5 AAEP) attributable to desmitis of branches of the suspensory ligament ($n = 3$), acute tendinopathy of the superficial digital flexor tendon ($n = 1$), and fetlock osteoarthritis (n = 3). Age ranged from 9 to 15 years; body mass from 167 to 193 kg.

PT and PB study

A pressure platform (EPS/R1, Loran Engineering, Bologne, Italy) with Biomech software (Loran Engineering, Bologne, Italy) was used. The device contained a total of 2304 pressure sensors (density 1 sensor/cm^2) distributed in an area of 48 × 48 cm, with an acquisition frequency of 100 Hz and a measuring range of 30–400 Kpa. The platform was placed in a purpose-built cavity to maintain it leveled with the floor. All the support surface, included the platform, was covered with a flexible leatherette mat of 2 mm thick; in this way, fore and hindlimbs were at the same level.

Animals were placed with both forelimbs on the platform while standing still for at least 20 s. A total of three trials were obtained from each animal. A trial was considered valid when no movement of the limbs, head, and/or neck was observed, and the handler did not had to have any physical contact to restraint the animal during the recording. The obtained PT data included statokinesiograms, Mean COP X and Y (mm), COP length (mm), LFS ratio, and mean COP velocity (mm/s). The obtained PB data included static pressure distribution, MP, and PP (Kpa).

Force platform analysis

The differences in static PB parameters (between contralateral limbs and between groups) obtained with the pressure platform were compared with the differences in PVF and VI obtained at a walk from the same animals with a 4-sensors force platform of 35 × 35 cm and 250 Hz of sample frequency (Pasco, California, USA) placed adjacently to the pressure platform. DataStudio software (Pasco, California, USA) was used to obtain

PVF (N) and VI (Ns) values from three valid trials. A trial was considered valid when ponies walked over the platform at a velocity range of 1.6 ± 0.3 m/s and had an acceleration of ≤0.3 m/s^2. These parameters were obtained by using a motion sensor (Pasco, California, USA).

PVF and VI mean values were normalized to body weight (% BW).

For comparison purposes, limbs with lower forces than the contralateral limb were considered as 'lame' limbs (LL), whereas the other limb was considered as 'control' limb (CL) in both groups. The difference in percentage between CL and LL was calculated using the following formula: Δ% = 200* (CL-LL)/(CL + LL) [33].

Statistical analysis

A linear mixed effects model was used for the analysis of data, using the following formula:

$$y_{ij} = \beta_i + b_i + \epsilon_{ij}$$

where y_ij is the value of the response variable in the jth measure made under status i (sound/lame).

Ninety-five percent confidence intervals (95% CI) were calculated for the model parameters and the differences between groups. Normality in the residuals was checked using the Shapiro-Wilk test. Homoscedasticity of the residuals was checked by the Levene test. For all tests, a significance level of 5% was used. The power of the statistical tests was evaluated by whether the estimates of the variances obtained in the model fit. For every test, we have calculated which difference value could be detected with a power of 90%. Statistical analysis was performed with 'R' statistical language and environment, version 3.3.2. (https://www.R-project.org/).

Results

Mean values of age (mean ± SD) were 11.61 ± 4.47 years; body mass 174 ± 6.31 kg, and height at the withers 1.20 ± 0.05 m. There was no statistically significant difference in the body mass of ponies in the control group vs. the study group ($P = 0.32$).

The mean (± SD) values and 95% CI of all obtained PT and PB parameters are shown in Tables 1 and 2, respectively. All data were normally distributed and homoscedastic ($p \geq 0.06$ and $p \geq 0.07$, respectively). Detectable differences with a statistical power of 90% are shown. The sample size used in this study (7 lame and 10 control ponies with three trials each) proved to be large enough for detecting significant differences, consisting of 90% statistical power for almost all variables.

Table 1 Mean ± SD, 95% confidence interval and difference between study and control groups for PT parameters. The 90% statistical power value when significant differences were found is also provided

Statokinesiogram (mm^2)		Difference	Δ 90%
Study			
	35.73 ± 19.61		
	24.85, 46.61		
Controls			
	3.33 ± 2.53	32.40 ± 6.30	22.60
	−5.63, 12.29	18.97, 45.84	
Mean X (mm)			
Study			
	1.33 ± 0.57		
	0.93, 1.72		
Controls			
	0.82 ± 0.41	0.51 ± 0.23	0.82[a]
	0.49, 1.15	0.02, 1.00	
Mean Y (mm)			
Study			
	0.43 ± 0.20		
	0.32, 0.55		
Controls			
	0.44 ± 0.25	0.01 ± 0.07	
	0.34, 0.55	0.01, 0.07	
Lenght (mm)			
Study			
	102.66 ± 39.98		
	81.36, 123.95		
Controls			
	46.08 ± 20.52	56.58 ± 11.53	34.49
	31.55, 60.60	32.01, 81.15	
LFS			
Study			
	32.44 ± 29.65		
	17.85, 47.02		
Controls			
	6.73 ± 4.03	25.70 ± 6.60	5.56
	4.39, 9.07	11.63, 39.78	
Mean V (mm/s)			
Study			
	6.09 ± 1.92		
	4.99, 7.18		
Controls			
	2.38 ± 1.12	3.70 ± 0.59	1.78
	1.65, 3.11	2.45, 4.96	

Difference with a 90% power value in Mean X ([a]) is higher than detected difference; this means that the parameter is unable to distinguish between lame and sound ponies

Table 2 Mean ± SD, 95% confidence interval, and % difference between CL and LL limbs in both study and control groups for PB parameters. The 90% statistical power value when significant differences were found is also provided

	LL	CL	% Difference	Δ 90%
Pressure distribution				
Study				1.2
	42.82 ± 1.49%	57.18 ± 1.49%	7.18 ± 1.49[a]	
	42.09, 43.55	56.45, 57.91	6.48, 7.88	
Controls				
	49.44 ± 3.32%	50.56 ± 3.32%	0.56 ± 3.32[a]	
	48.09, 50.80	49.20, 51.91	−0.84, 1.96	
MP				
Study				12.2
	83.23 ± 10.27	157.54 ± 17.50	47.2 ± 4.37[b]	
	77.86, 88.60	148.68, 166.39	41.67, 52.80	
Controls				
	109.33 ± 17.97	111.42 ± 18.33	1.9 ± 1.98[b]	
	97.78, 120.89	99.67, 123.18	1.70, 5.4	
PP				
Study				5.4
	310.73 ± 49.35	398.59 ± 18.14	22 ± 11.76[b]	
	284.39, 337.07	387.96, 409.22	16.07, 28.07	
Controls				
	335.44 ± 32.33	357.61 ± 63.19	6.02 ± 11.23[b]	
	316.34, 354.54	329.49, 385.73	0.10, 12.53	
PVF				
Study				11.8
	66.84 ± 6.94	91.01 ± 6.67	26.6 ± 1.26[b]	
	61.66, 72.02	86.06, 95.96	21.60, 26.74	
Controls				
	72.58 ± 3.53	72.80 ± 3.27	0.3 ± 0.86[b]	
	71.10, 74.06	71.41, 74.18	−1.95, 1.52	
VI				
Study				14.0
	31.05 ± 2.91	40.38 ± 4.93	23.1 ± 1.06[b]	
	28.98, 33.11	37.60, 43.17	17.95, 28.75	
Controls				
	35.48 ± 2.56	35.79 ± 2.65	0.9 ± 0.56[b]	
	34.11, 36.86	34.45, 37.14	−0.81, 1.43	

[a]In regards to the ideal symmetry (i.e., 50% for each limb); [b]In regards to CL value

PT data

Data from statokinesiograms (Fig. 1a, b), Mean X, length, LFS, and mean COP velocity showed significantly higher values ($p \leq 0.03$) in lame ponies compared with the control group, which is compatible with a higher COP sway (i.e. instability in the lame animals). Mean X failed to reach the required statistical power. Mean Y showed no significant differences between groups ($p = 0.88$) (Fig. 2).

PB data

Differences in static pressure distribution (Fig. 3), MP and PP values between LL and CL showed a significant difference in the lame group ($p \leq 0.023$), which is in contrast with the data from the control group ($p \geq 0.053$). Compared with the sound group, CL values were significantly higher in the lame group for all measured parameters, which proves a pressure redistribution to the sound contralateral limb in lame ponies.

Force platform data

In agreement with the PB data, PVF and VI values showed significant differences between LL and CL in the lame group when compared with the control group ($p \leq 0.0001$) (Fig. 4). All PB and force platform data reach the 90% statistical power.

Discussion

Building further on previous reports detailing stabilographic variables in sound horses [23], this study is the first to describe static PT and PB data for the detection of lameness in equids, specifically in ponies.

In the present study, almost all parameters proved suitable to detect lameness, similar to what has been described in humans [24] and dogs [22]. Among these variables, statokinesiograms provide the most reliable information, which confirms other reports [31]. These similarities may be explained because this value corresponds with the ellipse area containing 90% of COP sway points, while discarding the other 10% usually corresponding to unavoidable head tilts and nods.

Statokinesiogram values in lame ponies were similar to those reported in dogs, where values in cases of unilateral elbow dysplasia were under 45 mm^2 [22]. Surprisingly, these values are lower than those considered normal in humans ($\leq 100\ mm^2$) [34]. This is in agreement with previous results obtained in horses [23] and is probably related to the four limbs providing a larger base of support than in a bipedal situation [18].

Another surprising finding was that in sound ponies latero-lateral sway was much bigger compared with that cranio-caudal, in contrast to humans, where predominant COP sway is the anteroposterior axis [35]. The greater distance between ipsilateral limbs and contralateral limbs provides more stability in the cranio-caudal sense, as previously reported in horses [17, 18]. This could also explain why the only parameter that did not show statistical differences between sound and lame ponies was the Mean Y.

A statistically significant difference between lame and sound groups was found for Mean X; however, this

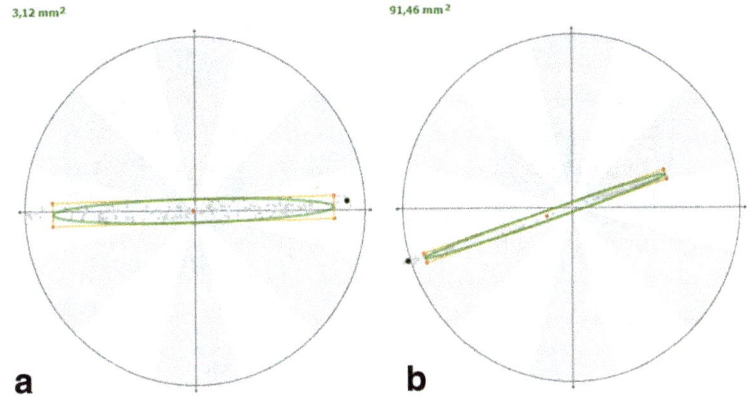

Fig. 1 Statokinesiograms obtained from a sound pony (**a**) and a pony with a right fore lameness (**b**). Compared with the sound animal, the ellipse in the lame pony is asymmetrically displaced to the left side due to the body COP being shifted to the left more frequently than to the right side. In addition, the area of the ellipse is much greater (3.12 mm^2 in the sound pony vs. 91.46 in the lame pony)

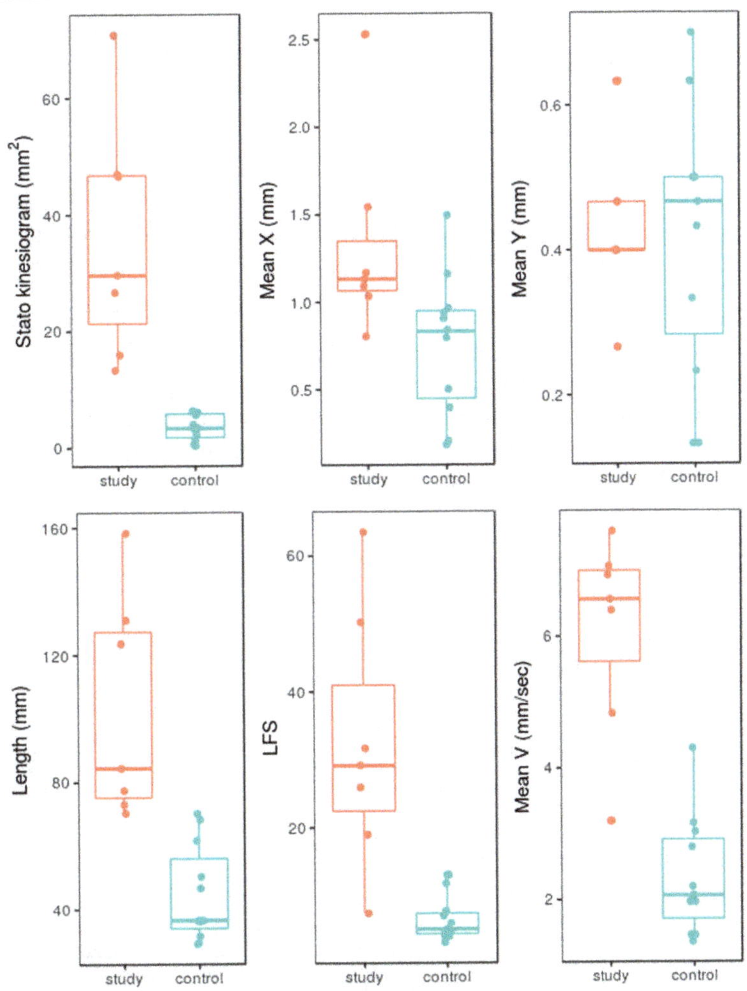

Fig. 2 Boxplots of the PT parameters. Except for Mean Y, all values in the lame group are significantly larger than in the sound group

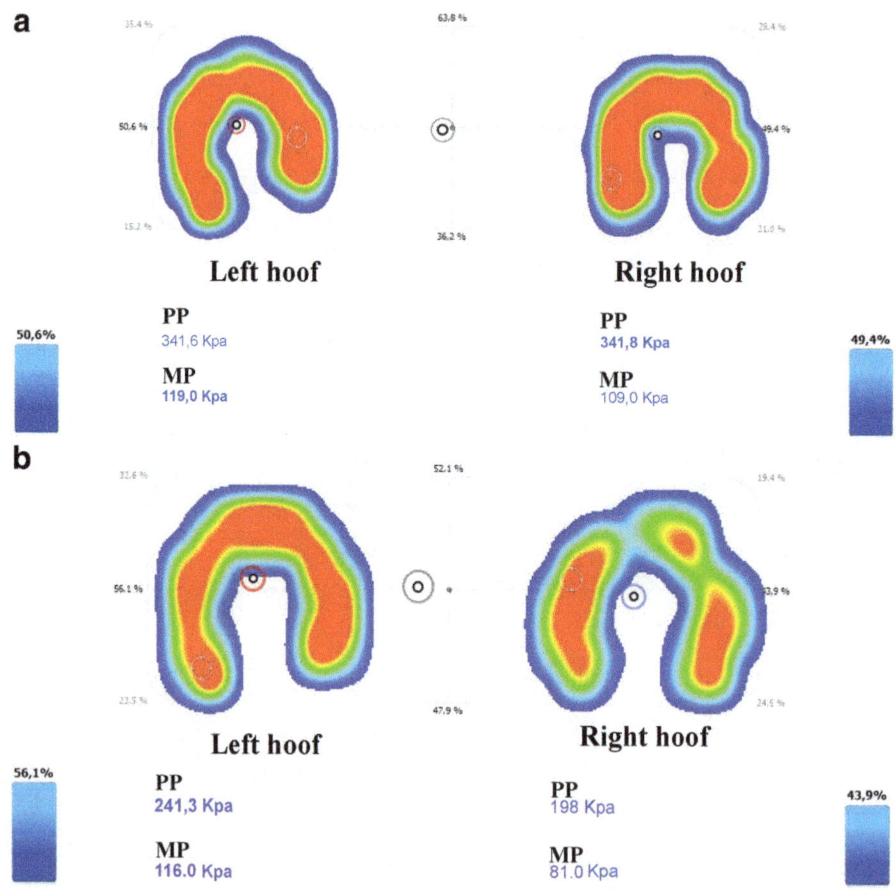

Fig. 3 Pedobarography in a sound pony (**a**) and in a pony with a right fore lameness (**b**). The differences in pressure distribution, MP, and PP between the left and right hooves are much higher in the lame group (**b**) than in the control group (**a**). A left displacement of the body COP can be also seen (black/grey circles)

difference was very small (less than 1 mm) and could not be detected with 90% statistical power. For this reason, we believe that the minimal differences observed in this parameter may be irrelevant and render it not as reliable as the other variables to detect mild lameness.

Previous studies in dogs have suggested the suitability of the Area of support for the detection of lameness [10] as paws expand, although not linearly, depending of the applied pressure [22]. However, the relative rigidity of the equine hoof when compared with dog pads do not

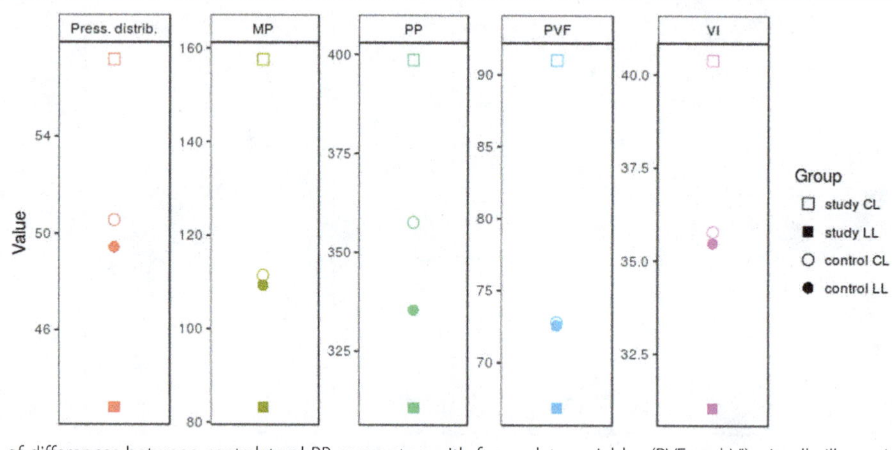

Fig. 4 Comparison of differences between contralateral PB parameters with force plate variables (PVF and VI), visually illustrating greater differences between LL and CL in the study group than in the control group of sound ponies

allow for the detection of acute changes in contact area. Until now, it has only been found useful to measure hoof size asymmetry, which can be observed, for example, in chronically lame limbs [36].

Notwithstanding their gold standard status in gait analysis [5], force plate analysis of GRF is limited to highly specialized labs or hospitals. This is not only because the installation is complicated and expensive, but also because gathering data is time-consuming and involves repeating many trials to record data of individual limbs. Moreover, trial repetition implies variations in velocity, which should be minimized. In contrast, static PT and PB analysis only requires a portable and rather inexpensive pressure platform and a minimum space to maintain the animal standing still, without the need to control speed.

However, in the veterinary field, static PT and PB studies have a main disadvantage in that, compared with humans, it is more difficult to maintain an animal completely immobile during a longer time. In humans, this time period has been classically set between 30 and 52 s [31, 34, 37]. In our study, we used a recording time of 20 s, which is an intermediate value compared with other postural equine studies [15, 17, 23, 25]. In our experience, extending the measurement beyond 20 s created problems because of animal movements, since the aim was to maintain the required steady position. It is important to note that this technique may be impossible to perform in certain nervous or fractious animals.

There are threelimitations of this study. First, as stated above, compensatory pressure redistribution in lame horses implies not only the contralateral limb [33, 38]; thus, it would be interesting to include data from hindlimbs in a subsequent study as well as determination if correlation exist between PT and PB values with lameness degree. Unfortunately, the relative small dimensions of the pressure platform impede the simultaneous analysis of more than two limbs. Second, direct comparison with previous studies using force or pressure platform equipment should be considered with caution, since different technology may alter the results [23]. Third, and last, besides its application for detecting lameness, this new technique may also serve for the detection of postural imbalances caused by neurological disorders as in humans, although further studies are required to distinguish between lame from ataxic animals. Should be also interesting to know what kind of correlation exist between our PB parameters in static animals with those obtained from ponies at walk or trot.

Conclusions

This study proves that static PT and PB parameters can be useful tools for the detection of equine lameness, especially in ponies.

Abbreviations

CL: Sound limb in the study group or the limb with the higher value in the control group; COP: Center of pressure; GRF: Ground reaction forces; LFS: Length/area ratio; LL: Lame limb in the study groups or limb with lesser value in the control group; MP: Mean pressure; PB: Pedobarography; PP: Peak pressure; PT: Posturography; PVF: Peak vertical force; VI: Vertical impulse

Acknowledgments

The authors thank Amanda Hand for translation and editing. We would also like to thank the ponies' owners for their collaboration. Thanks also to the Cátedra García Cugat for its technical support.

Authors' contributions

JMV, MO, JS, and JMC conceived and designed the experiments; MR performed the clinical and imaging analyses; JMV, LP and MLD performed the force and pressure platform analyses; AS analyzed the data; all authors read and approved the final manuscript.

Competing interests

The authors declare that they have no competing interests.

Author details

[1]Departamento de Patología Animal, Universidad de Las Palmas de Gran Canaria, Las Palmas de Gran Canaria, Spain. [2]Department of Surgery and Anaesthesiology of Domestic Animals, Faculty of Veterinary Medicine, Ghent University, Ghent, Belgium. [3]Departamento Medicina y Cirugía Animal, Cátedra García Cugat, Universidad CEU Cardenal Herrera, Valencia, Spain. [4]Departamento de Matemáticas, Universidad de las Palmas de Gran Canaria, Las Palmas, Spain. [5]Departamento de Patología Animal, Instituto Universitario de Investigaciones Biomédicas Y Sanitarias, Universidad de Las Palmas de Gran Canaria, Arucas, Spain.

References

1. Ishihara A, Reed SM, Rajala-Schultz PJ, Robertson JT, Bertone AL. Use of kinetic gait analysis for detection, quantification, and differentiation of hindlimb lameness and spinal ataxia in horses. J Am Vet Med Ass. 2009;234:644–51.
2. Kaido M, Kilborne AH, Sizemore JL, Reisbig NA, Aarnes TK, Bertone AL. Effects of repetition within trials and frequency of trial sessions on quantitative parameters of vertical force peak in horses with naturally occurring lameness. Am J Vet Res. 2016;77:756–65.
3. Maliye S, Marshall JF. Objective assessment of the compensatory effect of clinical hind limb lameness in horses: 37 cases (2011-2014). J Am Vet Med Assoc. 2016;249:940–4.
4. Olsen E, Fouchè N, Jordan H, Pfau T, Piercy RJ. Kinematic discrimination of ataxia in horses is facilitated by blindfolding. Equine Vet J. 2018;50:166–71.
5. Donnell JR, Frisbie DD, King MR, Goodrich LR, Haussler KK. Comparison of subjective lameness evaluation, force platforms and an inertial-sensor system to identify mild lameness in an equine osteoarthritis model. Vet J. 2015;206:136–42.
6. Silva MG, Moreira PVS, Rocha HM. Development of a low cost force platform for biomechanical parameters analysis. Res Biomed Eng. 2017;33:259–68.
7. Schnabl-Feichter E, Tichy A, Bockstahler B. Coefficients of variation of ground reaction force measurement in cats. PLoS One. 2017;12:e0171946.
8. Carr BJ, Canapp SO Jr, Zink MC. Quantitative comparison of the walk and trot of border collies and Labrador retrievers, breeds with different performance requirements. PLoS One. 2015;10:e0145396.
9. Bockstahler B, Tichy A, Aigner P. Compensatory load redistribution in Labrador retrievers when carrying different weights–a non-randomized prospective trial. BMC Vet Res. 2016;12:92.
10. Oosterlinck M, Bosmans T, Gasthuys F, Polis I, Van Ryssen B, Dewulf J, Pille F. Accuracy of pressure plate kinetic asymmetry indices and their correlation with visual gait assessment scores in lame and nonlame dogs. Am J Vet Res. 2011;72:820–5.

11. Van Heel MC, Moleman M, Barneveld A, Van Weeren PR, Back W. Changes in location of Centre of pressure and hoof-unrollment pattern in relation to an 8-week shoeing interval in the horse. Equine Vet J. 2005;37:536–40.
12. Moleman M, van Heel MC, van Weeren PR, Back W. Hoof growth between two shoeing sessions leads to a substantial increase of the moment about the distal, but not the proximal, interphalangeal joint. Equine Vet J. 2006;38:170–4.
13. Oosterlinck M, Pille F, Back W, Dewulf J, Gasthuys F. Use of a stand-alone pressure plate for the objective evaluation of forelimb symmetry in sound ponies at walk and trot. Vet J. 2010;183:305–9.
14. Oosterlinck M, Pille F, Huppes T, Gasthuys F, Back W. Comparison of pressure plate and force plate gait kinetics in sound warmbloods at walk and trot. Vet J. 2010;186:347–51.
15. Nauwelaerts S, Malone SR, Clayton HM. Development of postural balance in foals. Vet J. 2013;198(Suppl 1):e70–4.
16. Bialski D, Lanovaz JL, Bohart GV, Mullineaux DR, Clayton HM. Effect of detomidine on postural sway in horses. Comp Exerc Physiol. 2003;1:45–50.
17. Clayton HM, Nauwelaerts S. Effect of blindfolding on Centre of pressure variables in healthy horses during quiet standing. Vet J. 2014;199:365–9.
18. Clayton HM, Buchholz R, Nauwelaerts S. Relationship between morphological and stabilographic variables in standing horses. Vet J. 2013; 198(Suppl 1):e65–9.
19. Buchner HH, Obermuller S, Scheidl M. Body Centre of mass movement in the lame horse. Equine Vet J. 2001;33:122–7.
20. Rhodin M, Pfau T, Roepstorff L, Egenvall A. Effect of lungeing on head and pelvic movement asymmetry in horses with induced lameness. Vet J. 2013; 198(Suppl 1):e39–45.
21. Weishaupt MA, Wiestner T, Hogg HP, Jordan P, Auer JA. Compensatory load redistribution of horses with induced weight-bearing forelimb lameness trotting on a treadmill. Vet J. 2006;171:135–46.
22. Manera ME, Carrillo JM, Batista M, Rubio M, Sopena J, Santana A, Vilar JM. Static Posturography: a new perspective in the assessment of lameness in a canine model. PLoS One. 2017;12:e0170692.
23. Gomes-Costa M, Roupa I, Pequito M, Prazeres J, Gaivão M, Abrantes J, Clayton HM. The use of pressure plates for static Center of Pressure Analysis in horses. J Equine Vet Sci. 2015;35:315–20.
24. Baratto L, Morasso PG, Re C, Spada G. A new look at posturographic analysis in the clinical context. Sway-density versus other parameterization techniques. Mot Control. 2002;6:246–70.
25. Asseman F, Caron O, Cremieux J. Is there a transfer of postural ability from specific to unspecific postures in elite gymnasts? Neurosci Lett. 2004;358:83–6.
26. Clayton HM, Nauwelaerts S. Is a single force plate adequate for stabilographic analysis in horses? Equine Vet J. 2012;44:550–3.
27. Paillard T, Noe F. Techniques and methods for testing the postural function in healthy and pathological subjects. Biomed Res Int. 2015:891390. https://doi.org/10.1155/2015/891390.
28. Fabbri M, Martoni M, Esposito MJ, Brighetti G, Natale V. Postural control after a night without sleep. Neuropsychol. 2006;44:2520–5.
29. Lumbau A, Schinocca L, Chessa G. Influence of posture on swallowing. Eur J Paediatr Dent. 2011;12:171–4.
30. Duarte M, Freitas SM. Revision of posturography based on force plate for balance evaluation. Rev Bras Fisioter. 2010;14:183–92.
31. Sipko T, Chantsoulis M, Kuczynski M. Postural control in patients with lumbar disc herniation in the early postoperative period. Eur Spine J. 2010;19:409–14.
32. Marghitu DB, Swaim SF, Rumph PF, Cojonaru D, Gillette RL, Scardino MS. Dynamics analysis of ground contact pressure of English pointer dogs. Nonlinear Dyn. 2003;33:253–65.
33. Molsa SH, Hyytiainen HK, Hielm-Bjorkman AK, Laitinen-Vapaavuori OM. Long-term functional outcome after surgical repair of cranial cruciate ligament disease in dogs. BMC Vet Res. 2014;10:266.
34. Sulkowski WJ, Kowalska S, Sobczak Z, Jozwiak Z. The statokinesiometry in evaluation of the balance system in persons with chronic carbon disulphide intoxication. Pol J Occup Med Environ Health. 1992;5:265–76.
35. Clark RA, Bell SW, Feller JA, Whitehead TS, Webster KE. Standing balance and inter-limb balance asymmetry at one year post primary anterior cruciate ligament reconstruction: sex differences in a cohort study of 414 patients. Gait Posture. 2017;52:318–24.
36. Oosterlinck M, Pille F, Back W, Dewulf J, Gasthuys F. A pressure plate study on fore and hindlimb loading and the association with hoof contact area in sound ponies at the walk and trot. Vet J. 2011;190:71–6.
37. Scoppa F, Capra R, Gallamini M, Shiffer R. Clinical stabilometry standardization: basic definitions–acquisition interval–sampling frequency. Gait Posture. 2013;37:290–2.
38. Maliye S, Voute LC, Marshall JF. Naturally-occurring forelimb lameness in the horse results in significant compensatory load redistribution during trotting. Vet J. 2015;204:208–13.

13

The use of imepitoin (Pexion™) on fear and anxiety related problems in dogs

Kevin J. McPeake* and Daniel S. Mills

Abstract

Background: Fear and anxiety based problems are common in dogs. Alongside behaviour modification programmes, a range of psychopharmacological agents may be recommended to treat such problems, but few are licensed for use in dogs and the onset of action of some can be delayed. The low affinity partial benzodiazepine receptor agonist imepitoin (Pexion™, Boehringer Ingelheim) is licensed for treating canine epilepsy, has a fast onset of action in dogs and has demonstrated anxiolytic properties in rodent models. This case series reports on the use of imepitoin in a group of dogs identified as having fear/anxiety based problems. Twenty dogs were enrolled into the study, attended a behaviour consultation and underwent routine laboratory evaluation. Nineteen dogs proceeded to be treated with imepitoin orally twice daily (starting dose approximately 10 mg/kg, with alterations as required to a maximum 30 mg/kg) alongside a patient-specific behaviour modification plan for a period of 11–19 weeks. Progress was monitored via owner report through daily diary entries and telephone follow-up every two weeks. A Positive and Negative Activation Scale (PANAS) of temperament was also completed by owners during baseline and at the end of the study.

Results: The primary outcome measure was average weekly global scores (AWG) from the owner diaries. Average weekly reaction scores (AWR) for each type of eliciting context was used as a secondary outcome. Seventeen dogs completed the trial. Treatment with imepitoin alongside a behaviour modification programme resulted in owner reported improvement with reduced AWG and reduced AWR for anxiety across a range of social and non-social eliciting contexts including noise sensitivities. Significant improvement was apparent within the first week of treatment, and further improvements seen at the 11 week review point. There was a significant reduction in negative activation (PANAS) with 76.5% of owners opting to continue imepitoin at their own expense after completion of the study.

Conclusions: This study provides initial evidence indicating the potential value of imepitoin (Pexion™) alongside appropriate behaviour modification for the rapid alleviation of signs of fear and anxiety in dogs. Further research with a larger subject population and a placebo control would be useful to confirm the apparent efficacy reported here.

Keywords: Anxiety, Dog, Drug, Fear, GABA, Imepitoin

Background

Fear and anxiety-related problems in dogs are common. In the People's Dispensary for Sick Animals Pet Animal Welfare report [1] (2011) 82% of owners reported their dog was afraid of 'something'. Another study [2] found that 25% of owners considered their dogs to be fearful of noises, but 49% reported at least one behavioural sign suggestive of fear when exposed to loud noises. The Association of Pet Behaviour Counsellors in the UK [3] report that 8% of canine cases were referred for a specific fear or phobia, 6% for owner-absent problems (which includes "separation anxiety") and 64% for aggressive behaviour towards people and dogs (the extent to which fear or anxiety played a role in these cases was not stated). In the US, a study [4] found 10.3% of cases had a specific fear, anxiety or phobia, 14% separation anxiety and 22% fear-related aggression towards people.

* Correspondence: kmcpeake@lincoln.ac.uk
Animal Behaviour, Cognition and Welfare Group, School of Life Sciences, University of Lincoln, Lincoln, Lincolnshire, UK

Both fear and anxiety can occur in the context of the perception of increased threat to the individual [5]. Whereas fear occurs in response to the presence of a specific aversive trigger, anxiety develops when an animal anticipates a negative outcome such as in a location where they previously encountered an aversive trigger [6, 7]. In a novel or unpredictable environment, or in a situation of ambiguous threat, a dog may experience anxiety and uncertainty due to a conflict of approach and avoidance tendencies [8]. Dogs may also experience anxiety associated with the departure of the owners. These may arise from fear and anxiety related associations (e.g. fear of isolation, fear of stimuli occurring in the context of being separated) as well as problems related to separation from an attachment figure (PANIC sensu Panksepp, [9]). Different neurochemical networks are thought to underpin these different forms of anxiety [10, 11]. A further distinction may also be made between social and non-social stimuli that trigger a response [12].

The affective state of fear and anxiety can operate at the level of: a specific emotional reaction (i.e. in response to a specific aversive trigger); a mood change (longer lasting emotional changes that bias behaviour and cognition occurring in response to a series of related aversive events); or as a feature of temperament (behavioural predispositions arising from the interaction of genetic and early experiential factors). One method developed for assessing aspects of temperament in dogs is the Positive and Negative Activation Scale (PANAS) [13], a reliable and valid measure of positive activation/affect (mediates behavioural approach and neophilia) and negative activation/affect (mediating behavioural inhibition, withdrawal and avoidance (fear-anxiety)). Anxious emotional reactions, moods and temperament can all be problematic for an owner and are a cause for welfare concern.

Fear and anxiety related problems in dogs are principally resolved using behaviour modification techniques such as desensitisation and counter-conditioning (operant and classical) [14]. Various psychopharmacological agents have been suggested as potentially useful adjuncts in such cases, [15] including: tri-cyclic antidepressants (TCAs) e.g. amitriptyline [16] and clomipramine [17, 18]; tetra-cyclic antidepressants e.g. mirtazapine [14]; selective serotonin reuptake inhibitors (SSRIs) e.g. fluoxetine [19, 20]; monoamine oxidase inhibitors (MAO-Is) e.g. selegiline [21]; progestins e.g. megestrol acetate [22]; anticonvulsants e.g. phenobarbital [23]; benzodiazepines e.g. diazepam [24] and alprazolam [25]; alpha-2 adrenergic receptor agonists clonidine [26] and dexmedetomidine [27].

However, there are few psychopharmacological agents licensed for use in dogs. In the European Union (EU), where a licensed drug is not available, veterinary surgeons should follow the prescription cascade as outlined in the European Union Veterinary Medicines Directive (2001/82) [28]. Although this allows the use of the benzodiazepines listed above because they have a human licence, the prescription cascade regulations indicate that for a different condition in the same species should be given preference. In the United States (US), where a veterinary formulation does not exist informed consent can be obtained from a client to use human formulations "extra-label".

At the time of writing, clomipramine (Clomicalm, Novartis – EU and US), selegiline (Selgian, CEVA - EU; Anipryl, Zoetis, US), the progestogen megestrol acetate (Ovarid, Virbac – EU), fluoxetine (Reconcile – not currently available) and most recently dexmedetomidine (Sileo, Zoetis) all have veterinary licenses for dogs.

The effects of using medications such as SSRIs and TCAs can typically take around 3–5 weeks to become apparent [15]. Benzodiazepines have a faster onset of action [15, 29], but no benzodiazepines are licensed in any form for use in dogs in the EU nor available as veterinary formulations in the US.

Benzodiazepines exhibit their effects by binding to a specific benzodiazepine binding site on the inhibitory neurotransmitter GABA (ɣ-aminobutyric acid) receptor and they can exhibit anxiolytic properties [30]. One retrospective study in dogs explored the anxiolytic properties of diazepam as reported by owners, where the response was variable, where 53% of owners discontinued diazepam therapy due to lack of efficacy and 58% due to adverse effects [24]. In the same study in the group of dogs classed as having 'thunderstorm phobia' 100% of owners classed the treatment as effective. Dosages of diazepam varied widely in this study, which is important as the effects of benzodiazepines are dose dependent with moderate doses often needed for anxiolytic effects and higher doses more likely to cause adverse effects such as ataxia [15]. In addition, tolerance can develop with the use of benzodiazepines [15, 31]. However, as benzodiazepines can be highly effective there is value in further exploring the safety and reliability of using this class of drugs as anxiolytics in dogs.

Imepitoin (Pexion™, Boehringer Ingelheim) is a low affinity partial benzodiazepine receptor agonist [32, 33] licensed in the EU for the reduction of the frequency of generalised seizures due to idiopathic epilepsy in dogs [34]. When used in dogs, imepitoin appears to be well tolerated and safe [35, 36]. Pharmacokinetic studies in dogs show imepitoin has a fast onset of action of around 2–3 h after single oral dosing [37]. Fear and anxiety are common behavioural co-morbidities in canine epileptic patients [38]. During the development of imepitoin for the treatment of idiopathic epilepsy in dogs, it was reported anecdotally that some owners wanted to continue using imepitoin due to reported improvements in their dog's behaviour even when seizure frequency was unaffected [39]. In a variety of experimental rodent models, imepitoin has demonstrated anxiolytic properties [39–41]. In addition, being a low affinity partial agonist, the likelihood of developing reduced efficacy related to tolerance and potential for abuse are lower which may offer advantages over full agonist benzodiazepines [39].

The aim of the current study was to undertake an initial investigation of the potential value of imepitoin alongside an individualised behaviour modification programme for the treatment of a range of anxiety and fear related behaviour problems in dogs through a carefully monitored case series.

Methods

Subjects

Cases were recruited following a local publicity campaign via referral from the owner's regular veterinary surgeon. Clients were offered a free behaviour consultation, blood test, trial medication and follow up for a period of up to three months. Potential cases were screened using a series of inclusion and exclusion criteria (Table 1).

To be considered for the study, 4 initial documents had to be completed: a veterinary referral form to be completed by their referring vet and returned with a full medical history; the University of Lincoln Animal Behaviour Clinic standard client questionnaire; a Positive and Negative Activation Scale (PANAS); an individualised diary (Additional file 1) to be completed to provide one week of baseline data for their dog's reaction in eliciting context(s) established through a telephone discussion. The diary was adapted from The Lincoln Sound-Sensitivity Scale [10] to relate more broadly to recognisable signs of fear and anxiety in contexts other than noises. To do this an on-line forum of pet behaviour counsellors [42] was asked to provide signs they would attribute to fear and anxiety in dogs. As a result of this three signs were added to the diary – yawning; licking lips; moving away. This gave 20 specific signs with an additional 'others' category. The 'frequency' score was replaced by an 'Event Occurrence' box which could be marked 'yes' or 'no'. The severity score range was changed from '0–5' to '1–5'. A total score for the dog's reaction to that eliciting context on that occasion, could then be calculated by totalling each severity score for each sign/category (maximum score = 105). Examples of eliciting contexts included: encounters with strangers; noises; dogs etc. The same diary format was used during baseline and the follow up period to monitor the dog's reactions ('Event occurrence' and 'Severity') based on the owner's observation and scoring. For the single dog with separation related problems (Case 17), video footage was taken weekly whilst the dog was home alone and reviewed by the owner in order to complete the diary scoring. Of the initial 28 owners sent this information, 7 failed to return the complete paperwork and one dog was euthanized before the consultation for unrelated reasons. This left 20 dogs with suspected fear and anxiety related problems.

The clinician in immediate charge of the case (KM) under the supervision of a European and RCVS recognised specialist in behavioural medicine (DM) assessed all the documents completed at the enrolment stage.

Behaviour consultation

Each of the 20 dogs in the initial group was brought to the University of Lincoln Animal Behaviour Clinic for a behaviour consultation, typically lasting 2–3 h. The approach used to establish a diagnosis relating to fear-anxiety adopted the systematic and scientific evaluation of the four key components of emotion (as described by Mills et al., [10]) relating to context, physiological arousal, behavioural tendencies and communicative elements.

Clinical examination and blood sampling

During the consultation, a full clinical examination was performed on each dog and bodyweight was measured. Jugular venepuncture was performed to obtain a

Table 1 Inclusion and exclusion criteria

Inclusion criteria	Exclusion criteria
At least 6 months of age	Lactating or pregnant bitch
Greater than 5 kg bodyweight	Male breeding dog
Behavioural complaint related to fear-anxiety as diagnosed by a veterinary behaviourist	Dogs receiving phenobarbital treatment for epilepsy
Incidences of behavioural complaint apparent at least twice a week	Any current uncontrolled medical problem
Willing to attend a behaviour consultation at the University of Lincoln	Severely impaired hepatic function
Willing to commit to giving medication for up to a 3 month period if medication deemed to be of potential benefit to the case (owner has option of withdrawing from study at any time)	Severe renal disorders
Willing to have a blood sample taken from their dog for routine laboratory evaluation (at no expense to owner), prior to use of any medication	Severe cardiovascular disorders
Willing to complete all study paperwork including a daily diary referring to the animal's behaviour problem and more global behaviour	Significant family related risk factors affecting risk to individuals from the dog's behaviour identified (e.g. toddlers in the home in the case of aggressive behaviour towards people; aggression between dogs within home)

complete blood count, serum biochemistry, thyroid panel (fT4, TT4, cTSH) and basal cortisol values for each dog.

Behaviour modification programmes

Given the wide range of presenting problems, it was not desirable to standardise the treatment protocols for each dog. Behaviour modifications were tailored to the individual, taking into account the dog, the presenting problems, the owner and other factors relating to the dog's specific environment. Advice was given during the consultation on techniques, which were demonstrated where necessary, and owners were provided with an aide memoire of key points, followed up by a full written report within 7 days of the consultation.

Use of imepitoin

As imepitoin is licensed for use in dogs at a dose range of 10-30 mg/kg twice daily, all cases were commenced on a dose around 10 mg/kg twice daily. During the study, and depending on the individual's progress, dose alterations were made. Dose changes were made at intervals of no less than two week periods. The rationale for increasing the dose was twofold: 1) if there was no apparent improvement at the previous dose; 2) if improvement at the previous dose had plateaued and the behaviour problem was not resolved to the satisfaction of the owner and behaviour clinicians.

Monitoring during follow-up period

During the follow up period, owners completed an eliciting context diary sheet every time their dog was exposed to an eliciting context identified in the baseline period, and these were submitted to the investigators every two weeks. These diaries were scored and a telephone call to the owner was arranged to review progress.

End of study

All cases used in the final analysis were followed for at least 3 months including the one week of baseline monitoring before reaching the 'decision point' (this varied between 11 to 19 weeks depending on the availability of the owner to complete a telephone survey at the end of the study). At this time owners were asked to complete a second PANAS and questioned about various aspects of their experience of using imepitoin including: ease of administration; satisfaction with overall treatment success; whether they would use imepitoin at their own expense (and if so, tactically or continuously). They were also given the clinician's opinion on using imepitoin for their dog in the future and were offered further advice on behaviour modification as necessary. In those owners continuing imepitoin responsibility for prescribing imepitoin was passed to the referring veterinary surgeon. Imepitoin can be stopped abruptly, however for those owners stopping imepitoin, guidelines were given for weaning which was typically reducing each dose by 50% for 2 weeks before stopping completely

Statistical analysis

The data were analysed informally for evidence of a relationship between imepitoin dosing and owner report of changes in behaviour with statistical analysis undertaken using Minitab 17. Normality of distribution of data were assessed using Anderson-Darling normality tests. Effect sizes were calculated for all assessments of difference using Cohen's d [43].

Effects on reactions

Two main metrics were used to monitor efficacy on fear-anxiety reaction scores: average weekly fear-anxiety reaction scores (AWR) and average weekly global fear-anxiety scores (AWG). The equations were developed specifically for this study to use the owner's diary entry scores to assess response and control for the number of eliciting contexts.

In addition, given that the eliciting contexts did not occur every week, we adopted a method of conservative data imputation in order to avoid having missing scores. Imputations for responses in weeks when the eliciting context did not occur in a given week were made using the following rules: if a week of data was missing during the follow up, the average of the weeks on either side was taken and imputed (i.e. the value used for that week was estimated from the average of the week before and afterwards); if in the final week of the follow up period, there was no eliciting context, the last value obtained before this was imputed. This method probably provided a conservative estimate of the effect, potentially underestimating any effect, since it referred back to an earlier stage of treatment. At all the time points analysed (baseline, week 1, week 11 and decision point): for the primary measure of interest, average global weekly scores, 3 imputations were made out of 68 entries (3/68 = 4.4%); for the measure of secondary interest, average weekly reactions, 28 imputations were made out of 140 entries (28/140 = 20%). All these data related to an absence of the eliciting context in a given week (e.g. a week where there was no exposure to an eliciting context recorded by the owner) and not lost data from recorded responses.

Statistical analysis was stratified with AWR and AWG as the primary outcome measures and subsequent analyses post hoc based on the significance of the primary measures. As there were 2 measures a Bonferroni correction was applied to AWR and AWG only as to apply it to all post hoc calculations would risk a type II error.

Average weekly reactions scores The average weekly reaction score (AWR) (maximum score 105) was calculated for each dog for each eliciting context as shown in the example below for a dog with noise sensitivities:

$$AWR\,(individual\ noise) = \frac{Sum\ of\ diary\ scores\ for\ that\ individual\ noise\ that\ week}{Number\ of\ exposures\ to\ that\ individual\ noises\ that\ week}$$

$$AWR\,(noises) = \frac{Sum\ of\ all\ AWR\,(individual\ noises)\ that\ week}{Number\ of\ different\ individual\ noises\ exposed\ to\ that\ week}$$

Similar equations were used to calculate AWR scores for dogs with social fear-anxiety and also non-social fear-anxiety. To compare differences in the AWR in dogs between eliciting contexts grouped into noise sensitivities, social fear-anxiety and non-social fear-anxiety (excluding noise sensitivities at specific time points (week 1, week 11, decision point) whilst on treatment through the study, paired sample t-tests were used. The accepted level of significance after Bonferroni correction was $p < 0.025$.

Average weekly global scores The average weekly global score (AWG) (maximum score 105) was calculated for each dog using the following equation:

$$AWG = \frac{Sum\ of\ all\ AWR\ that\ week}{Number\ of\ eliciting\ contexts\ recorded\ that\ week}$$

To compare the average weekly global scores in dogs between baseline and specific time points (week 1, week 11, decision point) whilst on treatment through the study, paired sample t-tests were used. The accepted level of significance after Bonferroni correction was $p < 0.025$.

Effects on temperament

Positive and negative activation To compare the effects of treatment on owner reported positive and negative activation (from the PANAS) between baseline and the decision point of treatment, paired sample t-tests were used. A value of $p < 0.05$ was considered significant.

Owner satisfaction with treatment

A Spearman's correlation coefficient was computed to assess whether owner satisfaction with treatment success correlated with: i) changes in reactions (percentile reduction in average global weekly fear-anxiety reactions from baseline to decision point); ii) changes in temperament (percentile reduction in negative activation from baseline to decision point). A value of $p < 0.05$ was considered significant.

At the end of the study, owners were also asked about their interest in continuing treatment with imepitoin at their own expense and to rate the ease of administration of the imepitoin

Results

Demographics

The initial group was composed of 20 dogs (see Table 2): three dogs were withdrawn from the study: case 1 due to change in analgesia during the follow-up period whilst on imepitoin case 4 due to a reported adverse event whilst on imepitoin; case 18 due to abnormalities in initial laboratory evaluation results before imepitoin was commenced. This left 17 dogs in the final analysis (Table 3) comprising 11 females (64.7%) and 6 males (35.3%) (all dogs were neutered), of a range of breeds and ages ranging from 1 year 1 month to 10 years 7 months (average age of 4 years 6 months). Bodyweight ranged from 5.0 kg to 36.7 kg (average bodyweight 18.9 kg). All dogs had been owned for a minimum of 3 months by their owners prior to enrolment.

Clinical examination and laboratory evaluation findings

Clinical examination revealed abnormalities in 6 cases, with some cases having more than 1 abnormality: gait abnormalities/musculoskeletal problems (5 dogs), interdigital cyst (1 dog), entropion (1 dog), dental disease (1 dog). Further investigations/treatments were performed at the referring veterinary practices. Where this included the use of trial analgesia, or surgical correction (canine extraction, entropion correction) a new baseline week of diary entries was established after recovery/once deemed stable on analgesia for approximately 4 weeks. Laboratory evaluation revealed abnormalities in one dog (case 18) indicative of atypical hypoadrenocorticism and this dog did not proceed to the treatment group.

Adverse events

Among the 19 dogs treated with imepitoin, 7 adverse events were reported in 6 dogs, these were not necessarily associated with medication but are recorded here in accordance with best practice. Two dogs showed signs of ataxia, and 1 dog chewed some plastic and vomited. These three incidents resolved without specific treatment whilst continuing the imepitoin. Recurrence of a pre-existing lameness occurred in Case 1 resulting in withdrawal from the study by the investigators due to a change in analgesia regime by the referring veterinarian. Diarrhoea was seen in 1 dog (Case 17) which resolved on cessation of imepitoin at 10 mg/kg; when the drug was reintroduced at the lower dose of 5 mg/kg there was no recurrence in diarrhoea and the dog remained on this dose. Case 4 had 2 episodes of ataxia and muscle tremors, (including around the head) the first during week 7 and the second during week 8 of treatment with 10 mg/kg imepitoin. Both of these episodes occurred around the time where noises were audible which had historically resulted in a fearful response. The blood profile was repeated and no abnormalities were detected.

Table 2 Initial group and overview of clinical details and withdrawals

Case No.	Breed	Sex[a]	Age at clinic visit	Weight (kg)	Eliciting contexts recorded	Other treatments	Notes on other treatments	Adverse events	Reason for withdrawal
1	Cross-breed	MN	3 y 8mo	21.00	Noises; Carrying objects; Entering back door	Meloxicam SID	Changed to firocoxib during study	Y	Change of analgesia
2	Cross-breed	FN	6y	11.60	Noises	Carprofen SID	Continued during study	N	N/A
3	Cross-breed	MN	3y 7mo	21.30	Noises	None	-	N	N/A
4	Labrador Retriever	FN	7y	23.75	Noises; Visitors; Dogs	None	-	Y	Adverse events
5	Staffordshire Bull Terrier	FN	10y 7mo	18.45	Noises	Meloxicam SID	Trialled only, not used during study	N	N/A
6	Whippet	FN	3y 5mo	12.74	Noises; Walking	None	-	N	N/A
7	Staffordshire Bull Terrier	FN	2y 5mo	18.98	Noises; Walking	None	-	Y	N/A
8	Brittany Spaniel	FN	8y 4mo	12.78	Noises; Walking	None	-	N	N/A
9	English Bull Terrier	FN	2y 8mo	20.30	Visitors; Strangers; Noises; Moving from sofa	Firocoxib SID	Trialled only, not used during study	N	N/A
10	Labrador Retriever	MN	3y 9mo	25.75	Noises	None	-	N	N/A
11	German Wire-haired Pointer	MN	4y 1mo	31.60	Novel items; Strangers; Visitors; Postal delivery; Noises	Meloxicam SID	Trialled only, not used during study	Y	N/A
12	Tervuren Belgian Shepherd	MN	5y 1mo	23.40	Noises; Walking	Carprofen SID	Trialled only, not used during study	N	N/A
13	Cross-breed	FN	4y 10mo	20.20	Noises; Visitors	None	-	N	N/A
14	Cross-breed	FN	1y 1mo	20.00	Visitors; Strangers; Crowded areas; Dogs; New environments	None	-	N	N/A
15	Jack Russell Terrier	FN	5y	7.36	Noises; Walking	None	-	N	N/A
16	Cross-breed	FN	2y 3mo	18.48	Noises	None	-	N	N/A
17	Cross-breed	FN	2y 9mo	5.00	Home alone	None	-	Y	N/A
18	Border Collie	FN	6y 7mo	12.86	Noises	Firocoxib SID	-	N/A	Blood results
19	Cross-breed	MN	1y 7mo	15.40	Dogs; Strangers; Visitors	None	-	N	N/A
20	German Shepherd	MN	5y 1mo	36.70	Noises	Meloxicam SID	Continued during study	Y	N/A

[a]*M* male, *F* female, *N* neutered, *y* years, *mo* months, *Y* yes, *N* no, *N/A* not applicable

Table 3 Population used in final analysis, dose of imepitoin, AWG and PANAS at specific time points and owner satisfaction

Case No.	Baseline		Week 1		Week 11		Decision		Max. dose of imepitoin (mg/kg BID)	Score Reduction Negative Activation (Baseline to Decision)	% Score Reduction Negative Activation (Baseline to Decision)	Owner Satisfaction	Continuation of treatment at owner's expense – Y/N (C/T) = basis of use
	AWG	Dose (mg/kg)	AWG	Dose (mg/kg)	AWG	Dose (mg/kg)	AWG	Dose (mg/kg)					
2	46.70	0	26.50	8.6	9.00	30.2	4.00	30.2	30.2	−0.05	−6.25	S	Y (C)
3	11.57	0	2.50	9.4	0.50	19.8	2.50	19.8	19.8	−0.17	−22.67	S	Y (T)
5	32.33	0	24.50	10.8	11.00	21.6	0.00	21.6	21.6	−0.38	−47.50	VS	Y (C)
6	3.36	0	0.88	11.8	0.00	3.9	0.00	11.8	11.8	−0.04	−4.76	VS	Y (T)
7	20.94	0	4.36	10.5	5.00	10.5	5.00	10.5	10.5	−0.36	−46.15	VS	Y (C)
8	19.75	0	3.33	11.7	0.59	11.7	0.00	23.5	23.5	−0.04	−6.25	S	Y (T)
9	12.00	0	7.33	9.9	3.34	9.9	6.00	19.8	19.8	−0.18	−30.14	S	Y (C or T)
10	23.67	0	27.50	9.7	6.67	19.3	6.50	19.3	19.3	−0.16	−22.22	VS	Y (T)
11	28.07	0	13.38	12.7	9.00	19.0	9.67	19.0	19.0	−0.15	−21.13	S	Y (T)
12	34.75	0	34.00	10.7	9.64	19.2	17.58	29.9	29.9	−0.07	−8.54	PP	Y (C)
13	29.75	0	3.50	9.9	16.67	19.8	2.50	29.7	29.7	−0.31	−34.07	S	Y (C or T)
14	28.58	0	12.78	10.0	11.75	20.0	5.50	20.0	20.0	−0.15	−17.24	PP	N
15	34.91	0	21.00	13.6	8.00	30.5	1.00	30.5	30.5	−0.07	−8.54	VD	N
16	7.61	0	4.59	10.8	7.00	29.8	7.00	29.8	29.8	0.05	9.80	PP	N
17	28.00	0	21.00	10.0	1.00	5.0	1.00	5.0	10.0	−0.03	−5.88	VS	Y (C)
19	28.89	0	19.84	9.7	16.33	9.7	15.50	19.4	19.4	−0.16	−18.18	VS	Y (C or T)
20	6.33	0	3.33	10.9	8.00	21.8	9.50	21.8	21.8	−0.22	−30.14	PP	N

AWG Average weekly global score, *Baseline* Baseline week, *Decision* Decision point (11–19 weeks); *Y* yes, *N* no, VS very satisfied, *S* satisfied, *PP* partly satisfied/partly dissatisfied, *D* dissatisfied, *VD* very dissatisfied, *C* continuous use, *T* tactical use

Despite general improvements in behaviour in response to noise out with these events, the owner opted to stop the imepitoin and the dog was withdrawn from the study.

Fear-anxiety triggers

Of the 17 cases used in the final analysis 6 cases (35.3%) had a single eliciting context monitored, with the remaining 11 cases (64.7%) having 2 or more eliciting contexts each. This gave a total of 35 different eliciting contexts for fear-anxiety: 13 social (visitors, strangers, dogs, crowded areas, home alone) and 22 non-social (14 of which were noises, the remainder being: walking, moving from sofa, novel items, postal delivery, new environments).

Behaviour modification programmes

Behaviour modification recommendations generally included managing the dog's exposure to triggers which included environmental modifications and reinforcing appropriate behaviour. Other recommendations included introduction of a safe haven at home (12 cases); operant counterconditioning protocols with hand-touch to check-in with owner when the dog has heard a noise on walks (10 cases); desensitisation and counterconditioning protocols with sound CDs (9 cases – only 1 of the 9 used the sound CD during the follow up period); basket muzzle training (4 cases); teaching a 'go to mat' behaviour (3 cases); introduction of activity feeders (3 cases); introduction of front-attaching harness (2 cases); desensitisation and counterconditioning to vet practice (1 case); toilet training advice (1 case); cues for 'say hello, say goodbye' when meeting and disengaging from other dogs (1 case). The single case of separation related problems was advised on desensitisation to leaving rituals, introduction of safety signal when leaving dog alone, changing leaving/returning ritual and teaching increased independence from owner.

Use of imepitoin

During the study, of the 17 dogs in the final analysis, 4 received a maximum trial dose of around 30 mg/kg twice daily, 10 dogs received a maximum trial dose of around 20 mg/kg twice daily and 2 dogs remained on the initial dose of around 10 mg/kg twice daily, with 1 dog dropping down to and being maintained on 5 mg/kg twice daily. Mean doses of imepitoin being used at key time points were: week 1 (mean = 10.6 mg/kg, median = 10.5 mg/kg); week 11 (mean = 17.7 mg/kg, median = 19.3 mg/kg); decision point (mean = 21.3 mg/kg, median = 20.0 mg/kg).

Effects on reactions

Average weekly global scores

The primary measure of interest was the average weekly global scores (AWG). An Anderson-Darling normality test showed that the data distribution was not significantly different from normal across the 17 subjects at baseline (p = 0.306), week 11 (p = 0.463), decision point (p = 0.088) and mean (p = 0.064), but were significantly different to normal at week 1 (p = 0.037). In this situation, parametric tests can be used to examine effects within the population studied, but generalisation to the wider population should be more cautious [44] for the data relating to non-normally distributed data. Given the acknowledged preliminary nature of this study (case series), it is therefore acceptable to use parametric tests with this caution acknowledged. Summary effects are displayed in Table 4.

There was a statistically significant difference in the AWG between baseline and all specific time points whilst on treatment. These effect sizes are large and the results indicate that imepitoin alongside a behaviour modification programme had a useful effect on reducing AWG in dogs, with an initial meaningful effect being seen within the first week of treatment.

Average weekly reaction scores

The secondary measure of interest was the average weekly reaction scores (AWR) between the eliciting context groups previously described. An Anderson-Darling normality test showed that the data were normally distributed across the average weekly reactions for different eliciting contexts and subjects at baseline (p = 0.565), week 1 (p = 0.051) and week 11 (p = 0.139), but not at the decision point (p = <0.005).

Noise sensitive group For the noise sensitive group (n = 14), there was a significant difference in the AWR between: baseline and week 1; baseline and week 11;

Table 4 Average weekly global fear-anxiety reaction scores for all 17 dogs in final analysis

Week	Average weekly global fear-anxiety reaction score			t-value (16)	p-value	d_{Cohen}
	Mean +/– SD	Decrease from baseline (95% CI)	Median (range)			
Baseline	23.37 +/– 11.87	-	28.00 (3.36–46.70)	-	-	-
1	13.55 +/– 10.75	9.82 (5.76,13.88)	12.78 (0.88–34.00)	5.13	<0.001	–0.867
11	7.26 +/– 5.13	16.10 (10.88,21.32)	8.00 (0–16.67)	6.54	<0.001	–1.762
Decision	5.49 +/– 5.21	17.88 (11.48,24.28)	5.00 (0–17.58)	5.92	<0.001	–1.951

baseline and decision point. There was a larger effect size at week 11 and decision point compared to week 1. The data are displayed in Table 5.

Non-social fear-anxiety group For the non-social fear-anxiety group (excluding noise sensitivities) (n = 8), there was a significant difference in the average weekly reaction scores between: baseline and week 1; baseline and week 11; baseline and decision point. There was a larger effect size at week 11 and decision point compared to week 1. The data are displayed in Table 6.

Social fear-anxiety group For the social fear-anxiety group (n = 13), there was a significant difference in the average weekly reaction scores between: baseline and week 1; baseline and week 11; baseline and decision point. There was a larger effect size at week 11 and decision point compared to week 1. The data are displayed in Table 7.

These results indicate large effects in reducing average weekly reaction scores across dogs with noise sensitivities, social and non-social fears and anxieties, with significant effects being seen within the first week across all groups, and larger effects being seen at week 11 and decision points compared to week 1.

Effects on temperament

Negative activation

The paired sample t-test used to compare negative activation scores showed a significant difference in the mean scores between baseline and the decision point with a large effect size.

Positive activation

There was no significant difference in the mean positive activation scores between baseline and the decision point. Effect size was therefore not calculated. The data are displayed in Table 8.

These results suggest that imepitoin alongside a behaviour modification programme has a large statistically significant effect on reducing negative activation (i.e. fearfulness/anxiousness in dogs) as measured through the PANAS.

Owner satisfaction with treatment

Owners were also asked to rate their overall satisfaction with treatment success: 6 (35.3%) were very satisfied, 6 (35.3%) satisfied, 4 (23.5%) partly satisfied/partly dissatisfied, 0 dissatisfied and 1 (5.9%) very dissatisfied. The owner who was very dissatisfied (case 15) reported an improvement in anxiety on walks during treatment, but insufficient change in reactions to noises which was the main presenting problem.

There was no correlation between owner satisfaction with either percentile reduction in average global weekly fear-anxiety reactions (r_s = −0.288; p = 0.262) or percentile reduction in negative activation from baseline to decision point. (r_s = −0.201; p = 0.439).

Continuation of treatment at owners' expense

Of the 17 owners, 13 (76.5%) suggested they would use imepitoin at their own expense: 5 opted to use it on a continual basis from the end of the follow up period; 5 suggested they would consider using it on a tactical basis (e.g. leading up to and for the duration of periods during the year with increased risk of exposure to stressors); 3 suggested they would use it either continually or tactically depending on the outcome of discontinuing the imepitoin on their dog's behaviour – i.e. if improvements seen during the treatment period were not sustained, they would consider restarting the use of imepitoin. The remaining 4 owners (23.5%) suggested they would not consider using imepitoin again. In 3 of the 5 cases who opted to stop imepitoin on a continual basis and consider use on a tactical basis, the consulting clinician (KM) would have preferred using the imepitoin on a continuous basis given the reported improvements during the follow up period. In all other decisions the clinician was in complete agreement with the client's decision.

Ease of administration

At the end of the study, owners were asked to rate the ease of administration of imepitoin with the results being: 6 (35.3%) very easy, 9 (52.9%) easy, 2 (11.8%) moderately easy/moderately difficult. No owners rated administration as difficult or very difficult.

Table 5 Average weekly reaction score – noise sensitive group (n = 14)

Week	Noise sensitivities - Average weekly reaction score			t-value (13)	p-value	d_{Cohen}
	Mean +/− SD	Decrease from baseline (95% CI)	Median (range)			
Baseline	21.11 +/− 13.50	-	21.50 (4.92–46.70)	-	-	-
1	14.17 +/− 11.65	6.94 (3.07,10.81)	10.50 (0.25–34.00)	3.87	0.002	−0.5504
11	8.30 +/− 6.71	12.81 (6.55,19.08)	7.00 (0.50–26.50)	4.42	0.001	−1.2017
Decision	8.26 +/−11.11	12.85 (5.10,20.59)	5.75 (0.00–43.00)	3.58	0.003	−1.039

Table 6 Average weekly reaction score – non-social fear/anxiety group (excluding noise sensitivities) (n = 8)

Week	Non-Social - Average weekly reaction score			t-value (7)	p-value	d_{Cohen}
	Mean +/− SD	Decrease from baseline (95% CI)	Median (range)			
Baseline	18.57 +/− 10.20	-	19.02 (1.79–30.00)	-	-	-
1	9.76 +/− 6.59	8.81 (2.03,15.60)	10.17 (0.00–20.00)	3.07	0.018	−0.782
11	6.78 +/− 5.56	11.79 (6.07,17.51)	7.88 (0.00–15.00)	4.88	0.002	−2.786
Decision	6.51+/− 5.57	12.06 (4.75,19.38)	6.88 (0.00–15.00)	3.90	0.006	−2.824

Additional information

Owner reported improvements with change in dose of imepitoin

During the study, there were 7 owner reports of improvements in behaviour quickly following dose increases in imepitoin suggesting specific efficacy of imepitoin. Five cases where dose was increased from approximately 10 mg/kg to 20 mg/kg (Cases 5, 11, 12, 13, 16), and 2 cases where dose was increased from around 20 mg/kg to around 30 mg/kg (Cases 2, 12).

Owner reported reduction in recovery time during treatment with imepitoin

Three owners (Case 5, 12, 13) reported reduction in recovery time (i.e. quicker recovery) whilst on imepitoin following exposure to fireworks compared to previous years.

Owner reported deterioration on cessation of imepitoin

Two owners continued to keep diary entries through weaning, and behavioural deterioration on cessation of therapy with continuation of the behaviour modification programme suggests specific efficacy of imepitoin. In case 15 the owner reported an increase reluctance to go for walks which had improved during the period on imepitoin. In Case 3 the owner reported an increase in noise sensitivity and reactivity to other dogs at classes which had improved during the period on imepitoin.

Dog's responses from diaries

A total of 1210 individual diary forms were completed by owners during the study. Dog's responses for each of the options from the diary were assessed with mean scores between baseline ('off imepitoin) and the entire treatment period ('on imepitoin') with the percentage change shown in Table 9. There was a reduction in mean scores of all clinical signs across all eliciting contexts during treatment compared with baseline with the exception of one single episode of diarrhoea (under title of 'vomiting/urinating/defecating') when home alone reported for Case 17 which was reported as an adverse event.

Discussion

These results provide initial evidence of the potential value of using imepitoin alongside a behaviour modification programme in reducing the average weekly global scores reported by owners of dogs with fear-anxiety related problems. When grouped into noise sensitivity, social and non-social fear-anxiety based problems, a reduction in average weekly reaction scores were seen across all groups. These effects appeared to be quick acting (within a week of the onset of administration of treatment) but improve over time. In addition imepitoin alongside a behaviour modification programme significantly reduced owner report of fearfulness as a temperament trait in dogs. Therefore it may be of value in cases where dogs have been identified as having a generally fearful or anxious temperament and potentially to help prevent a recurrence of problems in such individuals, although this remains to be tested empirically. At the end of the study 76.5% of owners would consider using imepitoin at their own expense, 88.2% of owners found imepitoin very easy or easy to administer, and 70.6% of owners were satisfied or very satisfied with treatment success. This demonstrates that there were also clinically meaningful improvements being seen by dog owners during the treatment period, although owner satisfaction did not relate to the scale of improvement measured here. This might be because owner satisfaction may depend on a few signs that are of particular concern to them (e.g. destructiveness or vocalisation) [10] whereas

Table 7 Average weekly reaction score – social fear/anxiety group (including single case of separation related problems) (n = 13)

Week	Social - Average weekly reaction score			t-value (12)	p-value	d_{Cohen}
	Mean +/− SD	Decrease from baseline (95% CI)	Median (range)			
Baseline	25.68 +/− 7.82	-	27.20 (13.00–38.00)	-	-	-
1	15.48 +/− 8.97	10.20 (7.15,13.25)	19.00 (1.33–26.25)	7.28	<0.001	−1.112
11	8.48 +/− 6.11	17.20 (12.81,21.59)	7.00 (0.00–17.00)	8.54	<0.001	−2.451
Decision	8.22 +/− 6.38	17.46 (12.73,22.20)	7.00 (0.00–19.33	8.03	<0.001	−2.447

Table 8 Positive and negative activation scale scores

Week	Baseline Mean +/− SD	Baseline Median (range)	Decision Point Mean +/− SD	Decision Point Median (range)	Mean Decrease from baseline (95% CI)	t-value (16)	*p*-value	d_{Cohen}
Negative activation	0.7541 +/− 0.1148	0.78 (0.51–0.91)	0.6053 +/− 0.1216	0.58 (0.42–0.80)	0.1488 (0.0865,0.2111)	5.07	<0.001	−1.258
Positive activation	0.6653 +/− 0.1152	0.70 (0.52–0.84)	0.6665 +/− 0.1236	0.66 (0.52–0.87)	0.0012 (0.0303,0.0280)	−0.09	0.933	-

the metric used to assess improvement considers all signs even if not problematic to the owner.

Although case series provide a relatively low level of evidence among clinical studies [45] they can serve an important purpose in advancing medical knowledge [46]; for example, this report provides the first exploration of the potential application of imepitoin as an anxiolytic for clinical behaviour problems. The majority of dogs had multiple problems extending from fear-anxiety, and so two types of metric were used. One type of metric (average global weekly scores; negative activation scores) gave a measure of the overall response for the totality of problems. The other (average weekly reaction scores) focused on the response to treatment to particular types of problem, grouped by context into social, non-social or noise related fear-anxiety problems. This resulted in dogs being included in multiple evaluations for average weekly reaction scores according to which context(s) the problem(s) were apparent, however only data relating to the relevant eliciting contexts for that context were included in that assessment, and not the global problem data.

Table 9 Clinical signs as reported by owners across all eliciting contexts between baseline and whole period on imepitoin

Dog's response from eliciting context diary	Mean scores at baseline	Mean scores on imepitoin	% change in scores
Running around	0.802	0.412	−48.6
Drooling saliva	0.481	0.165	−65.7
Hiding	1.091	0.577	−47.1
Destructiveness	0.092	0.017	−81.5
Cowering	2.588	1.096	−57.7
Restlessness/pacing	1.344	0.570	−57.6
Aggressive behaviour	0.310	0.154	−50.3
"Freezing" to the spot	1.114	0.459	−58.8
Barking/whining/howling	0.786	0.608	−22.6
Panting	1.605	0.772	−51.9
Vomiting/defecating/ urinating	0.000	0.005	+0.50
Owner-seeking behaviour	1.277	0.750	−41.3
Vigilance/scanning of environment	2.128	1.406	−33.9
Bolts	0.939	0.460	−51.0
Exaggerated response when startled	2.273	1.063	−53.2
Shaking or trembling	1.567	0.482	−69.2
Self-harm	0.017	0.007	−58.8
Yawning	0.522	0.249	−52.3
Licking lips	1.693	0.683	−59.7
Moving away	1.661	0.477	−71.3

In the current study, baseline diary entries before commencing treatment meant each dog could acted as its own control, and although there was no control for dogs receiving imepitoin without behaviour modification advice, this is more typical of the recommended way of using medication in clinical behaviour cases. Medication is typically used as an adjunct to behaviour modification advice therefore this study replicates how imepitoin would likely be used in veterinary behavioural practice. However, given the rapid onset of effect within the first week, the finding that during the study there were 7 owner reports of improvements in behaviour quickly following dose increases, and the 2 owner reports of deterioration in their dogs behaviour on cessation of imepitoin, it seems likely that there is a specific effect of the drug in these cases and the results are not simply due to the behaviour modification programme.

These improvements seen within the first week of treatment, also raise the question of the potential to use imepitoin tactically. In the current study, this was important for those owners who saw benefits whilst their dog was on imepitoin but did not wish to use it continuously, but would consider using it at times of the year where there would be an increased risk of exposure to triggers for fear-anxiety (e.g. fireworks season, shooting season). For these cases it was advised to use imepitoin, in future, at the dose found to be effective during the current study, commencing 1 week before the anticipated onset of problematic triggers, and for the duration of this period (this could range from days to weeks depending on the trigger and level of exposure in the environment anticipated by the owner for the dog). Currently unlicensed benzodiazepines are often used tactically, given 30–60 min before the fear-anxiety trigger is expected, but responses to medication by individuals are often hard to predict [24, 25]. Further studies are required to investigate the potential benefits of using imepitoin in this way or in the context of individual dosing in relation to a specific event, in particular, the minimum period of time imepitoin can be given for an effect to be seen. Typically other anxiolytics such as SSRIs and TCAs may have an onset of action of around 3–5 weeks

[15], so in cases where a more rapid onset of action is required, imepitoin may be a valuable option.

There were significant differences in reports of reactions to noises between week 1 of treatment and both week 11 and decision point. It should be noted that the average dosage of imepitoin being administered across all dogs differed at these time points, as it was determined and increased on an individual basis. Mean dosage at week 1 was 10.6 mg/kg, at week 11 was 17.7 mg/kg, and at the decision point was 21.3 mg/kg. Reduction in reaction scores could therefore reflect a difference in dose being given, be the result of a longer duration of treatment or reflect the synergistic effect of imepitoin and behaviour modification therapy. However, in light of these findings 20 mg/kg imepitoin twice daily appears to be a reasonable recommended dose for anxiolytic effects with dose titration built around this dose according to effect.

The study used a standardised diary format to reduce subjectivity in owner responding, and self-reporting to gather data for analysis. There can be multiple limitations with this method - during the study there were 3 owners who suggested that they were failing to record all eliciting contexts resulting in 'no response' from their dog. This suggests that improvements may actually have been under-reported. The diary was used to record a summary of what the owner saw during the whole event their dog was exposed to the eliciting context, and there was no standardised duration of time each owner was required to observe their dog for. A caregiver placebo effect has been shown in dogs receiving treatment for osteoarthritis [47] and should also be considered when assessing the data from the study, which can potentially result in over-reporting of improvements by owners. The diary used did not include a section on recovery time after exposure to an eliciting context however 3 owners spontaneously reported reduced recovery times after exposure to noises compared to the time before treatment with imepitoin. Recovery time might therefore be a useful metric to include in future studies.

There were 6 dogs with 7 reported adverse events during the trial, with a high likelihood (as judged by the authors) of the imepitoin being implicated in 2 of these (mild ataxia, Case 11; diarrhoea, Case 17) but the likelihood of the drug's involvement in the other 3 is largely unknown although in one we consider it unlikely (Case 1).

Paradoxical excitement can occur in species (including dogs) receiving benzodiazepines [24, 31], and although a potential adverse effect of using imepitoin is transient hyperactivity [35], there were no dogs in the study where this was reported.

Tolerance to the effects of benzodiazepines can develop with ongoing use [15, 31] such as those demonstrated in anxiolytic models in mice [48]. The development of tolerance to the anticonvulsant effects of diazepam in dogs has also been documented [49]; however tolerance to the anticonvulsant effects of imepitoin has not been demonstrated [33, 37]. Additionally, when looking at anxiolysis, the results of this study showed significant effects within the first week of treatment with continued improvements seen at week 11 and decision points which is not suggestive of tolerance developing within this time frame.

Concerns have been raised over the potential for benzodiazepines disinhibiting and therefore increasing aggressive behaviour in dogs and other species [15, 31] and one study reported increased aggressive behaviour and new aggression in a small proportion of dogs treated with diazepam [24]. There were no dogs in the study where aggressive behaviour was reported in the diary entries where it had not been seen before, and overall, there was a 50.3% reduction in owner reported signs of aggressive behaviour across all dogs whilst on imepitoin compared to the baseline period.

In the human literature, there is conflicting evidence supporting or refuting the amnesic, memory and cognitive impairing effects of long term benzodiazepine use (for a meta-analysis and review see [50]). During the study there were no reports of adverse events suggestive of memory impairments such as loss of previously learned behaviours. In addition, all owners were asked to use operant and/or classical conditioning as part of their individualised behaviour modification programmes and subjectively there appeared to be no difficulty in implementation of such training protocols.

It is important to consider both the physical health and concurrent medical problems of any patient presenting with a behavioural complaint [51]. Although this study excluded dogs with a history of seizures, given that behavioural comorbidities are common in canine epilepsy [38], further studies could explore the value of using imepitoin in these patients. Musculoskeletal pain may cause or exacerbate behaviour problems such as aggressive behaviour [52, 53]. Fear and anxiety may also amplify pain [54]. For these reasons, it was important to establish that any medical abnormalities detected on clinical examination were investigated and treated prior to commencing imepitoin and a behaviour modification plan, which occurred in 6 of the 20 dogs enrolled in the study. Indeed 11 subjects were not enrolled in the study due to uncontrolled medical reasons, with 8 of these related to suspected musculoskeletal pain. In addition one dog (Case 1) was withdrawn from the analysis due to recurring lameness which resulted in increased general anxiety and required a change in analgesia. Pain remains an important differential and moderator of response in anxiety cases, and so all cases need careful medical evaluation.

Conclusions

This report provides the first exploration of the potential application of imepitoin as an anxiolytic for clinical behaviour problems. This study suggests that imepitoin may be an effective medication to aid the treatment of a range of fear-anxiety based problems when used alongside a behaviour modification programme. The current veterinary formulation of imepitoin licensed for long term use in dogs with epilepsy appears to be safe and well tolerated. A dose of 20 mg/kg imepitoin twice daily appears to be an appropriate starting dose for anxiolytic effects in most patients, with a fast onset of action with improvements being seen within the first week of commencing treatment, giving it an advantage over some other classes of anti-anxiety medication such as TCAs and SSRIs. Further research with a randomized, double-blind, placebo-controlled trial would be useful to confirm the apparent efficacy reported here.

Acknowledgements
We would like to thank Boehringer Ingelheim for funding this research after reviewing the protocol for the study design and allowing us to report our findings without comments or restrictions. We would also like to thank all the dogs and their owners for enrolling in the study and dedicating their time, particularly with keeping diary entries and regular communication with the Animal Behaviour Clinic.

Funding
The research was funded by Boehringer Ingelheim, producers of Pexion™. Boehringer Ingelheim reviewed the protocol for the study design, but were not involved with collection, analysis or interpretation of the data, nor with the writing of the manuscript.

Authors' contributions
The idea for the work was conceived by DM. The study was designed by DM and KM. The consultations were performed by KM. The data were analysed by DM and KM. The paper was written by DM and KM. Both authors read and approved the final manuscript.

Competing interests
The authors declare that they have no competing interests.

Consent for publication
Not applicable.

References
1. PDSA and YouGov. PDSA Animal Wellbeing (PAW) Report 2011 - The State of Our Pet Nation. 2011.
2. Blackwell EJ, Bradshaw JW, Casey RA. Fear responses to noises in domestic dogs: prevalence, risk factors and co-occurrence with other fear related behaviour. Appl Anim Behav Sci. 2013;145(1):15–25.
3. APBC - Association of Pet Behaviour Counsellors. Annual Review of Cases 2012. http://www.apbc.org.uk/system/files/apbc_annual_report_2012.pdf. Accessed 20 August 2016.
4. Bamberger M, Houpt KA. Signalment factors, comorbidity, and trends in behavior diagnoses in dogs: 1,644 cases (1991–2001). J Am Vet Med Assoc. 2006;229(10):1591–601.
5. Sherman BL, Mills DS. Canine anxieties and phobias: an update on separation anxiety and noise aversions. Vet Clin North Am Small Anim Pract. 2008;38(5):1081–106.
6. Casey R. Fear and stress. BSAVA manual of canine and feline behavioural medicine. 2002:144–53.
7. Levine E. Sound sensitivities. BSAVA manual of canine and feline behavioural medicine Quedgeley, Gloucester: British Small Animal Veterinary Association. 2009:159–68.
8. Mills DS. Marchant-Forde JN. The encyclopedia of applied animal behaviour and welfare: CABI; 2010.
9. Panksepp J. Affective neuroscience: the foundations of human and animal emotions: Oxford university press; 1998.
10. Mills DS, Dube MB. Zulch H. Stress and pheromonatherapy in small animal clinical behaviour: John Wiley & Sons; 2012.
11. Panksepp J, Fuchs T, Iacobucci P. The basic neuroscience of emotional experiences in mammals: the case of subcortical FEAR circuitry and implications for clinical anxiety. Appl Anim Behav Sci. 2011;129(1):1–17.
12. Serpell JA, Hsu Y. Development and validation of a novel method for evaluating behavior and temperament in guide dogs. Appl Anim Behav Sci. 2001;72(4):347–64.
13. Sheppard G, Mills DS. The development of a psychometric scale for the evaluation of the emotional predispositions of pet dogs. Int J Comp Psychol. 2002;15(2).
14. Landsberg GM, Hunthausen WL, Ackerman LJ. Behavior problems of the dog and Cat3: behavior problems of the dog and cat. Elsevier Health Sciences; 2012.
15. Overall K. Manual of clinical behavioral medicine for dogs and cats. Elsevier Health Sciences; 2013.
16. Takeuchi Y, Houpt KA, Scarlett JM. Evaluation of treatments for separation anxiety in dogs. J Am Vet Med Assoc. 2000;217(3):342–5.
17. King J, Simpson B, Overall K, Appleby D, Pageat P, Ross C, et al. Treatment of separation anxiety in dogs with clomipramine: results from a prospective, randomized, double-blind, placebo-controlled, parallel-group, multicenter clinical trial. Appl Anim Behav Sci. 2000;67(4):255–75.
18. Seksel K, Lindeman M. Use of clomipramine in treatment of obsessive-compulsive disorder, separation anxiety and noise phobia in dogs: a preliminary, clinical study. Aust Vet J. 2001;79(4):252–6.
19. Ibáñez M, Anzola B. Use of fluoxetine, diazepam, and behavior modification as therapy for treatment of anxiety-related disorders in dogs. Journal of Veterinary Behavior: Clinical Applications and Research. 2009;4(6):223–9.
20. Simpson BS, Landsberg GM, Reisner IR, Ciribassi JJ, Horwitz D, Houpt KA, et al. Effects of reconcile (fluoxetine) chewable tablets plus behavior management for canine separation anxiety. Vet Ther. 2007;8(1):18.
21. Pageat P, Lafont C, Falewee C, Bonnafous L, Gaultier E, Silliart B. An evaluation of serum prolactin in anxious dogs and response to treatment with selegiline or fluoxetine. Appl Anim Behav Sci. 2007;105(4):342–50.
22. Joby R, Jemmett J, Miller A. The control of undesirable behaviour in male dogs using megestrol acetate. J Small Anim Pract. 1984;25(9):567–72.
23. Walker R, Fisher J, Neville P. The treatment of phobias in the dog. Appl Anim Behav Sci. 1997;52(3):275–89.
24. Herron ME, Shofer FS, Reisner IR. Retrospective evaluation of the effects of diazepam in dogs with anxiety-related behavior problems. J Am Vet Med Assoc. 2008;233(9):1420–4.
25. Crowell-Davis SL, Seibert LM, Sung W, Parthasarathy V, Curtis TM. Use of clomipramine, alprazolam, and behavior modification for treatment of storm phobia in dogs. J Am Vet Med Assoc. 2003;222(6):744–8.
26. Ogata N, Dodman NH. The use of clonidine in the treatment of fear-based behavior problems in dogs: an open trial. Journal of Veterinary Behavior: Clinical Applications and Research. 2011;6(2):130–7.
27. Korpivaara M, Laapas K, Huhtinen M, Schöning B, Overall K. Dexmedetomidine Oromucosal gel for alleviation of acute anxiety and fear associated with noise in dogs. J Vet Intern Med. 2016;30(4):1493.
28. European Union Veterinary Medicines Directive (2001/82).
29. Dodman NH, Shuster D. Psychopharmacology of animal behaviour disorders. Blackwell Science, 350 Main Street.; 1998.
30. Sigel E, Buhr A. The benzodiazepine binding site of GABA a receptors. Trends Pharmacol Sci. 1997;18(11):425–9.
31. Crowell-Davis SL. Murray T. Veterinary psychopharmacology: John Wiley & Sons; 2008.
32. Löscher W, Hoffmann K, Twele F, Potschka H, Töllner K. The novel antiepileptic drug imepitoin compares favourably to other GABA-mimetic drugs in a seizure threshold model in mice and dogs. Pharmacol Res. 2013;77:39–46.
33. Löscher W, Potschka H, Rieck S, Tipold A, Rundfeldt C. Anticonvulsant efficacy of the low-affinity partial benzodiazepine receptor agonist ELB 138 in a dog seizure model and in epileptic dogs with spontaneously recurrent seizures. Epilepsia. 2004;45(10):1228–39.
34. National Office of Animal Health (NOAH) Compendium. 2016.
35. Rundfeldt C, Tipold A, Löscher W. Efficacy, safety, and tolerability of imepitoin in dogs with newly diagnosed epilepsy in a randomized controlled clinical study with long-term follow up. BMC Vet Res 2015;11(1):1.

36. Tipold A, Keefe T, Löscher W, Rundfeldt C, Vries F. Clinical efficacy and safety of imepitoin in comparison with phenobarbital for the control of idiopathic epilepsy in dogs. J Vet Pharmacol Ther. 2015;38(2):160–8.
37. Rundfeldt C, Gasparic A, Wlaź P. Imepitoin as novel treatment option for canine idiopathic epilepsy: pharmacokinetics, distribution, and metabolism in dogs. J Vet Pharmacol Ther. 2014;37(5):421–34.
38. Shihab N, Bowen J, Volk HA. Behavioral changes in dogs associated with the development of idiopathic epilepsy. Epilepsy Behav. 2011;21(2):160–7.
39. Rundfeldt C, Löscher W. The pharmacology of imepitoin: the first partial benzodiazepine receptor agonist developed for the treatment of epilepsy. CNS drugs. 2014;28(1):29–43.
40. Rostock A, Tober C, Dost R, Bartsch R, editors. AWD131–138 is a potential novel anxiolytic without sedation and amnesia: A comparison with diazepam and buspirone. NAUNYN-SCHMIEDEBERGS ARCHIVES OF PHARMACOLOGY; 1998: SPRINGER VERLAG 175 FIFTH AVE, NEW YORK, NY 10010 USA.
41. Rostock A, Tober C, Dost R, Rundfeldt C, Bartsch R, Egerland U, et al. AWD-131-138. Drugs Future. 1998;23(3):253–5.
42. Association of Pet Behaviour Counsellors (APBC). http://www.apbc.org.uk/.
43. Cohen J. Statistical power analysis for the behavioural sciences. Lawrence Earlbaum Associates: Hillside. NJ; 1988.
44. Kirk RERE. Statistical issues; a reader for the behavioral sciences; 1972.
45. Sackett DL, Richardson WS, Rosenberg W, Haynes RB. Evidence-based medicine: how to practice and teach. Edinburgh: EBM Second Edition Churchill Livingstone; 2000.
46. Vandenbroucke JP. In defense of case reports and case series. Ann Intern Med. 2001;134(4):330–4.
47. Conzemius MG, Evans RB. Caregiver placebo effect for dogs with lameness from osteoarthritis. J Am Vet Med Assoc. 2012;241(10):1314–9.
48. Stephens D, Schneider H. Tolerance to the benzodiazepine diazepam in an animal model of anxiolytic activity. Psychopharmacology. 1985;87(3):322–7.
49. Frey H-H, Philippin H-P, Scheuler W. Development of tolerance to the anticonvulsant effect of diazepam in dogs. Eur J Pharmacol. 1984;104(1–2):27–38.
50. Barker MJ, Greenwood KM, Jackson M, Crowe SF. Cognitive effects of long-term benzodiazepine use. CNS drugs. 2004;18(1):37–48.
51. Fatjó J, Bowen J. Medical and metabolic influences on behavioural disorders. BSAVA manual of canine and feline behavioural medicine 2nd ed Gloucester, England: British Small Animal Veterinary Association. 2009:1–9.
52. Barcelos A, Mills D, Zulch H. Clinical indicators of occult musculoskeletal pain in aggressive dogs. Vet Rec. 2015:vetrec-2014-102823.
53. Camps T, Amat M, Mariotti VM, Le Brech S, Manteca X. Pain-related aggression in dogs: 12 clinical cases. Journal of Veterinary Behavior: Clinical Applications and Research. 2012;7(2):99–102.
54. Hellyer P, Rodan I, Brunt J, Downing R, Hagedorn JE, Robertson SA, et al. AAHA/AAFP pain management guidelines for dogs and cats. J Feline Med Surg. 2007;9(6):466–80.

Rifaximin is an effective alternative to metronidazole for the treatment of chronic enteropathy in dogs

Alessandro Menozzi[1*], Manuel Dall'Aglio[2], Fausto Quintavalla[1], Luca Dallavalle[3], Valentina Meucci[4] and Simone Bertini[1]

Abstract

Background: A clinical trial was conducted in order to assess the efficacy of rifaximin, a broad-spectrum antibiotic with negligible gastrointestinal absorption, in comparison with metronidazole, a commonly employed antimicrobial drug, in dogs with chronic enteropathy. Twenty-four pet dogs were randomly enrolled into two different groups: MET group (10 dogs) and RIF group (14 dogs). Dogs of MET group received metronidazole 15 mg/kg q12h for 21 days by oral route, whereas dogs of RIF group, were given rifaximin 25 mg/kg q12h for 21 days by oral route. Clinical signs of disease were evaluated the day before the beginning of drug administration (D0), and at the end of treatment (D21), by means of Canine IBD Activity Index (CIBDAI). Blood levels of C-reactive protein (CRP) at D0 and D21 were also measured, as another parameter of treatment efficacy. The primary outcome measure of efficacy was the complete remission at D21, defined as a 75 % or greater decrease of CIBDAI; secondary outcome measures were the variation of mean CIBDAI scores, of mean CRP serum levels, and any observed adverse effect from D0 to D21.

Results: Treatment with metronidazole or rifaximin greatly improved the clinical signs of disease in each group: in MET group the complete remission was achieved in 8 of 10 dogs (80.0 %), and partial remission in 2 subjects (20.0 %). In RIF group, 12 of 14 dogs showed complete remission (85.7 %), and the remaining 2 dogs were in partial remission (14.3 %). There were also significant decreases of CIBDAI scores ($P = 0.002$ and $P = 0.0002$ for MET and RIF, respectively), and CRP levels ($P = 0.002$ and $P = 0.0001$ for MET and RIF, respectively) compared to pre-treatment values in both groups. No significant difference, however, was found when comparing MET and RIF groups. No relevant side-effect was reported during the trial with either drugs.

Conclusions: The present study showed, for the first time, that oral rifaximin could represent an effective alternative to metronidazole for the induction of clinical remission in dogs with chronic enteropathy.

Keywords: Dog, Chronic enteropathy, Rifaximin, Metronidazole, CIBDAI

Background

Inflammatory bowel disease (IBD) is a generic name which includes different chronic inflammatory disorders affecting the gastrointestinal tract in human patients, the most important of which are Crohn's disease (CD) and ulcerative colitis (UC). Dogs and cats are also susceptible of developing chronic gastro-intestinal inflammation which share several aspects with human IBD [1]. In these species the most frequent histological forms of chronic enteropathy are lymphocytic-plasmacytic enteritis (LPE) and eosinophilic gastroenteritis (EGE), and while the clinical and histological features of IBD in small animals are not always closely akin to those of CD and UC, the pathogenesis of such diseases is thought to be very similar. Indeed, it seems that an abnormal response of the immune system due to a loss of tolerance to different luminal antigens is the key pathogenetic event of both human and animal IBD [2–4]. Though the pathogenesis is still not fully understood, it is generally accepted that IBD has a multifactorial etiology, and that

* Correspondence: alessandro.menozzi@unipr.it
[1]Department of Veterinary Science, University of Parma, Strada Del Taglio 10, 43126 Parma, Italy
Full list of author information is available at the end of the article

genetic predisposition, together with environmental factors and a derangement of gut epithelial barrier, are all contributing to the generation and/or perpetuation of inflammation. Several studies suggest that a hyper-reactivity of the immune system in the gut against normally well-tolerated antigens, like food components or bacterial microbiota, ignites the inflammatory response which is then responsible for gastrointestinal damage [2, 3]. Moreover, the inflammation is carried on and exacerbated by various problems such as resistance to apoptosis of lymphocytes and recurrent exposure to luminal antigens due to an enhanced mucosal permeability [5–7].

The treatment of CD or UC in human patients, as well as in animals affected by IBD, is mainly based on the use of anti-inflammatory and immunosuppressant drugs (corticosteroids, 5-aminosalicylates, azathioprine, cyclophosphamide) in order to normalize the up-regulated immune response. Even though the drugs prescribed to dogs and cats affected by IBD are often the same employed in human patients, some forms of chronic enteritis in these species respond to simple diet modification or to probiotics and antimicrobial drugs [8, 9]. There are several evidences of the importance of bacterial microbiota in the pathogenesis or worsening of IBD [10–12] but, whereas antibiotics seem to ameliorate experimental bowel inflammation [13–15], the results obtained against CD or UC in clinical trials with antibacterial agents are not very encouraging, except for some positive effects obtained with metronidazole and ciprofloxacin [16, 17]. Metronidazole has proven to be effective also in small animal IBD [18], suggesting that bacteria may play a role in chronic gastrointestinal inflammation of dogs and cats, even if the real weight of antimicrobial action compared with the immunomodulating activity possessed by this drug has to be clarified yet.

Rifaximin (4-deoxy-4′-methylpyrido[1′,2′-1,2]imidazo-[5,4-c]-rifamycin SV) is a semisynthetic rifamycin endowed with a wide spectrum of antibacterial activity, and it is virtually non-absorbable by oral route [19], thus granting high efficacy and low incidence of side-effects [20]. Previous studies showed that rifaximin was more effective than other antibiotics in human patients with irritable bowel syndrome (IBS), and induced remission of moderately active CD in 2/3 of the subjects treated [21, 22]. Rifaximin was also more active than metronidazole in human patients with intestinal bacterial overgrowth [23]. Even though an efficacy of this drug in human IBD and in experimental models of intestinal inflammation [15, 24, 25] was demonstrated, as for metronidazole, the reasons underlying this beneficial activity are still unclear.

The aim of the present study was to investigate the therapeutic effects of oral rifaximin in dogs affected by chronic entheropathy, compared with those of metronidazole, an antimicrobial and antiprotozoal drug commonly employed in the therapy of chronic intestinal inflammation in small animals.

Methods

Animals

Thirty-six pet dogs, males and females, diagnosed with chronic enteropathy both by clinical and histological evaluation, were assessed for eligibility, and 25 of them, were enrolled in the clinical trial (Fig. 1). The sample size was determined on the basis of a previous similar study [26]. The study was conducted between September 2014 and March 2016, at the Veterinary Hospital of the University of Parma, apart from the histologic and biochemical analysis, which were performed at the Idexx Laboratories. The animals were included in the trial on the basis of the following criteria: clinical signs of gastrointestinal disease lasting for more than 3 weeks; lack of a relevant improvement after at least 4 weeks of a commercial elimination diet (with the recommendation to the owner to feed the dogs exclusively with the prescribed diet), or after the treatment with anthelmintic drugs, antibiotics (amoxicillin/clavulanic acid or enrofloxacin), spasmolytic and antidiarrhoeal agents; failure to detect other causes of disease after a thorough diagnostic protocol. The diagnostic evaluation for all dogs included at least CBC, serum biochemistry and urinalysis, three daily consecutive faecal examinations for endoparasites (both by direct smear and by flotation technique), faecal chymotrypsin and serum trypsin-like immunoreactivity, abdominal ultrasonography. Exclusion criteria were a previous treatment with immunosuppressant drugs or the presence of hypoalbuminemia (9 dogs); moreover, 2 dogs with a suspected diagnosis of primary lymphangiectasis were also not included in the study. The diagnosis of chronic enteropathy was confirmed in all subjects by means of endoscopy (Fujinon EG-250WR5), and subsequent histologic evaluation of multiple biopsies.

Trial design

The dogs were randomly assigned to two different groups, named MET (metronidazole) and RIF (rifaximin), with an allocation ratio of 1:1. MET group was composed by 10 dogs, while the dogs assigned to RIF group were 15. One of the dogs belonging to RIF group died before the conclusion of the treatment period, and was therefore excluded from the results. Each dog meeting the criteria for enrolment in the trial was assigned to MET group if its name was composed by an even number of letters, or to RIF group if the name was instead made of an odd number of letters.

Metronidazole was administered by oral route to the dogs of MET group, at the dose of 15 mg/kg q12h for 21 days, whereas rifaximin, at the dose of 25 mg/kg q12h for 21 days, was given by oral route to the dogs enrolled in RIF group. Metronidazole was administered

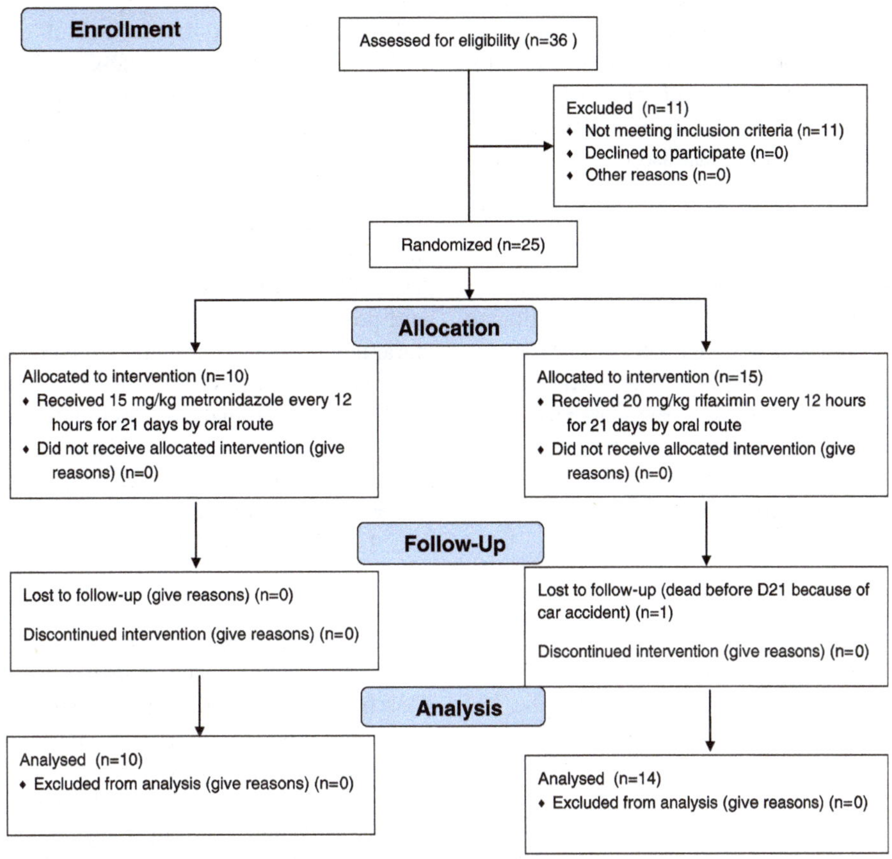

Fig. 1 Flow chart of trial enrolment and treatment protocol

at a dose in the range commonly employed in the therapy of IBD in dogs (10–25 mg/kg q12h) [18], whereas the dosage used for rifaximin was chosen on the basis of a previous work [15]. The dogs were examined for the assessment of the severity score of the disease by a member of our research group, blind to the treatment, the day before the beginning of drug administration (D0), at day 15, and at day 21 (D21), at the end of metronidazole or rifaximin administration period. All dogs received also ranitidine (2 mg/kg q12h), and metoclopramide (0.3 mg/kg q12h until day 15). A supplement of vitamin B_{12} (cyanocobalamin 250–1000 μg i.m. according to the weight) was administered once a week to the dogs. In order to exclude any influence of food on the evaluation of drug efficacy, all dogs were fed with a home-made diet which consisted exclusively of boiled chicken meat and rice.

Blood samples were collected from each dog at D0 (pre-treatment level) and at D21 (post-treatment level) for the measurement of C-reactive protein (CRP), which is an acute-phase protein produced by the liver in response to inflammation, infection and tissue injury, and whose decrease from pre-treatment serum level is considered a suitable marker of the improvement of the intestinal inflammatory status [27].

Drugs

A commercially available oral formulation of metronidazole, Flagyl® 250 mg tablets (Zambon Italia Srl, Milano, Italy) was employed in the study. Rifaximin 250 mg divisible tablets were kindly supplied by Ati Pets Srl, Fatro Group SpA, Ozzano dell'Emilia, Bologna, Italy.

Clinical evaluation and measures of outcome

The severity of the disease was scored by means of Canine IBD Activity Index (CIBDAI), which is a widely accepted index of mucosal inflammation in canine IBD [28]. Briefly, six salient clinical signs (attitude/activity, appetite, vomiting, stool consistency, stool frequency, weight loss) were assessed and scored 0 through 3, according to the degree of alteration from normal in each patient. The obtained scores were then summed in order to obtained a cumulative CIBDAI score, indicating the severity of the disease: clinically insignificant (0–3), mild (4–5), moderate (6–8) or severe (9 or greater).

The primary outcome assumed as therapeutic response to the treatment was clinical remission at D21, according to a previous study [27]. Complete remission, was defined as 75 % or greater decrease of CIBDAI score with respect to pre-treatment (D0), while a reduction of

CIBDAI <75 % but >25 % was considered as a partial remission. Secondary measures were the percent variation of mean CIBDAI score from D0 to D21 in both groups, and the modification of pre-treatment mean CRP serum concentration at the end of treatment. Any adverse effect observed during the trial was also considered as a secondary outcome.

Histology

Tissue samples collected during endoscopy, after fixation in 10 % buffered formalin, were processed according to an automatised method (Tissue-Tek Xpress 120, Sakura Finetek Europe B.V., Flemingweg, the Netherlands). Serial paraffin sections (2 μm) were then prepared, and stained with haematoxylin and eosin for morphological examination. Histologic evaluation was performed by two observers, blind to the treatment (Fig. 2).

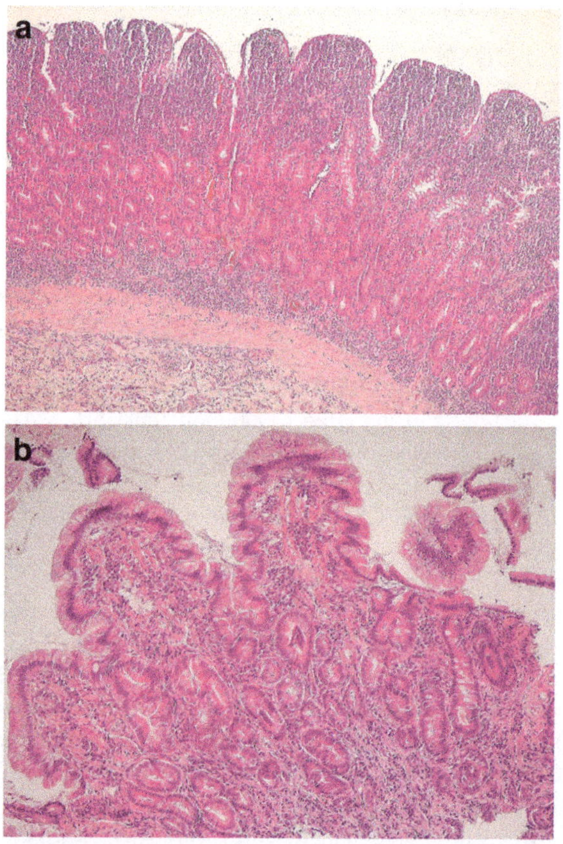

Fig. 2 Histologic features of small intestine sections of dogs with LPE. Panel **a**: Duodenal mucosa of a dog enrolled in MET group (CIBDAI score 11 at D0) with severe lymphoplasmacytic inflammation. The infiltrate of inflammatory cells is extending from the tip of the villi, through the lamina propria, to the muscularis mucosae (haematoxylin and eosin; 20×). Panel **b**: Duodenal mucosa of a dog enrolled in RIF group (CIBDAI score 3 at D0), with moderate lymphoplasmacytic inflammation. The villi are blunted, and the inflammatory cells are scattered into the lamina propria (haematoxylin and eosin; 40×)

C-reactive protein assay

CRP was measured by means of an immunoturbidimetric assay (Randox Canine CRP, Randox Laboratories Ltd., U.K.). The reference range for CRP level in healthy dogs measured with this assay is 0–10.7 mg/l.

Statistical analysis

The two different treatment groups were compared about two outcome results (CIBDAI and CRP serum level). Comparisons within the same group between pre- and post-treatment values were made by means of non-parametric Wilcoxon matched pairs signed rank tests; whereas when the differences between MET group and RIF group were analysed, cumulative distributions were compared with Kolmogorov-Smirnov unpaired tests. All statistical measures were performed using a commercial software (GraphPad Prism, ver. 6.05, GraphPad Software Inc., La Jolla, CA, U.S.A.).

Results

MET group consisted of 10 dogs (3 cross-breeds, 2 German Shepherds, 1 Rottweiler, 1 Boxer, 1 Golden Retriever, 1 Pinscher, 1 Épagneul Breton), whereas RIF group was composed by 14 dogs (5 cross-breeds, 2 German Shepherds, 1 Irish Setter, 1 Poodle, 1 Dachshund, 1 Boxer, 1 Dogo Argentino, 1 Maltese, 1 Bichon Frisè). Mean weight at D0 was 21.65 ± 11.61 kg (range: 6–45) for dogs of MET group, and 16.32 ± 8.47 kg (range: 5–28) for dogs belonging to RIF group.

Histologic features of biopsies of all dogs showed an inflammation with lymphocytic-plasmacytic infiltrate of small intestinal mucosa, ranging from mild to severe, often with alterations of the structure of villi (blunted or fused). In particular, in MET group the number of dogs with mild, moderate or severe inflammation, were 1, 6, and 3, respectively. In the same group 5 dogs presented blunted, and one dog fused villi. In RIF group, 4 dogs showed mild, 7 moderate, and 4 severe inflammation. In this group, 8 dogs showed blunted, and 2 fused villi.

At D21 in dogs of MET group the complete remission was achieved in 8 of 10 animals (80.0 %), while 2 subjects were in partial remission (20.0 %). In RIF group, 12 of 14 dogs showed complete remission (85.7 %), and the remaining 2 dogs were in partial remission (14.3 %) (Fig. 3).

Mean CIBDAI scores at D0 were 7.70 ± 2.41 (range: 4–11) and 7.29 ± 2.61 (range: 3–11) for MET and RIF group, respectively ($P = 0.921$). Treatment with metronidazole or rifaximin, along with diet change, greatly improved the clinical signs of disease in each group at D21, as shown by the significant decrease of CIBDAI values, compared to pre-treatment values (1.30 ± 1.83, $P = 0.002$, and 0.92 ± 1.11, $P = 0.0002$, respectively) (Fig. 3). There was, however, no significant difference between MET

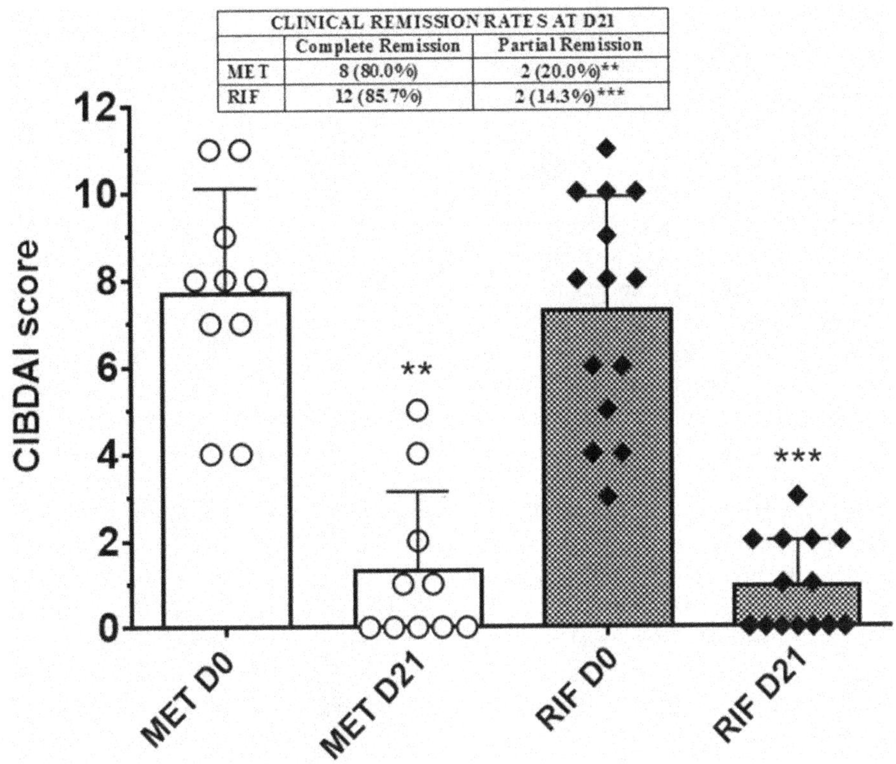

Fig. 3 Effect of metronidazole and rifaximin administration on clinical remission rates (*box*) and CIBDAI scores (*columns* and *symbols*) of dogs in both treatment groups. *Columns* in the graph represent mean ± SD, while *symbols* are individual CIBDAI scores of dogs in MET group and RIF group at D0 and at D21. $^{**}P < 0.001$ D21 vs D0; $^{***}P < 0.0001$ D21 vs D0

and RIF groups in the percent decrease of CIBDAI scores from pre-treatment level to D21 (85.84 vs 88.34 %, respectively, $P = 0.999$).

Mean CRP levels at D0 of dogs in MET group and RIF group were 9.95 ± 1.71 mg/l and 10.46 ± 1.80 mg/l, respectively ($P = 0.974$). After 3 weeks of both metronidazole and rifaximin administration (D21), mean CRP serum levels were significantly reduced (2.66 ± 1.42 mg/l, $P = 0.002$, and 2.23 ± 1.30 mg/l, $P = 0.0001$, respectively) (Fig. 4). The decrease, expressed in percentage, of mean CRP concentration in MET group was 74.07 ± 12.45 %, whereas it was 79.75 ± 10.00 %, in dogs of RIF group, without achieving, anyway, a significant difference ($P = 0.446$).

No significant adverse effect was observed during the treatment period in both groups of dogs. Raw data of CIBDAI scores, remission rates, dog weights, and CRP serum levels are reported in Additional file 1.

Discussion

Treatment of canine chronic enteropathies is often including antibacterial agents, based on the evidences of an efficacy of antibiotic therapy in ameliorating clinical signs of disease, and of a possible pathogenetic role of bacterial antigens in the generation and perpetuation of inflammatory status in the gastrointestinal mucosa [29, 30]. The present study was aimed to compare the clinical efficacy of rifaximin, a non-absorbable rifamycin, with respect to metronidazole, an antibiotic commonly prescribed against canine IBD, in dogs in which non-hypoproteinemic chronic enteropathy was diagnosed. After the administration of either antibiotic for 21 days, and diet modification, clinical signs were greatly improved, as shown by the number of

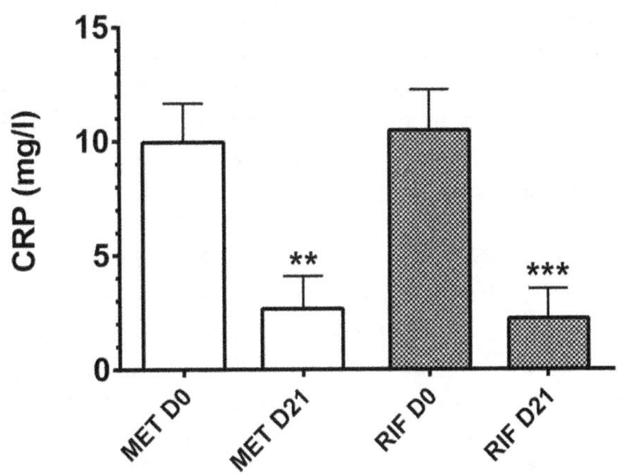

Fig. 4 Effect of metronidazole and rifaximin administration on CRP serum levels of dogs in MET group and RIF group. *Columns* in the graph represent mean ± SD. $^{**}P < 0.001$ D21 vs D0; $^{***}P < 0.0001$ D21 vs D0

dogs which achieved complete remission, and by the significant fall of mean CIBDAI scores in both groups. There was, however, no significant difference in efficacy between metronidazole and rifaximin, which demonstrated to be equally effective in this clinical trial.

The beneficial effect of metronidazole and rifaximin against intestinal inflammation was confirmed by the significant decrease of mean CRP serum concentration at D21 with respect to pre-treatment level in both groups, as the correlation of this acute-phase protein with inflammatory status in human and dog IBD has been observed in several studies [27, 31]. However, since CRP is a non-specific marker of inflammation, the interpretation of this result should be prudently considered without further studies.

To date, little is known about the species of microbiota which may play a role in the pathogenesis of canine IBD. Whereas many studies have shown that an alteration of gut microbiota takes place in dogs and cats with chronic intestinal inflammation, and that this dysbiosis is similar to those observed in human IBD or in animal models of intestinal inflammation, the composition of such abnormal bacteria population seems to be variable, thus making the choice of a selective antibiotic treatment a very difficult task [32]. In the present study, rifaximin, a broad spectrum antibiotic, was effective as metronidazole, whose activity is directed only against anaerobes. This result seems to suggest that anaerobic bacteria could be particularly important in the pathogenesis of chronic diarrhoea in dogs; as a matter of fact, a recent study [33] evidenced an increased number of anaerobic species in the mucosa of dogs with chronic enteropathies. By contrast, other studies conducted in dogs with IBD, found either a reduction of anaerobic bacteria [32] or no significant alterations compared to healthy subjects [26]. Interestingly, it was observed that rifaximin was able to enhance the growth of beneficial bacteria such as *Bifidobacteria* or *Faecalibacterium praunsnitzii* [34], and that a reduced population of *Faecalibacterium* in particular, which seems to exert a protective activity against intestinal inflammation [35], is usually present in human patients and dogs with IBD [26, 36, 37]. However, metronidazole, which resulted effective as rifaximin in this clinical trial, is by contrast known to decrease anaerobes such as *Faecalibacterium*, and thus the protective role of some intestinal microbiota against inflammation remains to be clarified.

Metronidazole, a nitroimidazole antibiotic, is widely used for the treatment of IBD in dogs, both alone or in combination with corticosteroids or immunosuppressant drugs, even though its efficacy was investigated only in few published studies [26, 27, 38, 39], and the mechanisms by which it improves the clinical signs of the disease are still to be fully understood. Likewise, although abundant experimental evidence supports the hypothesis that bacteria participate to the pathogenesis of IBD in humans, and metronidazole was shown to be effective in reducing disease severity in patients with CD [16, 40], and equal or even superior to sulphasalazine in another study [41], the real utility of this drug, or the reasons underlying its beneficial activity, remain controversial. It has been proposed that metronidazole could be effective for its immuno-modulating properties rather than for a simple antibacterial activity, since this drug is able to suppress cell-mediated immunity [42, 43].

As for rifaximin, an open-label study on IBD patients demonstrated an efficacy in decreasing disease activity index [44], and a significant advantage of a 12-week treatment with this antibiotic over placebo in inducing clinical remission in mild-to-moderate CD [22]. Furthermore, rifaximin was proved to be effective in preventing bacterial translocation into mesenteric lymph nodes, and to ameliorate experimental colitis in mice [15].

Recently, a protective role by nuclear receptors like pregnane X receptor (PXR), peroxisome proliferator-activated receptor-γ and liver X receptor in IBD was suggested by some studies [45–47]. In particular, PXR ligand pregnenolone-16α-carbonitrile was able to ameliorate dextran sodium sulfate (DSS)-induced colitis in mice, and such effect was related to a reduced expression of NF-kB transcription factor [48]. Through NF-kB inhibition, a repression of its target genes is obtained, leading to a decrease in the production of pro-inflammatory mediators like TNF-α, IL-1β and IL-6. Rifampicin and rifaximin are known agonists at PXR [49], and the latter has been recently investigated for its effects on experimental colitis in the mouse, showing to protect against DSS-induced damage by inhibiting NF-kB signaling inflammatory cascade [24]. Since NF-kB activation has been observed in dogs affected by LPE [50, 51], it is possible that rifaximin efficacy could be due, at least in part, to its anti-inflammatory activity. It is interesting to note that, tylosin, a macrolide antibiotic employed in the treatment of chronic diarrhoea in dogs [38], and which was effective against experimental colitis in rats [52], is also endowed with anti-inflammatory properties [53], thus strengthening the hypothesis that antimicrobic agents which are effective against chronic intestinal inflammations in dogs, might aim at two distinct targets, the bacteria in the bowel lumen, which trigger the immune response, and the immune response itself.

In this clinical trial, no significant side-effect was observed with either antibiotic treatment during the 21-days administration. Several adverse effects are nevertheless reported in literature following metronidazole administration, and neurological toxicity is frequently reported [54, 55]. Even though data about rifaximin safety in dogs are thus far lacking, this drug was devoid of adverse effects when administered to rats up to 100 mg/kg for 6 months [56], and was shown to be safe and effective in children with IBD [57], most probably because of its negligible intestinal absorption through healthy or inflamed mucosa. Indeed, rifaximin absorption was not modified by intestinal inflammation in indomethacin-induced enteropathy in rats [58]. However, a long-term evaluation of potential adverse effects in dogs caused by rifaximin administration is necessary in order to thoroughly assess the safety of this antimicrobic drug. Negative effects due to antibiotic-induced alteration of intestinal microbiota cannot be in fact excluded, since, for instance, it was observed in a recent study that antibiotic-responsive dogs with chronic enteropathies have worse outcome compared to those treated only with diet modification [59].

A limitation of this clinical trial could be the relatively small number of dogs evaluated, which might have not allowed to unveil small differences of efficacy between the two antibiotic treatments; moreover, a single dosage for both rifaximin and metronidazole was employed, thus possibly clouding the evidence of a dose-dependent effect. Metronidazole, however, was administered at a commonly employed dose, whose efficacy and relative lack of major side-effects is generally accepted; as for rifaximin instead, possible dose-related differences in efficacy or adverse effects could not be ruled out. Another limitation of the present study is represented by the possible therapeutic role played by the home-made diet, as it is a low-fat, highly digestible one, and some of the dogs could have responded to diet modification. A future clinical trial including a group of dogs treated only with this kind of home-made diet, in comparison with antibiotic administration, would be useful to better enlighten the therapeutic effect of rifaximin. Furthermore, a contribution of antiemetic drugs to the improvement of CIBDAI scores cannot be excluded. It would also have been very important to include in the study the effects of drug treatment in a longer period of time, as chronic enteropathies are commonly relapsing after therapy is discontinued; the evaluation at the conclusion of the 3 weeks of treatment is, anyway, usually adequate to assess the response to drugs, at least to evaluate the ability to induce the remission of clinical signs [28]. Further studies with different doses of rifaximin, and over a longer period of time, will allow to better understand the efficacy and safety profile of this new therapeutic approach to chronic intestinal inflammation in dogs. Moreover, supplementary studies about rifaximin activity on different intestinal microbiota could be crucial to broaden the knowledge on the clinical potential of this antibiotic against chronic enteropathies in dogs.

Conclusions

This study suggests, for the first time, that rifaximin may indeed represent an attractive alternative to metronidazole for the therapy of chronic intestinal inflammations in dogs.

Abbreviations

CBC: Complete blood count; CD: Crohn's disease; CIBDAI: Canine IBD activity index; CRP: C-reactive protein; DSS: Dextran sodium sulfate; EGE: Eosinophilic gastroenteritis; IBD: Inflammatory bowel disease; IBS: Irritable Bowel Syndrome; IL-1β: Interleukin-1β; IL-6: Interleukin-6; LPE: Lymphocytic plasmacytic enteritis; MET: Metronidazole group; NF-kB: Nuclear factor kappa-light-chain-enhancer of activated B cells; PXR: Pregnane X receptor; RIF: Rifaximin group; TNF-α: Tumour necrosis factor alpha; UC: Ulcerative colitis

Acknowledgments

The authors would like to thank Idexx Laboratories Italia for the histologic analysis.

Funding

There was no external funding support for this study. ATI Pets Srl supplied rifaximin tablets used in the trial but otherwise did not provide any financial support.

Authors' contributions

AM and SB equally contributed to the study design, data interpretation, and to the writing of the manuscript. MD performed the clinical and endoscopic evaluation of the animals; MD, FQ and VM equally contributed to the statistical analysis and data interpretation. LD contributed to the trial design. All authors have read and approved the final manuscript.

Competing interests

LD is an employee of ATI Pets Srl but did not contribute to data analysis and interpretation or to manuscript writing. All the other authors have no competing interests to declare.

Consent for publication

Not applicable.

Author details

[1]Department of Veterinary Science, University of Parma, Strada Del Taglio 10, 43126 Parma, Italy. [2]Veterinary Practitioner, Parma, Italy. [3]ATI Pets Srl, Fatro Group SpA, Ozzano dell'Emilia, Bologna, Italy. [4]Department of Veterinary Science, University of Pisa, Pisa, Italy.

References

1. Cerquetella M, Spaterna A, Laus F, Tesei B, Rossi G, Antonelli E, Villanacci V, Bassotti G. Inflammatory bowel disease in the dog: differences and similarities with humans. World J Gastroenterol. 2010;16:1050–6.
2. Pirzer U, Schonhaar A, Fleischer B, Hermann E, Zumbuschenfelde KHM. Reactivity of infiltrating lymphocytes-T with microbial antigens in Crohns-disease. Lancet. 1991;338:1238–9.
3. Fiocchi C. Inflammatory bowel disease: etiology and pathogenesis. Gastroenterology. 1998;115:182–205.
4. Guarner F, Malagelada JR. Gut flora in health and disease. Lancet. 2003;361:512–9.
5. Elson CO, Sartor RB, Tennyson GS, Riddell RH. Experimental-models of inflammatory bowel-disease. Gastroenterology. 1995;109:1344–67.
6. Neurath MF. Regulation of T-cell apoptosis in inflammatory bowel disease: to die or not to die, that is the mucosal question (vol 22, pg 21, 2001). Trends Immunol. 2001;22:225–25
7. Dandrieux JR, Bornand VF, Doherr MG, Kano R, Zurbriggen A, Burgener IA. Evaluation of lymphocyte apoptosis in dogs with inflammatory bowel disease. Am J Vet Res. 2008;69:1279–85.
8. Allenspach K, Wieland B, Grone A, Gaschen F. Chronic enteropathies in dogs: evaluation of risk factors for negative outcome. J Vet Intern Med. 2007;21:700–8.
9. Jergens AE, Moore FM, Haynes JS, Miles KG. Idiopathic inflammatory bowel disease in dogs and cats: 84 cases (1987–1990). J Am Vet Med Assoc. 1992;201:1603–8.

10. Giaffer MH, Holdsworth CD, Duerden BI. The assessment of faecal flora in patients with inflammatory bowel disease by a simplified bacteriological technique. J Med Microbiol. 1991;35:238–43.
11. Taurog JD, Richardson JA, Croft JT, Simmons WA, Zhou M, Fernandez-Sueiro JL, Balish E, Hammer RE. The germfree state prevents development of gut and joint inflammatory disease in HLA-B27 transgenic rats. J Exp Med. 1994;180:2359–64.
12. Blaser MJ, Miller RA, Lacher J, Singleton JW. Patients with active Crohn's disease have elevated serum antibodies to antigens of seven enteric bacterial pathogens. Gastroenterology. 1984;87:888–94.
13. Madsen KL, Doyle JS, Tavernini MM, Jewell LD, Rennie RP, Fedorak RN. Antibiotic therapy attenuates colitis in interleukin 10 gene-deficient mice. Gastroenterology. 2000;118:1094–105.
14. Khan KJ, Ullman TA, Ford AC, Abreu MT, Abadir A, Marshall JK, Talley NJ, Moayyedi P. Antibiotic therapy in inflammatory bowel disease: a systematic review and meta-analysis. Am J Gastroenterol. 2011;106:661–73.
15. Fiorucci S, Distrutti E, Mencarelli A, Barbanti M, Palazzini E, Morelli A. Inhibition of intestinal bacterial translocation with rifaximin modulates lamina propria monocytic cells reactivity and protects against inflammation in a rodent model of colitis. Digestion. 2002;66:246–56.
16. Sutherland L, Singleton J, Sessions J, Hanauer S, Krawitt E, Rankin G, Summers R, Mekhjian H, Greenberger N, Kelly M, et al. Double-blind, placebo controlled trial of metronidazole in Crohns-disease. Gut. 1991;32:1071–5.
17. Arnold GL, Beaves MR, Pryjdun VO, Mook WJ. Preliminary study of ciprofloxacin in active Crohn's disease. Inflamm Bowel Dis. 2002;8:10–5.
18. Jergens AE. Inflammatory bowel disease–current perspectives. Veterinary Clinics of North America-Small Animal Practice. 1999;29:501–21.
19. Venturini AP. Pharmacokinetics of L/105, a new rifamycin, in rats and dogs, after oral administration. Chemotherapy. 1983;29:1–3.
20. Ojetti V, Lauritano EC, Barbaro F, Migneco A, Ainora ME, Fontana L, Gabrielli M, Gasbarrini A. Rifaximin pharmacology and clinical implications. Expert Opin Drug Metab Toxicol. 2009;5:675–82.
21. Yang J, Lee HR, Low K, Chatterjee S, Pimentel M. Rifaximin versus other antibiotics in the primary treatment and retreatment of bacterial overgrowth in IBS. Dig Dis Sci. 2008;53:169–74.
22. Prantera C, Lochs H, Grimaldi M, Danese S, Scribano ML, Gionchetti P, Retic Study G. Rifaximin-extended intestinal release induces remission in patients with moderately active Crohn's disease. Gastroenterology. 2012;142:473–81. e4.
23. Lauritano EC, Gabrielli M, Scarpellini E, Ojetti V, Roccarina D, Villita A, Fiore E, Flore R, Santoliquido A, Tondi P, et al. Antibiotic therapy in small intestinal bacterial overgrowth: rifaximin versus metronidazole. Eur Rev Med Pharmacol Sci. 2009;13:111–6.
24. Cheng J, Shah YM, Ma XC, Pang XY, Tanaka T, Kodama T, Krausz KW, Gonzalez FJ. Therapeutic role of rifaximin in inflammatory bowel disease: clinical implication of human pregnane X receptor activation. J Pharmacol Exp Ther. 2010;335:32–41.
25. Ciobanu L, Taulescu M, Prundus R, Diaconu B, Andreica V, Catoi C, Pascu O, Tantau M. Effects of rifaximin on indomethacin-induced intestinal damage in guinea-pigs. Eur Rev Med Pharmaco. 2014;18:344–51.
26. Rossi G, Pengo G, Caldin M, Piccionello AP, Steiner JM, Cohen ND, Jergens AE, Suchodolski JS. Comparison of microbiological, histological, and immunomodulatory parameters in response to treatment with either combination therapy with prednisone and metronidazole or probiotic VSL#3 strains in dogs with idiopathic inflammatory bowel disease. Plos One. 2014;9:e94699.
27. Jergens AE, Crandell J, Morrison JA, Deitz K, Pressel M, Ackermann M, Suchodolski JS, Steiner JM, Evans R. Comparison of oral prednisone and prednisone combined with metronidazole for induction therapy of canine inflammatory bowel disease: a randomized-controlled trial. J Vet Intern Med. 2010;24:269–77.
28. Jergens AE, Schreiner CA, Frank DE, Niyo Y, Ahrens FE, Eckersall PD, Benson TJ, Evans R. A scoring index for disease activity in canine inflammatory bowel disease. J Vet Intern Med. 2003;17:291–7.
29. German AJ, Hall EJ, Day MJ. Chronic intestinal inflammation and intestinal disease in dogs. J Vet Intern Med. 2003;17:8–20.
30. Burgener IA, Konig A, Allenspach K, Sauter SN, Boisclair J, Doherr MG, Jungi TW. Upregulation of toll-like receptors in chronic enteropathies in dogs. J Vet Intern Med. 2008;22:553–60.
31. Solem CA, Loftus Jr EV, Tremaine WJ, Harmsen WS, Zinsmeister AR, Sandborn WJ. Correlation of C-reactive protein with clinical, endoscopic, histologic, and radiographic activity in inflammatory bowel disease. Inflamm Bowel Dis. 2005;11:707–12.
32. Honneffer JB, Minamoto Y, Suchodolski JS. Microbiota alterations in acute and chronic gastrointestinal inflammation of cats and dogs. World J Gastroenterol. 2014;20:16489–97.
33. Cassmann E, White R, Atherly T, Wang C, Sun YX, Khoda S, Mosher C, Ackermann M, Jergens A. Alterations of the ileal and colonic mucosal microbiota in canine chronic enteropathies. Plos One. 2016;11
34. Maccaferri S, Vitali B, Klinder A, Kolida S, Ndagijimana M, Laghi L, Calanni F, Brigidi P, Gibson GR, Costabile A. Rifaximin modulates the colonic microbiota of patients with Crohn's disease: an in vitro approach using a continuous culture colonic model system. J Antimicrob Chemother. 2010;65:2556–65.
35. Sellon RK, Tonkonogy S, Schultz M, Dieleman LA, Grenther W, Balish E, Rennick DM, Sartor RB. Resident enteric bacteria are necessary for development of spontaneous colitis and immune system activation in interleukin-10-deficient mice. Infect Immun. 1998;66:5224–31.
36. Loh G, Blaut M. Role of commensal gut bacteria in inflammatory bowel diseases. Gut Microbes. 2012;3:544–55.
37. Suchodolski JS, Markel ME, Garcia-Mazcorro JF, Unterer S, Heilmann RM, Dowd SE, Kachroo P, Ivanov I, Minamoto Y, Dillman EM, et al. The fecal microbiome in dogs with acute diarrhea and idiopathic inflammatory bowel disease. Plos One. 2012;7:e51907.
38. Craven M, Simpson JW, Ridyard AE, Chandler ML. Canine inflammatory bowel disease: retrospective analysis of diagnosis and outcome in 80 cases (1995–2002). J Small Anim Pract. 2004;45:336–42.
39. Garcia-Sancho M, Rodriguez-Franco F, Sainz A, Mancho C, Rodriguez A. Evaluation of clinical, macroscopic, and histopathologic response to treatment in nonhypoproteinemic dogs with lymphocytic-plasmacytic enteritis. J Vet Intern Med. 2007;21:11–7.
40. Rutgeerts P, Hiele M, Geboes K, Peeters M, Penninckx F, Aerts R, Kerremans R. Controlled trial of metronidazole treatment for prevention of Crohn's recurrence after ileal resection. Gastroenterology. 1995;108:1617–21.
41. Ursing B, Alm T, Barany F, Bergelin I, Ganrot-Norlin K, Hoevels J, Huitfeldt B, Jarnerot G, Krause U, Krook A, et al. A comparative study of metronidazole and sulfasalazine for active Crohn's disease: the cooperative Crohn's disease study in Sweden. II. Result. Gastroenterology. 1982;83:550–62.
42. Grove DI, Mahmound AA, Warren KS. Suppression of cell-mediated immunity by metronidazole. Int Arch Allergy Appl Immunol. 1977;54:422–7.
43. Fararjeh M, Mohammad MK, Bustanji Y, Alkhatib H, Abdalla S. Evaluation of immunosuppression induced by metronidazole in Balb/c mice and human peripheral blood lymphocytes. Int Immunopharmacol. 2008;8:341–50.
44. Shafran I, Johnson LK. An open-label evaluation of rifaximin in the treatment of active Crohn's disease. Curr Med Res Opin. 2005;21:1165–9.
45. Langmann T, Moehle C, Mauerer R, Scharl M, Liebisch G, Zahn A, Stremmel W, Schmitz G. Loss of detoxification in inflammatory bowel disease: dysregulation of pregnane X receptor target genes. Gastroenterology. 2004;127:26–40.
46. Jakobsson T, Vedin LL, Hassan T, Venteclef N, Greco D, D'Amato M, Treuter E, Gustafsson JA, Steffensen KR. The oxysterol receptor LXRbeta protects against DSS- and TNBS-induced colitis in mice. Mucosal Immunol. 2014;7:1416–28.
47. Terc J, Hansen A, Alston L, Hirota SA. Pregnane X receptor agonists enhance intestinal epithelial wound healing and repair of the intestinal barrier following the induction of experimental colitis. Eur J Pharm Sci. 2014;55:12–9.
48. Shah YM, Ma X, Morimura K, Kim I, Gonzalez FJ. Pregnane X receptor activation ameliorates DSS-induced inflammatory bowel disease via inhibition of NF-kappaB target gene expression. Am J Physiol Gastrointest Liver Physiol. 2007;292:G1114–22.
49. Ma X, Shah YM, Guo GL, Wang T, Krausz KW, Idle JR, Gonzalez FJ. Rifaximin is a gut-specific human pregnane X receptor activator. J Pharmacol Exp Ther. 2007;322:391–8.
50. Okanishi H, Kabeya H, Maruyama S, Kagawa Y, Watari T. Activation of nuclear factor-kappa B and cell adhesion molecule mRNA expression in duodenal mucosa of dogs with lymphocytic-plasmacytic enteritis. Vet Immunol Immunop. 2013;154:145–52.

51. Luckschander N, Hall JA, Gaschen F, Forster U, Wenzlow N, Hermann P, Allenspach K, Dobbelaere D, Burgener IA, Welle M. Activation of nuclear factor-kappaB in dogs with chronic enteropathies. Vet Immunol Immunopathol. 2010;133:228–36.
52. Menozzi A, Pozzoli C, Poli E, Lazzaretti M, Cantoni A, Grandi D, Giovannini E, Coruzzi G. Effect of the macrolide antibacterial drug, tylosin, on TNBS-induced colitis in the rat. Pharmacology. 2005;74:135–42.
53. Culic O, Erakovic V, Parnham MJ. Anti-inflammatory effects of macrolide antibiotics. Eur J Pharmacol. 2001;429:209–29.
54. Dow SW, LeCouteur RA, Poss ML, Beadleston D. Central nervous system toxicosis associated with metronidazole treatment of dogs: five cases (1984–1987). J Am Vet Med Assoc. 1989;195:365–8.
55. Stein RB, Hanauer SB. Comparative tolerability of treatments for inflammatory bowel disease. Drug Saf. 2000;23:429–48.
56. Borelli G, Bertoli D. Acute, subacute, chronic toxicity and mutagenicity studies of rifaximin (L/105) in rats. Chemioterapia. 1986;5:263–7.
57. Muniyappa P, Gulati R, Mohr F, Hupertz V. Use and safety of rifaximin in children with inflammatory bowel disease. J Pediatr Gastroenterol Nutr. 2009;49:400–4.
58. Scarpignato C, Pelosini I. Experimental and clinical pharmacology of rifaximin, a gastrointestinal selective antibiotic. Digestion. 2006;73 Suppl 1:13–27.
59. Allenspach K, Culverwell C, Chan D. Long-term outcome in dogs with chronic enteropathies: 203 cases. The Veterinary record. 2016;178:368.

15

Safety and efficacy of targeted hyperthermia treatment utilizing gold nanorod therapy in spontaneous canine neoplasia

Elizabeth M. Schuh[4], Roberta Portela[2], Heather L. Gardner[5], Christian Schoen[3] and Cheryl A. London[1*]

Abstract

Background: Hyperthermia is an established anti-cancer treatment but is limited by tolerance of adjacent normal tissues. Parenteral administration of gold nanorods (NRs) as a photosensitizer amplifies the effects of hyperthermia treatment while sparing normal tissues. This therapy is well tolerated and has demonstrated anti-tumor effects in mouse models. The purpose of this phase 1 study was to establish the safety and observe the anti-tumor impact of gold NR enhanced (plasmonic) photothermal therapy (PPTT) in client owned canine patients diagnosed with spontaneous neoplasia.

Results: Seven dogs underwent gold NR administration and subsequent NIR PPTT. Side effects were mild and limited to local reactions to NIR laser. All of the dogs enrolled in the study experienced stable disease, partial remission or complete remission. The overall response rate (ORR) was 28.6% with partial or complete remission of tumors at study end.

Conclusions: PPTT utilizing gold nanorod therapy can be safely administered to canine patients. Further studies are needed to determine the true efficacy in a larger population of canine cancer patients and to and identify those patients most likely to benefit from this therapy.

Keywords: Hyperthermia, Plasmonic photothermal therapy, Gold nanorod, Dog, Tumor

Background

The emerging field of nanoparticles holds promise for a variety of applications including but not limited to imaging contrast enhancement, cancer treatment, drug and gene delivery, fluorescent labeling and tissue engineering [1]. Specifically, gold nanorods (NRs) have been identified as an optimal nanoparticle as they may be synthesized in bulk, have broadly tunable plasmon resonance and exhibit absorption coefficients 10^4–10^6-fold higher than conventional organic fluorochromes typically used for photodynamic therapy [2, 3]. While both spherical and rod gold nanoparticles exhibit a specific plasmon frequency according to their size and shape [4], only gold NRs can be engineered to near-infrared (NIR) plasmon resonance for biomedical in vivo uses [5, 6]. The critical NIR wavelength window between 650 and 900 nm allows for absorption and scatter in the optical light range making gold nanorods an excellent choice for high sensitivity photoacoustic contrast and thermal ablation of solid tumors [7, 8].

More recently, NRs have received attention as a potential photothermal agent for targeted hyperthermia with a wide safety range [3, 7]. The NRs have the ability to passively accumulate within tumors due to the chaotic and poorly developed framework of most tumor blood vessels. When administered by intravenous injection a proportion of the NRs are cleared by the reticuloendothelial system while the remaining NRs tend to become lodged

* Correspondence: london.20@osu.edu
[1]College of Veterinary Medicine, The Ohio State University, Columbus OH AND Cummings School of Veterinary Medicine, Tufts University, North Grafton, MA, USA
Full list of author information is available at the end of the article

in tumors. This enhanced permeability and retention or "EPR" effect is critical for both therapeutic and imaging techniques [9, 10]. One study shows that non-coated gold NRs clear the bloodstream almost immediately while polyethyleneglycol (PEG) polymers applied to the NR surface extends their half-life to 19 h due to immune system evasion, with the spleen showing the highest collection of NRs [11]. When gold NRs are coupled with visible and NIR-absorbing molecules, the pairing results in Surface-Enhanced, Resonant Raman Scattering (SERS) creating a unique spectral multiplexing density far superior to alternate methods, making them a highly suitable tool for targeted photothermal ablation [3].

A key safety concept while utilizing SERS NRs is ensuring specific targeting of tumors. For effective ablation to occur through hyperthermia in vivo, the enhanced NRs must demonstrate significant EPR effects to maximize anti-tumor efficacy while sparing normal tissues. Multiple mouse models have now demonstrated aggregation of NRs in xenogeneic tumors following intravenous administration [3, 12, 13]. In vivo, SERS-coated NRs permit remote photothermal tumor heating to ablative temperatures via ex vivo NIR diode lasers [3]. When these NRs are treated from an external laser source, varying degrees of success (25–57%) have been achieved in shrinking xenogeneic tumors dependent on the route in which the NRs are administered [12, 14]. Intratumoral NR administration followed by computationally derived quantitative photothermal modeling and NIR photothermal heating has recently been successfully used to treat tumors in mouse models of cancer without evidence of systemic toxicity with a 100% response rate that was durable over 50 days [13]. These data support the notion that notion that SERS NRs represent an alternative approach to traditional hyperthermia based cancer therapies. While the SERS nanorods have been studied extensively in mouse models of cancer, they have not been extensively tested in the setting of spontaneous disease. As such, the objectives of this clinical trial were to assess the adverse event profile of SERS NRs administered intravenously to dogs with solid tumors and to evaluate the anti-tumor activity of SERS NRs in dogs with solid tumors following treatment with a NIR diode laser.

Methods

Eligibility

This clinical trial was approved by the Clinical Research and Advising Committee at the College of Veterinary Medicine and the Institutional Animal Care and Use Committee (IACUC) at the Ohio State University. Informed consent was obtained from all owners prior to study enrollment and the clinical trial was performed in compliance with guidelines for conducting clinical trials in client owned animals at the College of Veterinary Medicine. Canine patients presenting to the Ohio State University Veterinary Medical Center Oncology service diagnosed with a solid tumor (carcinoma, sarcoma or mast cell tumor) that was at least 2 cm in size and amenable to repeat biopsy were eligible for enrollment. The patient may have failed standard therapy or had no other known effective therapeutic options. Alternately, the owners may have elected to enter the patient in lieu of standard of care. Prior to enrollment dogs underwent complete blood count, chemistry, urinalysis and thoracic radiograph testing. Patients were required to be over 1 year of age with adequate organ function (ALT and AST <4 times upper limit of institutional normal, bilirubin within normal limits and serum creatinine <2.5 mg/dL) and have an estimated life expectancy of at least 6 weeks. Exclusion criteria included evidence of metastatic disease, underlying cardiac disease/arrhythmias or any other serious systemic disorder incompatible with the study. Patients were required to be at least 3 weeks post any surgical intervention and not currently using any other investigational drug. If the patient was treated with prior radiation or chemotherapy, it also must have been completed these treatments at least 3 weeks prior to enrollment and be completely recovered from any acute toxicities.

Investigational drug product and concomitant medication

The gold nanorods were supplied by Nanopartz Inc. (Loveland, CO), and were a formulation of gold nanorods with a methyl terminated polyethylene glycol coating suspended in deionized water to a concentration of 10 mg/ml. These NRs were engineered to a surface plasmon resonance of 800 nm for photothermal heating. Concomitant medications permissible for use in prevention or managing adverse events included metoclopramide, ondansetron, maropitant, famotidine, ranitidine, omeprazole, metronidazole, bismuth subsalicylate, loperamide, butorphanol, tramadol, fentanyl, diphenhydramine. Patients were eligible to receive either an NSAID (non-steroidal anti-inflammatory drug) or prednisone as needed for pain relief or swelling associated with treatment at the discretion of the primary investigator.

Study design

A total of 7 dogs were enrolled in this study and each patient had a single tumor that was undergoing evaluation. Following screening, a baseline tumor biopsy was obtained with a 14 g needle core biopsy, processed in formalin and histopathologically evaluated through the Ohio State University Anatomic Pathology service. SERS NRs were administered intravenously at a dose of 10 mg/kg. Both plasma and serum absorbance was performed to assess NR levels at the following time points: pre-treatment, 15 min post administration, and 72 h post administration.

Dogs underwent NIR diode laser treatment 72 h post administration to ensure maximal clearance of the NRs and thus reduce the possibility of off-target effects. The tumor was then heated to a minimum of 40 °C for 1–2 min; an infrared camera was used to track the heating process. Dogs were evaluated 7 days following treatment with a physical examination and on day 14 after treatment a physical examination, CBC, serum biochemistry profile. An assessment of adverse events was performed at each visit. At Day 14, dogs were eligible to undergo tumor removal. If this was not elected, then a second needle core biopsy was performed at this time point. Dogs that had surgical resections of their tumor were evaluated 2 weeks post-operatively; dogs that had second needle core biopsies were evaluated at 2 and 6 weeks post-biopsy for evidence of adverse events secondary to NR treatment.

NR administration and assessment of serum and plasma concentrations

Gold nanorods were provided at a concentration of 10 mg/ml in 0.9% NaCl and stored at 4 °C. Prior to administration, the gold nanorod concentrate was diluted in 0.9% NaCl to a final concentration of 5 mg/ml. Nanorods were given as an intravenous infusion at a fluid rate of 50 ml/h or 250 mg nanorods/h. For example, a 25 kg dog would receive 250 mg of gold nanorods diluted in 50 ml of 0.9% NaCl given over 1 h. This dose (10 mg/kg) was based on clinical evaluation of NRs in normal beagle dogs in which doses up to 32 mg/kg (unpublished data, CARE Research LLC) were given with no adverse events. A portable UV/Vis (ultraviolet visible) spectrometer (Nanopartz fiber-optically modified Thor Labs CCS175 Compact UV/Vis spectrometer, Loveland CO 80537) was utilized to measure nanorods in the bloodstream and compared to a standard curve to estimate nanorod concentration. Briefly, serum and plasma were obtained from each patient through routine blood draw and centrifugation. The intensity of light passing through the sample was compared to the intensity of light before passing through the sample in order to calculate the absorbance. The UV/Vis spectrometer was calibrated against known standards, with a longitudinal absorption profile ranging from 700 to 950 nm. Nanorod concentration was assessed pretreatment, 15 min post treatment and 72 h post treatment in both plasma and serum. The analysis from the UV VIS was used to confirm nanorod concentration at the 72 h time point prior to NIR laser application to determine if the NRs had cleared the bloodstream prior to laser application.

Laser application and thermal imaging

Following administration of the NRs, dogs returned 72 h later to ensure that they had cleared the bloodstream. Dogs were then sedated with butorphanol (0.2 mg/kg) and acepromazine (0.02 mg/kg) by intramuscular injection 30 min prior to application of the laser. Once sedated, dogs were positioned to provide maximal access to the tumor. The normal tissues surrounding the target area were covered and exposure to laser was minimized. Appropriate personal protective equipment including safety glasses were utilized by staff members applying the laser and observing laser application (Jenoptik laser, JOLD-30 FC-14 30 W 400 μm fiber output, 808 nm Jena, Germany 07743). The laser was then applied to the tumor until the tumor has reached a sustained temperature of 40C for 1–2 min. The temperature assessment was performed using a thermal imaging camera (RAZ-IR, Las Vegas NV 89113). It was anticipated that the total treatment time to achieve a temperature of 40 °C for 1–2 min would be approximately 5 min. The dogs were then allowed to recover from sedation and be returned to the owner.

Evaluation of response

Determination of antitumor efficacy was based on objective tumor assessments made according to the RECIST (response evaluation criteria in solid tumors) guidelines consistent with the current guidelines [15]. Briefly, a complete response (CR) was defined as the complete disappearance of the target lesion and partial response (PR) was defined as a ≥ 30% decrease in the longest dimension of the target lesion taking as a reference the baseline longest dimension. Stable disease (SD) is defined as neither sufficient shrinkage to qualify for PR nor sufficient increase to qualify for PD taking as a reference the baseline longest dimension. The time interval to qualify for stable disease was the duration of the study (14 days). Progressive disease (PD) was defined as a ≥ 20% increase in the longest dimensions of the target lesion taking as a reference the baseline longest dimension or the appearance of 1 or more new lesions. Tumor assessments were obtained prior to treatment then day 7 and 14 post NIR laser treatment via caliper measurement of the longest diameter with photographic documentation.

Assessment of adverse events

Dogs were evaluated for adverse events (AEs) at every study visit. AEs were defined and graded according to the published VCOG-CTCAE criteria [16].

Results

Demographics

Seven dogs were enrolled into this clinical trial. The median age was 9 years (range 6–13 years) and the median weight was 28.2 kg (9.1–42.1). There were 4 spayed females and 3 neutered males enrolled, with several breeds represented including two Beagles and one of each of the following: Labrador Retriever, Golden Retriever, Boston Terrier, Greyhound, and Mixed Breed. Most dogs had undergone no prior therapy (n = 5) while one had recurrence of disease following surgery and another had recurrence following surgery and radiation therapy. The majority of dogs had a soft tissue sarcoma (n = 5) and the remaining 2 dogs had a mast cell tumor (Table 1).

Nanorod dosing, measurement and clearance

Nanorod dosage was standardized at 10 mg/kg and the total dose given ranged from 91 to 410 mg reflecting variation in patient size. Nanorod absorption was measured in plasma and serum and found to be comparable between the two samples (Fig. 1). Both samples showed minimal background scatter in the pre-treatment samples, a reliable peak at 800 nm 15 min post treatment and minimal to no residual nanorod detection 72 h post administration. The nanorod concentration 15 min post treatment was variable ranging from 60 to 192 μg/ml (Table 2). Most patients showed near complete clearance of circulating nanorods by 72 h post administration (Table 2). Interestingly, one dog had evidence of persistent high plasma levels of nanorods (97 μg/ml) at 72 h post administration although NIR laser application was completed without incident.

NIR laser application

After clearance of nanorods from the bloodstream was established, the NIR laser was applied to the tumors. The median treatment time was 2 min with therapy times ranging from 40 s to 4 min. All patients achieved a minimum tumor temperature of 40 °C (range 40–110 °C, Table 3) as assessed using real time monitoring with the infrared camera (Fig. 2).

Treatment outcome

All patients completed the study as expected with a varied follow up after the study period. Patients 1 and 7 experienced objective response with a CR and PR respectively showing a 28.6% objective response rate (both soft tissue sarcomas). After experiencing stable disease and having a needle core biopsy performed at the end of the study period, Patient 1 experienced a durable CR that lasted for approximately 8 months post treatment (Fig. 3a). No further surgical intervention was pursued for Patient 1. Patient 7 showed partial response for 77 days at which point the tumor showed mild enlargement from the previous visit and a surgical excision was elected (Fig. 3b). The patients that experienced stable disease (Patients 2, 3, 4, 5 and 6) had their tumors surgically removed at or near the end of the study period.

Histopathology

Baseline and post treatment histopathology were obtained in all dogs enrolled in this study (Table 4). Tumors from Patients 1, 3, 4 and 5 showed moderate changes in response to PPTT including coagulation, edema, hemorrhage and skin necrosis evident in their post treatment biopsies. The soft tissue sarcoma from Patient 1 demonstrated necrosis involving 20% of the submitted biopsy; this dog went on to achieve a complete response to therapy. The soft tissue sarcoma from Patient 3 showed approximately 60% microscopic tumor necrosis in response to treatment but the tumor remained unchanged grossly. Patient 4's mast cell tumor showed 40–50% necrosis with fibrin and hemorrhage in the center of the tumor and moderate to severe skin necrosis microscopically but also remained unchanged grossly. Lastly, the soft tissue sarcoma from Patient 5 showed moderate microscopic tumor necrosis (<50%) in response to treatment but also remained unchanged in size. Patients 2 and 6 both showed no tumor necrosis grossly post treatment and no tumor necrosis or cell death on histopathologic evaluation following resection. Patient 7 achieved a partial remission over time despite having no microscopic evidence of necrosis in the post-treatment biopsy sample.

Adverse events

All study related adverse events were considered mild (Table 5 - grade 1, n = 10; grade 2, n = 5) and generally did not require intervention with supportive care or concomitant medications. Skin/tumor ulceration over the treated area was the primary clinical effect observed in all dogs.

Skin adverse events

Nine adverse events confined to the tumor or surrounding tissues occurred. Erythema, skin ulceration, tumor

Table 1 Patient demographics

Patient	Breed	Age (yr)	Sex	Wt (kg)	Disease	Prior Treatment
1	Greyhound	12	MN	28.2	STS	Surgery
2	Mixed Breed	8	MN	37.8	STS	None
3	Boston Terrier	6	FS	11.7	STS	None
4	Beagle	9	MN	17.0	MCT	None
5	Beagle	13	FS	9.1	STS	None
6	Labrador Retriever	10	FS	38.3	MCT	None
7	Golden Retriever	7	FS	42.1	STS	Surgery and radiation

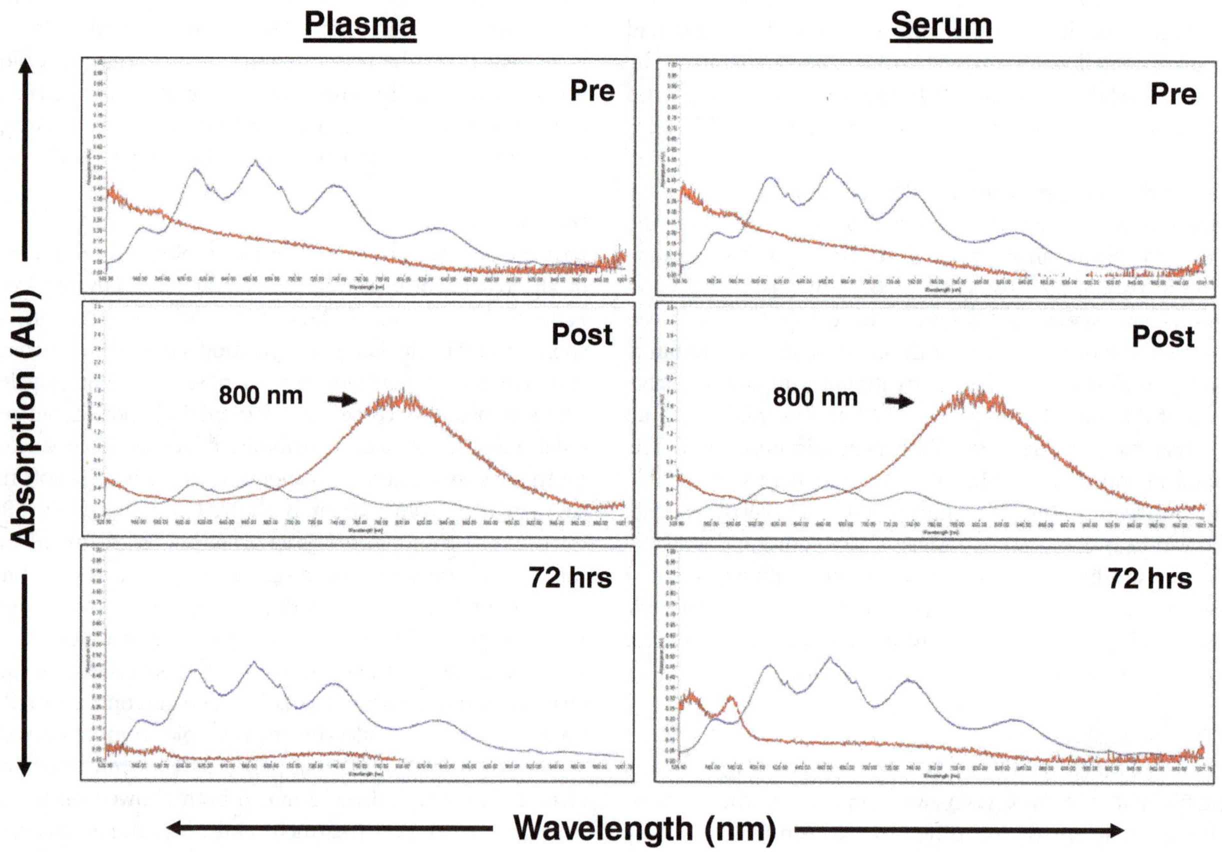

Fig. 1 Plasma and serum NR concentrations before and after treatment. The NR absorption peaks in Patient 7 are noted by the red line; background from blood components is noted with the blue line. A reliable peak is present at 800 nm (red) 15 min post NR infusion. Clearance of the NRs from serum and plasma is seen by 72 h

necrosis and swelling/edema were observed all occurred following NIR laser application.

Systemic adverse events

Six systemic adverse events were noted. In all cases, causality with either nanorod administration or laser application could neither be definitively confirmed nor completely ruled out. These included anemia, ALT elevation, CK elevation, nausea and lethargy. Patient 4 experienced a grade 1 CK elevation possibly attributable to tissue damage following NIR laser applications and a grade 2 ALT elevation of unknown etiology. Patient 7 experienced grade 1 nausea and lethargy the day following NIR laser application, which could have been secondary to laser application and subsequent tissue damage or the sedation from the procedure. This patient recovered from both of the adverse events within a 24 h time period. Finally, two patients developed a grade 1 anemia while on study that could have been related to study procedures, although anemia of chronic disease

Table 2 Plasma concentrations of NRs immediately and 72 h post treatment

Patient	NR Post Treatment (μg/ml)	NR 72 h (μg/ml)
1	108	12
2	120	0
3	192	97
4	160	0
5	60	6
6	72	0
7	168	0

Table 3 Thermal dose during NIR Diode laser treatment

Patient	Thermal Dose
1	75–100 ° C for 1 min
2	40–60 °C for 2 min
3	53–66 °C for 3 min
4	63–70 °C for 1 min
5	45–55 °C for 4 min
6	78–110 °C for 40 s
7	45–65 °C for 3 min

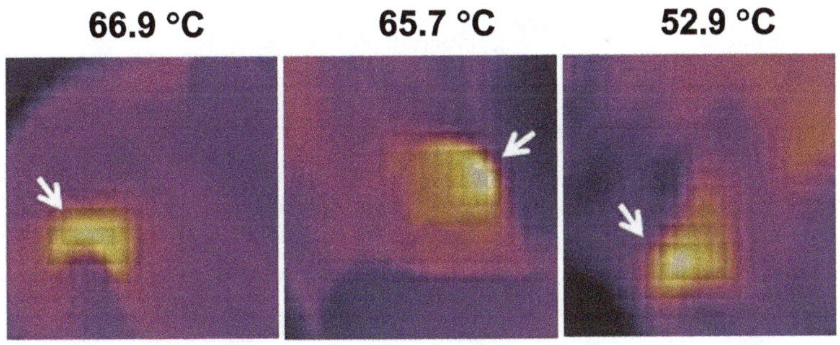

Fig. 2 Infrared imaging of tumors during NIR laser therapy. Shown are representative images of infrared imaging performed during treatment, with the associated intratumoral temperatures as assessed by the infrared camera

and pre-existing conditions such as hypothyroidism could not be ruled out as the primary causes.

Discussion

Photodynamic therapy (PDT) has been used in human medicine for decades primarily to treat superficial skin lesions. Major hurdles for the continued success of this treatment modality are specificity of targeting tumors while avoiding toxicity to normal tissues and adverse events related to photosensitizers. Photothermal therapy (PTT) is a therapeutic modality used in human cancer in which intratumoral heating is used to kill tumors through application of a light source specific for the thermal agent. In general, such agents are on the nanoscale given the enhanced permeability and retention effect observed with particles in a certain size range (typically 20–300 nm) [8, 17]. Molecules in this range preferentially accumulate in tumor tissue that typically possesses a disorganized, leaky vasculature and poor lymphatic drainage, different properties as compared to regular blood vessels, such as poor lymphatic drainage and a disorganized, leaky vasculature, promoting this selectivity. The agents used for PTT include gold nanorods (NRs), gold nanoshells, graphene and graphene oxide. Gold NRs have been identified as an optimal nanoparticle as they may be synthesized in bulk, have broadly tunable plasmon resonance and exhibit absorption coefficients 10^4–10^6-fold higher than conventional organic fluorochromes typically used for photodynamic therapy [2, 3]. The Surface-Enhanced, Resonant Raman Scattering (SERS) effect created by coupling gold NRs with visible and NIR-absorbing molecules results in enhanced capacity for PTT induced tumor ablation [3].

Multiple methods currently are under investigation to exploit the unique property of SERS NRs to passively collect into tumors [18]. Early in vitro work demonstrated that SERS NRs can be linked with specific monoclonal antibodies to target antigens overexpressed in cancer cells.

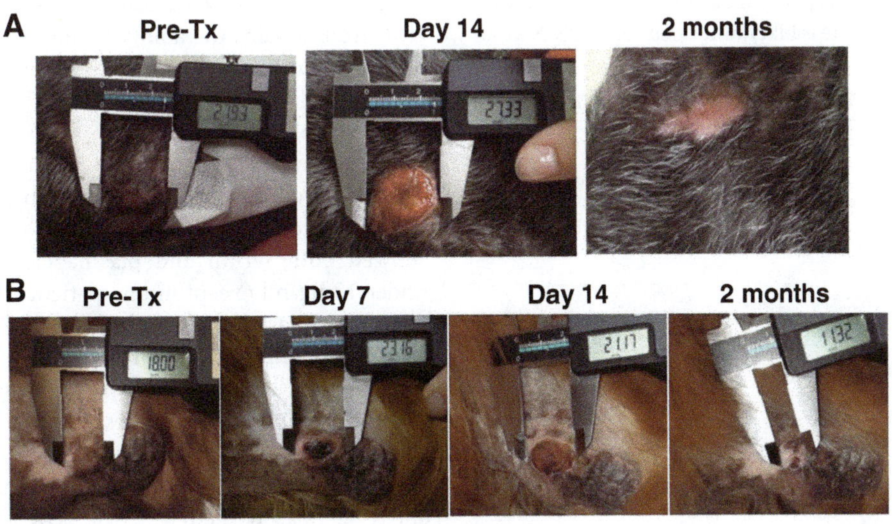

Fig. 3 Response to NIR therapy. **a** Patient 1 experienced a durable response that lasted for approximately 8 months post treatment. **b** Patient 7 showed partial response for 77 days at which point the tumor showed mild enlargement from the previous visit and a surgical excision was elected (**b**)

Table 4 Patient response and post-treatment histopathology

Patient	Response	Histopath pre-treatment	Histopath post treatment	Post-treatment biopsy
1	CR	10% tumor necrosis, no individual cell death	20% necrosis, coagulation and edema	Needle core
2	SD	no necrosis or individual cell death	no evidence of tumor cell death	Excisional
3	SD	<5% necrosis with rare individual cell death	60% necrosis with hemorrhage	Excisional
4	SD	no necrosis or individual cell death	40–50% necrosis and hemorrhage with moderate to severe skin necrosis	Excisional
5	SD	no necrosis and moderate cell death	Less than 50% multifocal mild hemorrhage and necrosis	Excisional
6	SD	no necrosis or individual cell death	no necrosis or individual cell death	Excisional
7	PR	no necrosis or individual cell death	no necrosis or individual cell death	Excisional

When exposed to both malignant and non-malignant epithelial cell lines, the SERS NRs showed preferential binding to malignant cell lines that subsequently caused cell death post irradiation at the appropriate spectrum [8]. Recent in vivo work in mouse models with xenograft tumors, which receive IV NRs and 5 min of heating to 70 degrees Celsius with an 810 nm laser, showed destruction of all tumors and durable response for up to 50 days [13]. In addition, gold NRs can be coated with a thermo-sensitive shell that includes dispersed drug molecules that when heated release drug in a targeted area [19]. The synergistic effects of heat and chemotherapy can be quite significant and thus warrant further investigation to allow for maximum efficacy of the PTT effect while potentially reducing toxicity associated with systemic chemotherapy administration [20].

Based on the published data suggesting both safety and efficacy of SERS NRS in the treatment of tumors in laboratory animals, the purpose of this clinical trial was to confirm these findings in a large animal model of cancer that more closely recapitulates the natural evolution of tumors. Therefore, we used dogs with spontaneous tumors in a pilot study setting to evaluate the feasibility and safety of SERS NRs administration combined with NIR diode laser application. A secondary objective of the study was to determine if this therapeutic approach had potential for clinical benefit as assessed by response to therapy. We predicted that the treatment would be safe and associated with a limited adverse event profile, and that most dogs would derive clinical benefit from participation in the study.

Table 5 Patient cutaneous and systemic adverse events

Patient	Cutaneous adverse events	Systemic adverse events
1	Grade 1 erythema; grade 2 skin ulceration	None
2	Grade 2 skin ulceration	Grade 1 anemia
3	Grade 1 skin ulceration	None
4	Grade 2 skin ulceration	Grade 2 ALT elevation; Grade 1 CK elevation
5	Grade 2 skin ulceration	Grade 1 anemia
6	Grade 1 edema and swelling	None
7	Grade 1 erythema and grade 1 tumor necrosis	Grade 1 nausea; Grade 1 lethargy

Administration of NRs and the subsequent NIR treatment laser treatment were well tolerated by all patients enrolled in this study. Although the number of dogs treated was small, a diverse set of breeds was represented and the size ranged from 9.1 to 42.1 kg. The reported adverse events were expected and related to the extreme intratumoral heating resulting in local cutaneous reactions, swelling, edema and redness. These were self-limiting and nearly all had resolved within 14 days. One of the challenges encountered was the difficulty in achieving consistent and even heating within the treated tumors. In most cases, the tumors developed specific hot spots within 10–20 s of NIR application and effectively moving the laser to evenly distribute the heating was affected by tumor size, tumor shape, and to some degree, operator proficiency. It is likely that this would improve over time with continued experience using the NIR. Additionally, the ability to adjust the circumference of NIR exposure would reduce the need to continually move the laser and thus reduce the development of intratumoral hot spots.

In this study, clearance and processing of the SERS NRs appeared relatively uniform with the exception of a single outlier. Dogs given a dose of 10 mg/kg NRs showed both serum and plasma clearance at 72 h to under 12 μg/ml except in one patient who had a 50% reduction of plasma and serum levels (192 μg/ml immediately after administration to 97μg/ml 72 h later). It is uncertain at this point what might have contributed to this occurrence but changes in either absorption or clearance due to neoplasia, concurrent comorbidities or idiosyncratic causes are all potential etiologies. Importantly, all dogs treated with the NIR laser at 72 h that had detectable NR plasma levels exhibited no additional adverse events when compared to those dogs with undetectable levels. However, as this was a pilot study, the safety threshold for highest potential NR plasma concentration during NIR laser treatment was not determined.

There was no correlation between residual circulating plasma NR levels and response to treatment (Tables 2, 4) supporting the notion that intratumoral accumulation and trapping of the NRs occurred by 72 h post dosing, permitting the observed NIR induced heating to occur.

Two dogs enrolled in this study experienced an objective response to therapy (1 PR, 1 CR). The remaining dogs had stable disease over the 14 day period of study evaluation. When the histopathologic results of dogs experiencing SD versus PR/CR were compared, there appeared to be no differences in the degree of treatment induced necrosis, coagulation and edema. For example, biopsies from dogs 3 and 5 that experienced SD demonstrated 60% and 50% necrosis and hemorrhage, respectively. In contrast, biopsies from dogs 1 (CR) and 7 (PR) had 20% and 0% necrosis and hemorrhage. The authors recognize that the relative amount of necrosis and hemorrhage in the pre treatment samples may not be an accurate representation of the entire tumor, given inherent intra-tumoral heterogeneity. As 6/7 tumors were removed in their entirety, intra tumor heterogeneity in the post treatment samples was minimized as much as possible.

Although all tumors were treated to at least 40 °C, there was a wide range of temperatures achieved during NIR application (from 40 to 110 °C). Time to minimum temperature of 40 °C varied greatly among patients and the authors hypothesize this is likely due to a variety of factors including vascularity, accumulation of NRs in tumors and potentially tumor type. Interestingly, higher temperatures did not appear to correlate with an enhanced induction of necrosis or hemorrhage. Further studies are necessary to determine factors that might be associated with response to therapy, such as in combination with chemotherapy, in order to maximize tumor necrosis.

The limitations of this study are similar to most phase 1 trials including a small non-uniform sample size of patients of varied tumor type and prior therapeutic interventions. Additionally, dose escalation of the NRs was not performed to interrogate a possible link between dose and response to therapy. Dogs were only treated once and it is possible that additional treatments may have enhanced response by promoting further intratumoral accumulation of NRs and thus enhancing the photothermal effect. Lastly, most tumors (5/7) were removed in their entirety at the conclusion of the brief study and another tumor was removed a short time after the study, making it difficult to draw meaningful conclusions regarding clinical benefit from the PTTT. It would have been ideal to allow tumors to be removed after PD was observed; however, the study was designed as a pilot trial with safety as one of the primary endpoints and the intention was not to delay standard of care therapy to patients that were enrolled.

Conclusions

SERs coated gold NRs are safe for parenteral administration to dogs and the application of NIR treatment following NR administration may hold potential for clinical benefit in dogs with solid tumors. Expansion to a larger cohort of dogs affected with a variety of neoplastic diseases than those enrolled in this pilot study is warranted to truly define the therapeutic potential of this approach. Opportunities exist to combine NR/NIR therapy with other standard treatment modalities such as chemotherapy and immunotherapy to maximize clinical benefit.

Abbreviations

AEs: Adverse events; ALP: Alkaline Phosphatase; ALT: alanine aminotransferase; AST: aspartate aminotransferase; BUN: blood urine nitrogen; CB: clinical benefit; CBC: complete blood count; CR: complete response; CT: computerized tomography; FS: female spayed; GI: gastrointestinal; IAUCUC: Institutional Animal Care and Use Committee; IV: intravenous; MCT: mast cell tumor; Ml: milliliter; MN: male neutered; NIR: near-infrared; NR: nanorod; NSAID: non-steroidal anti-inflammatory; ORR: overall response rate; PD: progressive disease; PDT: photodynamic therapy; PEG: polyethyleneglycol; PR: partial response; SD: stable disease; SERS: Surface-Enhanced, Resonant Raman Scattering; STS: soft tissue sarcoma; μg: microgram; ULN: upper limit of normal; UV/Vis: ultraviolet visible; VCOG-CTCAE: veterinary cooperative oncology group common terminology criteria for adverse events

Acknowledgements

The Blue Buffalo Veterinary Clinical Trials Office (BBVCTO) at the Ohio State University College of Veterinary Medicine coordinated all aspects of this study including generation of case report forms, collection of samples, collation of data, quality assurance and final quality control on all data.

Funding

SERS gold nanorods were provided by Nanopartz Inc. for this clinical trial. Funding for the study was provided by Concurrent Analytical, Inc. This project was also supported by the following grants: UL1TR001070 from the National Center for Advancing Translational Sciences and P30CA016058 from the National Cancer Institute to The Ohio State University.

Authors' contributions

CAL designed the clinical trial and supervised enrollment of all cases, quality assurance, writing of the manuscript and final edits. EMS was responsible for evaluation of patient data, data analysis, and writing of the manuscript. RP was the clinical trial intern primarily responsible for coordination of study recruitment. HG assisted in editing the final manuscript. CS contributed the concept for the study and assisted in study design. All authors read and approved the final manuscript.

Consent for publication

Not applicable.

Competing interests

Christian Schoen is an employee of Nanopartz, the company that provided the SERS gold nanorods for this clinical trial. None of the authors have any other competing interests.

Author details

[1]College of Veterinary Medicine, The Ohio State University, Columbus OH AND Cummings School of Veterinary Medicine, Tufts University, North Grafton, MA, USA. [2]Premier Veterinary Group, 3927 W. Belmont Ave, Chicago,

IL 60618, USA. [3]Nanopartz Inc., 146 Barberry Place, Loveland, CO 80537, USA. [4]Veterinary Cancer Group, 2887 Edinger Ave, Tustin, CA 92780, USA. [5]Sackler School at Tufts University, Boston, MA, USA.

References

1. Salata O. Applications of nanoparticles in biology and medicine. J Nanobiotechnology. 2004;2(1):3.
2. Hu M, Chen J, Li ZY, Au L, Hartland GV, Li X, Marquez M, Xia Y. Gold nanostructures: engineering their plasmonic properties for biomedical applications. Chem Soc Rev. 2006;35(11):1084–94.
3. von Maltzahn G, Centrone A, Park JH, Ramanathan R, Sailor MJ, Hatton TA, Bhatia SN. SERS-coded gold Nanorods as a multifunctional platform for densely multiplexed near-infrared imaging and Photothermal heating. Adv Mater. 2009;21(31):3175–80.
4. Anker JN, Hall WP, Lyandres O, Shah NC, Zhao J, Van Duyne RP. Biosensing with plasmonic nanosensors. Nat Mater. 2008;7(6):442–53.
5. El-Sayed MA. Some interesting properties of metals confined in time and nanometer space of different shapes. Acc Chem Res. 2001;34(4):257–64.
6. Orendorff CJ, Gearheart L, Jana NR, Murphy CJ. Aspect ratio dependence on surface enhanced Raman scattering using silver and gold nanorod substrates. Phys Chem Chem Phys. 2006;8(1):165–70.
7. Hahn MA, Singh AK, Sharma P, Brown SC, Moudgil BM. Nanoparticles as contrast agents for in-vivo bioimaging: current status and future perspectives. Anal Bioanal Chem. 2011;399(1):3–27.
8. Huang X, El-Sayed IH, Qian W, El-Sayed MA. Cancer cell imaging and photothermal therapy in the near-infrared region by using gold nanorods. J Am Chem Soc. 2006;128(6):2115–20.
9. Maeda H. The enhanced permeability and retention (EPR) effect in tumor vasculature: the key role of tumor-selective macromolecular drug targeting. Adv Enzym Regul. 2001;41:189–207.
10. Maeda H, Fang J, Inutsuka T, Kitamoto Y. Vascular permeability enhancement in solid tumor: various factors, mechanisms involved and its implications. Int Immunopharmacol. 2003;3(3):319–28.
11. Lankveld DP, Rayavarapu RG, Krystek P, Oomen AG, Verharen HW, van Leeuwen TG, De Jong WH, Manohar S. Blood clearance and tissue distribution of PEGylated and non-PEGylated gold nanorods after intravenous administration in rats. Nanomedicine (Lond). 2011;6(2):339–49.
12. Dickerson EB, Dreaden EC, Huang X, El-Sayed IH, Chu H, Pushpanketh S, McDonald JF, El-Sayed MA. Gold nanorod assisted near-infrared plasmonic photothermal therapy (PPTT) of squamous cell carcinoma in mice. Cancer Lett. 2008;269(1):57–66.
13. von Maltzahn G, Park JH, Agrawal A, Bandaru NK, Das SK, Sailor MJ, Bhatia SN. Computationally guided photothermal tumor therapy using long-circulating gold nanorod antennas. Cancer Res. 2009;69(9):3892–900.
14. Smith BR, Kempen P, Bouley D, Xu A, Liu Z, Melosh N, Dai H, Sinclair R, Gambhir SS. Shape matters: intravital microscopy reveals surprising geometrical dependence for nanoparticles in tumor models of extravasation. Nano Lett. 2012;12(7):3369–77.
15. Nguyen SM, Thamm DH, Vail DM, London CA. Response evaluation criteria for solid tumours in dogs (v1.0): a Veterinary Cooperative Oncology Group (VCOG) consensus document. Vet Comp Oncol. 2015;13:176–83.
16. Veterinary cooperative oncology group. common terminology criteria for adverse events (VCOG-CTCAE) following chemotherapy or biological antineoplastic therapy in dogs and cats v1.0. Vet Comp Oncol. 2004;2:195–213.
17. Maeda H, Wu J, Sawa T, Matsumura Y, Hori K. Tumor vascular permeability and the EPR effect in macromolecular therapeutics: a review. J Control Release. 2000;65(1–2):271–84.
18. Alkilany AM, Thompson LB, Boulos SP, Sisco PN, Murphy CJ. Gold nanorods: their potential for photothermal therapeutics and drug delivery, tempered by the complexity of their biological interactions. Adv Drug Deliv Rev. 2012;64(2):190–9.
19. Kawano T, Niidome Y, Mori T, Katayama Y, Niidome T. PNIPAM gel-coated gold nanorods for targeted delivery responding to a near-infrared laser. Bioconjug Chem. 2009;20(2):209–12.
20. Hauck TS, Jennings TL, Yatsenk T, Chan WCW. Ehancing the toxicity of cancer chemotherapeutics with gold nanorod hyperthermia. Adv Mater. 2008;20(20):3832–8.

16

Investigating the potential of the anti-epileptic drug imepitoin as a treatment for co-morbid anxiety in dogs with idiopathic epilepsy

Rowena M. A. Packer[1*], Luisa De Risio[2] and Holger A. Volk[1]

Abstract

Background: Behavioural changes associated with idiopathic epilepsy (IE) have been identified in dogs, with fear and anxiety-related problems seen in both drug-naïve dogs and dogs treated with anti-epileptic drugs (AEDs). Treating anxiety-related behaviour in dogs with IE may be challenging, as seizures are a contraindication for many conventional anxiolytic drugs. In addition, many dogs with IE are already treated with AEDs to reduce their seizure frequency, which may have negative effects if used in polytherapy. Imepitoin is low-affinity partial agonist at the benzodiazepine (BDZ) site of the $GABA_A$ receptor, and has been demonstrated to have both anticonvulsant and anxiolytic effects in laboratory rodents. Imepitoin has been developed for the treatment of IE in dogs, with demonstrated anticonvulsant effects and high tolerability and safety. To date, imepitoin's potential to reduce anxiety in dogs with IE has not been investigated. An online survey was conducted to investigate the effect of imepitoin on fear and anxiety-related behaviours in dogs with IE. Eighty-five valid responses were received from owners of dogs with IE currently treated with imepitoin. Anxiety-related behaviour was quantified before and during imepitoin treatment using a validated questionnaire tool (C-BARQ).

Results: No differences were observed in the five fear/anxiety-related measures between the two time periods (before vs. during treatment) for dog directed fear, stranger directed fear, non-social fear, pain sensitivity and separation related behaviour. A median 45% reduction in seizure frequency/month was observed following imepitoin treatment; however, imepitoin did not appear effective in reducing seizure frequency in a minority of cases. Polyphagia was the most common chronic side effect, and more side effects were reported in polytherapy cases.

Conclusions: Imepitoin does not appear to improve anxiety-related behaviour in dogs with IE treated with this medication for its anti-epileptic effects. Investigating the effects of imepitoin upon the behaviour of dogs with recognised behavioural anxiety-related problems (e.g. specific fears and phobias, separation related behaviours), in both healthy dogs and dogs with epilepsy is required to further explore any potential anxiolytic effects of this medication.

Keywords: Canine, Epilepsy, Anxiolytic, Anxiety, Fear, Behaviour, Seizure, Idiopathic

* Correspondence: rpacker@rvc.ac.uk
[1]Department of Clinical Science and Services, Royal Veterinary College, Hatfield, Hertfordshire AL9 7TA, UK
Full list of author information is available at the end of the article

Background

There is mounting evidence that epilepsy is not simply a seizure disorder, with the prevalence of psychiatric disorders in people with epilepsy higher than in either the general population or patients with other chronic medical diseases [1–4]. The most common co-morbid psychiatric disorders of epilepsy in people are anxiety and depression [2, 5–8]. Comorbidities may be a cause of epilepsy, a consequence of epilepsy, or a separate condition that is associated with epilepsy because there is a common cause for the epilepsy and the comorbidity [9]. The impact of co-morbid psychiatric disorders upon patient quality of life (QoL) may be severe, with interictal anxiety and depression found to have greater adverse effects on QoL than those of seizure frequency, severity and chronicity [10]. As such, treatment that does not simply focus upon seizure control may be beneficial to the QoL of patients with epilepsy [9].

Co-morbid anxiety has recently been recognised in dogs with idiopathic epilepsy (IE) [11], with behavioural changes including increases in fear and anxiety associated with the development of IE [11]. Increased fear and anxiety were observed in drug-naïve dogs as well as those treated with AEDs, indicating these behavioural changes were not merely a treatment side effect [11]. For example, in a recent study of epilepsy in the Italian Spinone, 55% of dogs developed behavioural abnormalities (commonly associated with anxiety) at epilepsy onset, before the initiation of AEDs [12]. Due to the potentially severe impact of anxiety upon QoL, addressing this behavioural change alongside managing seizures is desirable.

There are few psychopharmacological agents licensed for use in dogs, and treating anxiety-related behaviour in dogs with IE may be additionally challenging, as epilepsy or a history of seizures are a contraindication for many anxiolytic drugs. This includes the tri-cyclic antidepressant (TCA) clomipramine, buspirone, and the selective serotonin reuptake inhibitors (SSRI) fluoxetine, imipramine, paroxetine, sertraline, amitriptyline and fluvoxamine [13]. As such, there is a need for anxiolytic drugs that:

(i) Reduce anxiety without reducing the seizure threshold in dogs with IE;
(ii) Have the potential to be administered as a polytherapy alongside existing AEDs; and
(iii) Have a favourable side effect profile to allow their long-term administration, if required.

Imepitoin is low-affinity partial agonist at the benzodiazepine (BDZ) binding site of the $GABA_A$ receptor. Partial activation of the GABA receptors by imepitoin has been demonstrated to have pronounced anti-seizure activity and anxiolytic activity in rodent models, with a high tolerability [14]. The anxiolytic effects of imepitoin have been demonstrated in the rat in three experimental paradigms, the Vogel conflict test, the elevated plus maze and the light-dark box [15]. Imepitoin has been developed as an antiepileptic drug for canine idiopathic epilepsy (IE), with multiple studies indicating that it is well tolerated in dogs, with antiepileptic effects observed in both newly diagnosed IE cases as monotherapy and in drug-resistant dogs as add-on treatment to phenobarbital [16–20]. The anxiolytic effects of imepitoin have yet to be demonstrated in detail in the dog; however, anecdotal evidence from the first clinical studies of imepitoin indicated that owners perceived that their dog's epilepsy-related behavioural changes had improved during imepitoin treatment, an effect not previously seen with other anti-epileptic drugs (AEDs) such as phenobarbital [21]. Imepitoin has potential benefits over existing anxiolytics with a fast onset of action ~2–3 h post oral dosing [14, 22], compared to around 3–5 weeks for SSRIs and TCAs [23]. To date, the only behavioural effect of imepitoin that has been reported is hyperactivity [18], which may be expected as paradoxical excitement can occur in dogs treated with benzodiazepines (e.g. diazepam) [24].

Whether imepitoin, a BDZ partial agonist, can be both an effective anticonvulsant and anxiolytic in dogs with IE requires further investigation. The purpose of this study was to investigate the effect of imepitoin upon owner-reported indicators of fear and anxiety-related behaviour in dogs treated with imepitoin for IE, to investigate imepitoin's impact when administered as a polytherapy alongside other AEDs, and to quantify imepitoin's side effect profile when used as a mono- or polytherapy.

Methods

Recruitment

A web-based questionnaire study was conducted to investigate behavioural effects of imepitoin in dogs treated with this medication for IE. Owners of dogs currently being treated with imepitoin for IE were recruited online via online (canine epilepsy forums, Twitter, Facebook pages, the Royal Veterinary College and Animal Health Trust websites) and via posters and leaflets at local veterinary practices and breed association groups. To be included in the study, dogs must have:

(1) Been diagnosed with IE either:

i. By a first opinion vet due to recurrent seizures for more than 1 year, with the first seizure having occurred while aged between 6 months to 6 years, with no identifiable cause found (Tier I confidence level for the diagnosis of IE [25]); OR

ii. By a specialist in veterinary neurology with the aid of blood tests (minimum data base blood tests [25]) and MRI of the brain

(2) Been treated with imepitoin for IE for a minimum of 4 weeks (28 days).

All dogs currently being treated with imepitoin were eligible for this study, regardless of AED history to include a breadth of cases. No pre-screening of anxiety levels was conducted prior to inclusion in the study, to allow the investigation of imepitoin's effects upon dogs with a wide spectrum of anxiety levels. Consent was gained via a statement at the start of the questionnaire, after the purpose of the study and potential use of the results had been explained to the owner.

Questionnaire content

The survey was entitled "A questionnaire study of the impact of Pexion (Imepitoin) on canine behaviour and welfare" as not to bias responses towards owners of dogs with anxiety problems, or dogs who had experienced marked changes in anxiety following imepitoin treatment. The survey was structured into four sections: clinical history, behavioural changes, treatment efficacy and side effects profile.

Clinical history

Owners reported their dog's signalment, pedigree, age at first seizure, seizure history, diagnostic tests performed to diagnose IE, seizure frequency, experience of cluster seizures, and frequency of cluster seizures and status epilepticus (as defined by [26]), seizure semiology and seizure recovery characteristics. AED treatment history including the use of other anti-epileptic drugs was recorded, and whether the dog was currently being treated with imepitoin as a monotherapy or polytherapy. Owners were asked to report their dog's current dose of imepitoin (mg) and their dog's weight (kg).

Behavioural changes

Behavioural traits were quantified using a validated questionnaire tool, the Canine Behavioral Assessment and Research Questionnaire (C-BARQ) [27]. Owners were questioned on their dog's anxiety-related behaviour before and during imepitoin treatment using five of the eleven C-BARQ behavioural measures: 'Dog directed fear', 'Stranger directed fear'; 'Non-social fear'; 'Pain sensitivity' and 'Separation related behaviour'. The C-BARQ has previously been used to quantify neurobehavioral changes in dogs with neurological disease, including IE and syringomyelia [11, 28] and to quantify the impact of a ketogenic dietary therapy upon the behaviour of dogs with IE in a placebo-controlled crossover trial [29].

Treatment efficacy

The effect of imepitoin on seizure activity was recorded via owner reports of the following measures both *before* and *during* imepitoin treatment:

(i) Mean number of seizures/month;
(ii) Mean number of seizure days/month;
(iii) Mean number of cluster seizures/month (how many times their dog experienced more than one seizure in a 24 h period per month).

Owners were asked to estimate these measures from the 3 months prior to imepitoin use, and for the entire length of time they had been treated with imepitoin for. The percentage change in the number of seizures/month was calculated from measure (i) compared before and during imepitoin treatment.

Side effects profile

Owners were questioned on the presence and severity of 11 AED side effects in the first 2 weeks of imepitoin treatment, and after 2 weeks of imepitoin treatment: polyphagia, polydipsia, polyuria, weight gain, increased sleeping, ataxia, restlessness, pruritus, vomiting, diarrhoea and coughing. Owners were asked to report the severity of these side effects on a five point scale of very mild (1), mild (2), moderate (3), severe (4), and very severe (5). Composite side effect scores were compiled for the initial 2 weeks of treatment and after 2 weeks of treatment by adding the scores of each of the 11 signs (out of 55).

Statistical analysis

The five C-BARQ measures were calculated for each dog using weighted scores, calculated using the loading factors for each question established in the original C-BARQ validation study multiplied by the owner's response to each question. Descriptive statistics were calculated for each behavioural measure. Effects of treatment protocol (dogs receiving mono or polytherapy with imepitoin), cluster seizures, signalment and seizure frequency before treatment were investigated for each behavioural trait, measures of drug response and side effect profiles. Data were visually examined for normality of distribution using histograms. The Wilcoxon test was used to compare continuous paired data e.g. C-BARQ measures before and during imepitoin use, the Mann-Whitey (U) tests for comparing continuous independent data between two groups, and the Kruskall-Wallis (KW) test for comparing continuous independent data between more than two groups. Chi-squared (X^2) analysis was used to investigate associations between categorical variables. All tests were two-sided and $P < 0.05$ was considered to be significant. Data are presented as mean (±SD), or median (25th–75th quartile), where appropriate.

Results

Responses

Responses were received from 176 owners of which 85 were valid responses. Responses were deemed invalid (n = 91) for the following reasons: n = 74 were incomplete and could not be analysed, n = 9 dogs were deceased at the time of response, n = 4 dogs were not receiving imepitoin at the time of response, n = 2 dogs were over the limit of age at first seizure (without further veterinary diagnostics to increase the confidence of an IE diagnosis), and n = 2 had been diagnosed with structural epilepsy (caused by identified cerebral pathology) [26].

Demographics - Owner

The majority of the owners responding were female (77%, n = 65), with the most common age group being 46–60 years old (47.6%, n = 40), followed by 31–45 (32.1%, n = 27). The majority of responses were from the UK (92.9%, n = 78), with 3.6% from Germany (n = 3), 1.2% (n = 1) from Belgium, Spain, Sweden and n = 1 owner did not disclose their location. The majority of owners had heard about the survey via social media (60.7%, n = 51), followed by web searches (21.4%, n = 18), their regular vet (7.1%, n = 6) and their specialist vet (6.0%, n = 5). Nearly one third of dogs had experienced a seizure within a week of their owner completing the survey (31.8%, n = 27), and a further 28.2% 1–3 weeks prior to completion.

Demographics - dog

Nearly two thirds of dogs were male (male neutered: 55.3%, n = 47, male entire: 10.6%, n = 9), with around one third female (female neutered: 30.6%, n = 26, female entire 3.5%, n = 3). The mean age (months) ± SD was 57.7 ± 29.6 months and mean weight (kg) ± SD was 23.1 ± 12.3. The majority of dogs were pure bred (78.8%, n = 67), with 34 different breeds represented, and 21.2% were cross-bred (n = 18). Almost half of all dogs were Kennel Club registered (48.2%, n = 41). The most common breeds represented were the Labrador Retriever (12.9%, n = 11), Border Collie (10.6%, n = 9), Beagle (3.5%, n = 3), Golden Retriever (3.5%, n = 3) and Italian Spinone (3.5%, n = 3).

Epilepsy phenotype

The median age (months) at first seizure (25th–75th percentile) was 28.5 (18–46.3) months. The median total number of seizures a dog had experienced was 12 (8–30). Over half of dogs (55.3%, n = 47) had experienced cluster seizures (more than one fit within 24 h), with 43.5% only experiencing single seizures (n = 37) and 1.2% (n = 1) of owners unsure.

Anti-epileptic drug treatment

The median time in days from first seizure to imepitoin treatment was 275.0 (105.0–743.0). Imepitoin was started after 2–5 seizures in the majority of dogs (41.2%, n = 35), and after the first seizure in only 9.4% (n = 11) of dogs. The median duration of imepitoin treatment was 263.9 days (106.3–478.4). The mean dose of imepitoin was 23.37 mg/kg (SD: 6.43). The lowest dose was 10.0 mg/kg and the highest was 35.7 mg/kg, with the majority of dogs receiving a dose between 20 and 30 mg/kg (53.5%).

Imepitoin was the first anti-epileptic medication received for 65.9% of dogs (n = 56), with the other third of dogs (32.9%, n = 28) having already received other anti-epileptic drugs (AEDs). The majority of these dogs had already been treated with phenobarbital (PB) (n = 22), followed by potassium bromide (KBr) (n = 8), and levetiracetam (LEV) (n = 3). At the time of the survey, two thirds of dogs were being treated with imepitoin as a monotherapy (65.9%, n = 56) and one third were being treated as a polytherapy (34.1%, n = 29) (Fig. 1). Of those dogs receiving polytherapy, n = 21 were being treated with PB, n = 13 with KBr and n = 8 with LEV. Nearly one quarter of owners used rectal diazepam as an emergency treatment (23.5%, n = 20).

Of the monotherapy cases (n = 56), imepitoin was the first AED they were treated with for 76.8% of cases (n = 43), with the remaining 21.4% (n = 13) having previously been treated with other AED (s) whose use had since been discontinued. Of the polytherapy cases (n = 29), 44.8% (n = 13) had received imepitoin as their dogs first AED with additional AEDs added at a later date, and 55.2% (n = 16) received imepitoin as an add-on to existing AED medication. There was a significant association between cluster seizures and therapy type, with dogs that only experienced single seizures more likely to be treated with imepitoin as a monotherapy (83.6%) than as a polytherapy (16.2%) ($X^2 = 9.81, p = 0.002$).

Behavioural effects

No significant effect of imepitoin treatment was found on the five behavioural measures, in either the whole population (Table 1) or when only monotherapy cases were considered ($p > 0.05$) (Fig. 2).

When only those monotherapy cases that were drug-naive (had received no AED treatment prior to imepitoin treatment, n = 43) were analysed, there was still no difference observed in any of the five behavioural measures before and during treatment ($p > 0.05$). As dogs were not selected based on high anxiety levels, to investigate

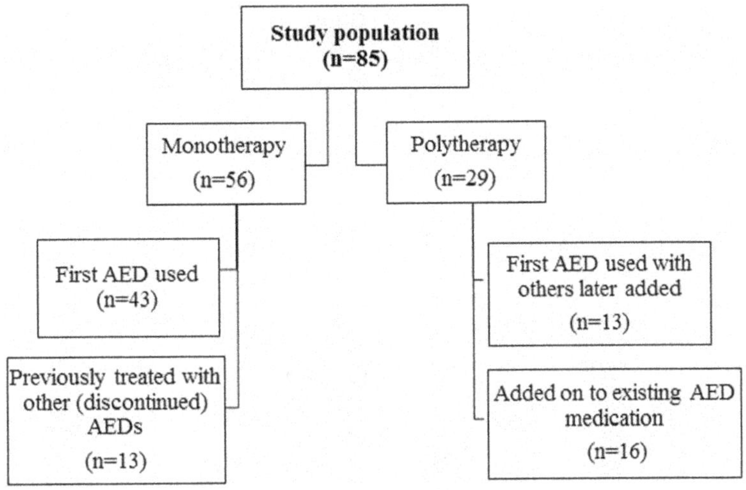

Fig. 1 Different uses of imepitoin as a monotherapy or a polytherapy in a study population of 85 dogs treated with imepitoin for idiopathic epilepsy

the effect of imepitoin on only those dogs with higher levels of anxiety within this population, analyses were repeated including only those dogs with CBARQ scores above the population median for each factor (Dog directed fear: 0.543, Stranger directed fear: 0.203, Non-social fear: 0.351, Pain sensitivity: 0.680, Separation related behaviour: 0.088). Again, no effect of imepitoin treatment upon the five measures was found in this sub-population ($p > 0.05$).

There was no effect of signalment (sex, neuter status or breed) on any of the five behavioural measures before or during imepitoin treatment ($p > 0.05$). There was no correlation between changes in any of the five behavioural measures before or during imepitoin treatment and drug response (as quantified by percentage change (%) in seizure frequency; $p > 0.05$), or with the side effects scores observed in either the first 2 weeks, or after 2 weeks of treatment ($p > 0.05$).

Impact on seizure frequency

Significant reductions in seizures/month and clusters/month were reported by owners while their dog was treated with imepitoin compared to before imepitoin treatment; however no significant change was seen in the number of seizure days/month (Table 2). The median reduction in seizure frequency following imepitoin treatment (number of seizures/month) was −1 (−2 to 0), and the median percentage change in seizure frequency was a 45% reduction (−89.6% - 0%) across all cases.

There was no significant difference in % reduction in seizure frequency between dogs with or without cluster seizures (Clusters median: 0% (−73.2% – 0%) vs. single seizures median: −58.3% (−100% - 0%); Mann-Whitney U = 863, $p = 0.073$). There was no significant difference in % reduction in seizure frequency between dogs being treated with imepitoin as a monotherapy or polytherapy (Monotherapy median: −50% (−100% - 0%) vs. polytherapy median: 0% (−76.3%- +100%); Mann-Whitney $U = 820.5$, $p = 0.058$). There was no association between the number of seizures before initiation of imepitoin treatment and the percentage change (%) in seizure frequency (KW = 3.11, $p = 0.375$), or any effect of sex, neuter status or breed on percentage change (%) in seizure frequency ($p > 0.05$).

Side effects profile

The most common and severe side effect reported in both the first 2 weeks and after 2 weeks of imepitoin treatment was polyphagia. There was a significant reduction in the

Table 1 Five C-BARQ behavioural measures before and after imepitoin treatment in dogs treated with imepitoin with or without other anti-epileptic drugs

Behavioural measure	Before imepitoin treatment	During imepitoin treatment	Wilcoxon (W)	N	p
Dog directed fear	0.40 (0–1.09)	0.54 (0–1.09)	265.5	83	0.660
Stranger directed fear	0.19 (0–0.81)	0.19 (0–0.99)	206.0	84	0.946
Non-social fear	0.36 (0.09–0.78)	0.38 (0.11–0.85)	505.0	84	0.108
Pain sensitivity	0.62 (0–1.29)	0.62 (0.24–1.33)	307.0	83	0.125
Separation related behaviour	0.0 (0–0.33)	0.09 (0–0.47)	268	80	0.058

Data are presented as the median accompanied by 25th–75th percentiles

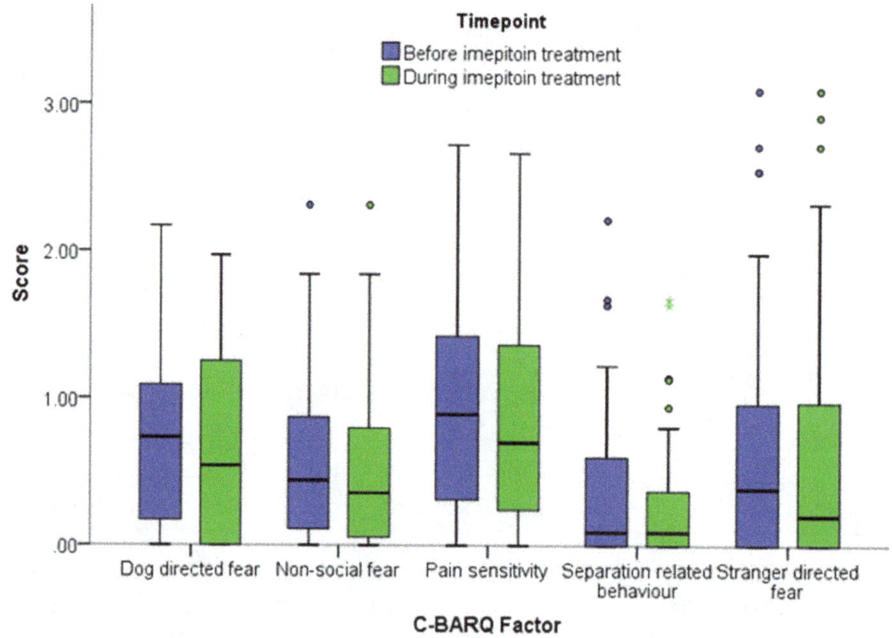

Fig. 2 Box and whisker plot of the five C-BARQ behavioural measures before and after imepitoin treatment in dogs in dogs treated with only imepitoin as a monotherapy (n = 56). The top and bottom lines of the boxes represent the 25th and 75th percentiles, the central line indicates the median, and the whiskers represent the range. Filled circles represent outliers and stars represent extreme outliers

side effect score before and after 2 weeks of treatment, with the median side effect score in the first 2 weeks 13 out of 55 (4–19.5) and after the initial 2 weeks 9 out of 55 (1.5–15.5) (W = 247.5, $p < 0.001$) (Table 3).

The side effect score was greater in polytherapy cases than in monotherapy cases in both the initial 2 weeks (median monotherapy 10 (2–16) vs. median polytherapy 18 (8–24.5); Mann-Whitney U = 1098.5, p = 0.008) and after the initial 2 weeks (median monotherapy 7 (1–13.75) vs. median polytherapy 12 (7–18); Mann-Whitney U = 1044.5, p = 0.030). In the first 2 weeks, differences in side effect frequencies between monotherapy and polytherapy cases were observed for: increased urinating (X^2 = 18.1, p = 0.03) and ataxia (X^2 = 12.7, p = 0.026) which were more common in polytherapy cases. After 2 weeks, differences in side effect frequencies between monotherapy and polytherapy cases were observed for: increased appetite (X^2 = 11.5, p = 0.04), increased urinating (X^2 = 11.4, p = 0.04), increased sleeping (X^2 = 11.6, p = 0.04) and ataxia (X^2 = 14.7, p = 0.01) which were all more common in polytherapy cases.

There was no correlation between treatment efficacy (percentage change (%) in seizure frequency) or the seizure frequency before imepitoin treatment was initiated and the side effect score in either period ($p < 0.05$). There was no relationship between side effect score and any aspect of signalment ($p > 0.05$).

Discussion

This study for the first time investigated the impact of an anti-epileptic drug used to treat seizures on fear and anxiety-related behaviour in dogs with IE. The results indicated that none of the five fear and anxiety-related behavioural measures changed significantly following treatment with imepitoin. It is possible that despite being a partial $GABA_A$ agonist, imepitoin does not have the same anxiolytic effects as other BDZ receptor agonists or partial agonists, or that this effect does not occur in dogs with IE. In line with previous reports, anti-epileptic effects were seen in the majority of dogs, with a median reduction in seizure frequency of 45%. Imepitoin side effects were generally mild and

Table 2 Changes in seizure frequency following imepitoin treatment in both monotherapy and polytherapy cases

Seizure frequency measure	Before imepitoin treatment	During imepitoin treatment	Wilcoxon (W)	N	P
Seizures/month	3.11 ± 4.02	1.93 ± 2.86	1256.0	76	0.002
Seizure days/month	2.31 ± 3.47	1.92 ± 3.30	802.5	74	0.105
Cluster seizure episodes/ month	0.91 ± 1.23	0.65 ± 1.34	461.0	77	0.038

Data are presented as the median accompanied by 25th–75th percentiles

Table 3 Side effect score (out of 5) in the first 2 weeks and after 2 weeks of treatment with imepitoin in dogs treated with imepitoin with or without other anti-epileptic drugs

Side effect	All cases (*n* = 85) (Median (25th–75th percentile)		Just imepitoin monotherapy cases (*n* = 56) (Median (25th–75th percentile)	
	Initial 2 weeks	After 2 weeks	Initial 2 weeks	After 2 weeks
Eating more / would like to eat more	3 (0–4)	2 (0–4)	2 (0–4)	1 (0–4)
Gaining weight	0 (0–3)	0 (0–2)	0 (0–3)	0 (0–2)
Drinking more	2 (0–3)	1 (0–3)	1 (0–3)	1 (0–2.75)
Urinating more	1 (0–3)	0 (0–2.5)	0 (0–3)	0 (0–2)
Sleeping more than before	1 (0–3)	0 (0–2)	1 (0–3)	0 (0–2.75)
Wobbly / not coordinated when walking	0 (0–3)	0 (0–1)	0 (0–1.75)	0 (0–0)
Restlessness / pacing	0 (0–3)	0 (0–2)	0 (0–2)	0 (0–1)
Itchiness or skin rash	0 (0–0)	0 (0–0)	0 (0–0)	0 (0–0)
Vomiting	0 (0–0)	0 (0–0)	0 (0–0)	0 (0–0)
Diarrhoea	0 (0–0)	0 (0–0)	0 (0–0)	0 (0–0)
Coughing	0 (0–0)	0 (0–0)	0 (0–0)	0 (0–0)
OVERALL SCORE (out of 55)	13 (4–19.5)	9 (1.5–15.5)	10 (2–16)	7 (1–13.75)

Side effects were rated by owners on a six point scale from side effect not present (0), very mild (1), mild (2), moderate (3), severe (4), and very severe (5)

short-lived, with a significant reduction in the number and severity of side effects observed after the initial 2 weeks of treatment. Ataxia, a common AED side effect [30] was mild or not present in the majority of cases, in line with recent objective evidence demonstrating reduced levels in IE patients treated with imepitoin compared to phenobarbitone [31]. A greater number of side effects were seen in dogs treated with imepitoin alongside other AEDs, which is in line with recent studies; for example, when imepitoin was used as an add-on therapy to phenobarbital, or vice versa, the number of side effects increased [32]. In addition, a recent study of imepitoin polytherapy found that 69% of dogs treated with imepitoin and KBr, and 79% of dogs treated with imepitoin and phenobarbital experienced side effects [33].

The lack of behavioural effects seen in this study may be due to the IE study population not exhibiting a severe enough initial anxiety level to allow for a significant effect to be seen. Investigating the effects of imepitoin upon the behaviour of dogs with recognised behavioural anxiety-related problems (e.g. specific fears and phobias, separation-related behaviours) +/− behavioural management steps (e.g. desensitisation and counter-conditioning [34]) is required to further explore any potential anxiolytic effects of this medication in general. This may extend beyond dogs, with imepitoin recently tested in clinically healthy cats in a randomised, controlled, blinded study, and found to be well tolerated [35]. In a case study of a 15 year old Persian cat with night-time vocalisation, 8 months of imepitoin treatment was found to control the screaming which may indicate anxiolytic effects [36]. Further placebo-controlled studies on a larger scale are required to confirm this effect in both species.

Studying the anxiolytic effects of imepitoin in healthy dogs and cats without epilepsy may provide further insights into imepitoin's efficacy as a behavioural medicine, due to the potential differences between the healthy and epileptic brain. It is possible that imepitoin may be an effective anxiolytic in the 'normal' brain, but ineffective in the epileptic brain (particularly in drug-resistant patients). The majority of studies of the anxiolytic effects of imepitoin have used either healthy animals or induced models of epilepsy. Imepitoin has shown mixed results in tests of anxiety in experimental animals (rats and mice) [15, 37–45]. In rats, although anxiolytic activity was shown in the elevated plus maze, Vogel conflict test, light-dark chamber tests and social interaction test, these effects were not seen in the Geller conflict test, a model in which prior food-deprived rats have to choose between consuming food and avoiding the punishment associated with this consumption. In mice, anxiolytic activity was shown in the elevated plus maze and light-dark chamber tests, but not in the four-plate test, where mice are punished upon crossing the border between four plates.

It is possible that behavioural changes such as anxiety may be a sign of the natural progression of IE that becomes worse over time. Imepitoin may have reduced the progression of these changes in the current study (hence the lack of change in the measured behavioural traits); however, without a control group of dogs with IE that were not treated with imepitoin or other AEDs over a comparable period, this could not be detected in the

22. Heinecke K. Thiel W. Identity and physicochemical properties of 1-(4-chlorophenyl)-4-morpholinoimidazolin- 2-one, AWD 131–138. Pharmazie. 2001;56:458–61.
23. Overall KM. Manual of clinical behavioral medicine for dogs and cats. St Louis: Elsevier Health Sciences; 2013.
24. Herron ME, Shofer FS, Reisner IR. Retrospective evaluation of the effects of diazepam in dogs with anxiety-related behavior problems. J Am Vet Med Assoc. 2008;233(9):1420–4.
25. De Risio L, Bhatti S, Munana K, Penderis J, Stein V, Tipold A, Berendt M, Farqhuar R, Fischer A, Long S, et al. International veterinary epilepsy task force consensus proposal: diagnostic approach to epilepsy in dogs. BMC Vet Res. 2015;11(1):148.
26. Berendt M, Farquhar R, Mandigers P, Pakozdy A, Bhatti S, De Risio L, Fischer A, Long S, Matiasek K, Munana K, et al. International veterinary epilepsy task force consensus report on epilepsy definition, classification and terminology in companion animals. BMC Vet Res. 2015;11(1):182.
27. Hsu Y, Serpell JA. Development and validation of a questionnaire for measuring behavior and temperament traits in pet dogs. J Am Vet Med Assoc. 2003;223(9):1293–300.
28. Rutherford L, Wessmann A, Rusbridge C, Mcgonnell IM, Abeyesinghe S, Burn CC, Volk HA. Questionnaire-based behaviour analysis of cavalier king Charles spaniels with neuropathic pain due to Chiari-like malformation and syringomyelia. Vet J. 2012;194:294–8.
29. Packer R, Law T, Davies E, Zhangi B, Pan Y, Volk H. Effects of a ketogenic diet on ADHD-like behaviour in dogs with idiopathic epilepsy. Epilepsy & Behavior. 2016;55:62–8.
30. Charalambous M, Shivapour SK, Brodbelt D, Volk HA. Antiepileptic drugs' tolerability and safety – a systematic review and meta-analysis of adverse effects in dogs. BMC Vet Res. 2016;12:79.
31. Suiter EJ, RMA P, Volk HA. Comparing the effects of first-line antiepileptic drugs on the gait of dogs with idiopathic epilepsy. Vet Rec. 2016;178:652.
32. Neßler J, Rundfeldt C, Löscher W, Kostic D, Keefe T, Tipold A. Clinical evaluation of a combination therapy of imepitoin with phenobarbital in dogs with refractory idiopathic epilepsy. BMC Vet Res. 2017;13(1):33.
33. Royaux E, Van Ham L, Broeckx BJG, Van Soens I, Gielen I, Deforce D, Bhatti SFM. Phenobarbital or potassium bromide as an add-on antiepileptic drug for the management of canine idiopathic epilepsy refractory to imepitoin. Vet J. 2017; 220:51–4.
34. Landsberg G, Hunthausen W, Ackerman L. Behavior problems of the dog and cat. 3rd ed. Philadelphia: Elsevier Health Sciences; 2012.
35. Engel O, Mueller J, FD V. Imepitoin is well tolerated by healthy cats. In: 28th ESVN-ECVN Congress: 2015; Amsterdam; 2015.
36. Dubé MB: The use of the drug Pexion® (Imepitoin) in a cat with night-time vocalisation. In: AWSELVA-ECAWBM-ESVCE Congress: 2015; Bristol, UK; 2015.
37. Rundfeldt C, Löscher W. The Pharmacology of Imepitoin: The First Partial Benzodiazepine Receptor Agonist Developed for the Treatment of Epilepsy. CNS Drugs. 2013;28:29–43.
38. Rostock A, Tober C, Dost R, Bartsch R. AWD 131-138 is a potential novel anxiolytic without sedation and amnesia: a comparison with diazepam and buspirone. Naunyn Schmiedeberg's Arch Pharmacol. 1998;358(1):35.
39. Grunwald C, Rundfeldt C, Lankau H-J, Arnold T, Höfgen N, Dost R, Egerland U, Hofmann H-J, Unverferth K. Synthesis, pharmacology, and structure–activity relationships of novel Imidazolones and Pyrrolones as modulators of GABAA receptors. J Med Chem. 2006;49(6):1855–66.
40. Dost R, Langen B, Rundfeldt C: The a-3 subunit selective benzodiazepine agonist ELB139 does not induce tolerance in animal models for anxiety and epilepsy. Soc Neurosci Abstr 2005, 678(1).
41. Langen B, Rundfeldt C, Dost R, Lüddens H, Rabe H: Method of treating or preventing central nervous system disorders with compounds having selectivity for the alpha 3 subunit of the benzodiazepine receptor. 2005.
42. Tober C, Rostock A, Bartsch R. Anticonvulsant profile of AWD 131-138 a derivative of a series of imidazolinones. Naunyn Schmiedebergs Archiv Pharmacology. 1998;357(4):98.
43. Tober C, Rostock A, White HS, Wolf HH, Bartsch R. Anticonvulsant activity of AWD 131-138 in genetic animal models of epilepsy. Naunyn Schmiedebergs Archiv Pharmacology. 1999;359(3):97.
44. Tober C, Rostock A, Bartsch R. AWD 131-138: a derivative of a series of imidazolinones with anticonvulsant activity. Naunyn Schmiedeberg's Arch Pharmacol. 1998;358(1):35.
45. Langen B, Rundfeldt C, Dost R, Lüddens H, Rabe H. Patent application: method of treating or preventing central nervous system disorders with compounds having selectivity for the alpha 3 subunit of the benzodiazepine receptor (WO 2005/004867 A2). 2005. Available at: https://www.google.ch/patents/US20080114032.
46. Tami G, Gallagher A. Description of the behaviour of domestic dog (*Canis familiaris*) by experienced and inexperienced people. Appl Anim Behav Sci. 2009;120(3–4):159–69.
47. Bahlig-Pieren Z, Turner DC. Anthropomorphic interpretations and ethological descriptions of dog and cat behavior by lay people. Anthrozoös. 1999; 12(4):205–10.
48. Gallucci A, Gagliardo T, Menchetti M, Ruffini A, Bianchi E, Milici A, Tosolini P, Cauduro A, Gandini G. Efficacy of imepitoin as first choice drug in the treatment of 53 naïve dogs affected by idiopathic epilepsy. In: 28th ESVN-ECVN Congress: 2015; Amsterdam; 2015.
49. Packer RMA, Shihab NK, Torres BBJ, Volk HA. Clinical risk factors associated with anti-epileptic drug responsiveness in canine epilepsy. PLoS One. 2014;9(8):e106026.
50. Packer RMA, Shihab NK, BBJ T, Volk HA. Responses to successive anti-epileptic drugs in canine idiopathic epilepsy. Vet Rec. 2015;176:203.
51. Wessmann A, Volk HA, Packer RMA, Ortega M, Anderson TJ. Quality-of-life aspects in idiopathic epilepsy in dogs. Vet Rec. 2016;179:229.
52. Kato M, Miyajo K, Ohtani N, Ohta M. Effects of prescription diet on dealing with stressful situations and performance of anxiety-related behaviours in privately owned anxious dogs. J Vet Behav Clin Appl Res. 2012;7:21–6.
53. Cannas S, Scagli E, Maltese F, Michelazzi M. Evaluation of a diet supplement on anxiety signs on dog. J Vet Behav Clin Appl Res. 2013;8(4):e29.
54. Packer RMA, Law TH, Davies E, Zanghi B, Pan Y, Volk HA. Effects of a ketogenic diet on ADHD-like behavior in dogs with idiopathic epilepsy. Epilepsy Behav. 2016;55:62–8.

17

A new age in AquaMedicine: unconventional approach in studying aquatic diseases

Michael Gotesman[1], Simon Menanteau-Ledouble[2], Mona Saleh[2], Sven M. Bergmann[3] and Mansour El-Matbouli[2*]

Abstract

Background: Marine and aquaculture industries are important sectors of the food production and global trade. Unfortunately, the fish food industry is challenged with a plethora of infectious pathogens. The freshwater and marine fish communities are rapidly incorporating novel and most up to date techniques for detection, characterization and treatment strategies. Rapid detection of infectious diseases is important in preventing large disease outbreaks.

Main text: One hundred forty-six articles including reviews papers were analyzed and their conclusions evaluated in the present paper. This allowed us to describe the most recent development research regarding the control of diseases in the aquatic environment as well as promising avenues that may result in beneficial developments. For the characterization of diseases, traditional sequencing and histological based methods have been augmented with transcriptional and proteomic studies. Recent studies have demonstrated that transcriptional based approaches using qPCR are often synergistic to expression based studies that rely on proteomic-based techniques to better understand pathogen-host interactions. Preventative therapies that rely on prophylactics such as vaccination with protein antigens or attenuated viruses are not always feasible and therefore, the development of therapies based on small nucleotide based medicine is on the horizon. Of those, RNAi or CRISPR/Cas- based therapies show great promise in combating various types of diseases caused by viral and parasitic agents that effect aquatic and fish medicine.

Conclusions: In our modern times, when the marine industry has become so vital for feed and economic stability, even the most extreme alternative treatment strategies such as the use of small molecules or even the use of disease to control invasive species populations should be considered.

Keywords: Aquaculture, Virus, Bacteria, Nanotechnology, RNAi, CRISPR/Cas

Background

Fish and aquatic industry

The global annual per capita fish consumption of fish was 20.1 kg for the year 2013; with an average consumption of 26.8 kg in industrialized countries and 18.1 kg in developing countries, respectively [1]. Fish protein accounted for up to 20% or more of the total animal protein consumed in low-income food-deficient countries and around 17% globally in the year 2013 [1]. In addition to producing a critical part of nutrition, food production through the marine industry also represents a major form of employment which harvested nearly 160 billion US dollars in 2014 and employed 56.6 million people [1]. Of the total 167.2 million tonnes of food products that the marine industry produced in 2014, the aquaculture accounted for 44.1% (73.8 million tonnes) production [1]. Carp (*Cyprinidae*) makes up a significant portion of the total freshwater cultured fish supply and is an especially important food in China and the remainder of East Asia, which produced 61.3 and 26.7% of cultured carp, respectively in 2010 [1, 2]. Salmon and shrimp are considered high-value species that are heavily traded and are also significant members of the aquaculture industry [1].

* Correspondence: Mansour.El-Matbouli@vetmeduni.ac.at
[2]Clinical Division of Fish Medicine, Department for Farm Animals and Veterinary Public Health, University of Veterinary Medicine, Veterinärplatz 1, 1210 Vienna, Austria
Full list of author information is available at the end of the article

Viral diseases of fish and crustaceans in the aquatic industry

Diseases of aquatic products, such as viral infection of aquatic animals, have become more problematic and are causing significant economical losses to the aquaculture industry [3–7]. The most serious viruses affecting cyprinid fish including koi and common carp (*Cyprinus carpio L.*) are: 1) Cyprinid herpesvirus 3 (CyHV-3), a member of the *Alloherpesviridae* family of viruses, which is the aetiological agent of a highly contagious disease termed Koi herpesvirus disease (KHVD) and 2) spring viraemia of carp virus (SVCV), which is a member of the *Rhabdoviridae* family of viruses. In addition, outbreaks of KHVD and SVC in cultured common carp caused significant economic losses in recent years. KHVD has been a major research topic in aquatic medicine and has been listed as a notifiable disease in Germany since 2005, in England and by the World Organization of Animal Health (OIE) since 2007 [8–13]. Similarly, the SVC is a major topic of aquatic research and is listed as a notifiable disease in the USA, and has been listed by the OIE since 1997 [14, 15]. Hemorrhagic septicemia virus (VHSV) is another pathogenic member of *Rhabdoviridae* known to infect northern pike, *Esox lucius* fry [16]. Members of the *Rhabdoviridae* family of viruses that code for the non-virion protein (NV) are subtyped into their own genus termed *Novirhabdovirus;* such as infectious hematopoietic necrosis virus (IHNV), which causes an OIE notifiable disease and is an economically important in a wide variety of salmonid species [17]. Infectious salmon anemia virus (ISAV) the causative agent of the ISA and White Spot Syndrome Virus (WSSV) the causative agent of White Spot Disease are of major economic importance in the respective salmon and crustacean aquaculture sector [18, 19]. *Iridoviridae* comprises a family of double stranded DNA virus that infect a wide variety of invertebrate and marine organisms, such as the genus *Megalocytivirus,* represented by red sea bream iridovirus (RSIV) [20, 21]. *Ranavirus,* another representative genus in the *Iridovirdae* family, is a global emergent pathogen capable of infecting fish, amphibians, and reptiles in both captive and wild animals causing hemorrhagic disease [22]. *Betanodaviruses,* which are non-enveloped single stranded RNA viruses, comprise an additional important family of viruses impacting the aquaculture industry [23, 24].

Bacterial pathogens

Among the most note-worthy bacterial aquatic pathogens is the warmwater bacterium *Aeromonas hydrophila* as well as its cold water relative *Aeromonas salmonicida,* which infect a variety of fish species in both the freshwater and marine environment. Among these susceptible fish species, tilapia, cyprinid [25, 26] and salmonid (salmon and trout) fish [26] are of particular economic importance. A bacterium that has mostly been studied in infecting salmonid is the enterobacterium *Yersinia ruckeri,* causative agent of then enteric redmouth disease, salmonid which has been associated with haemorrhages and petechial lesions in infected fish (Fig. 1; from personal archives) [27–29]. Moreover, the enterobacterium *Edwardsiella ictaluri* is considered one of the most important bacterial pathogen affecting the culture of catfish, in particular the channel catfish *Ictalurus punctatus* in the Southern United States [26] and, as it has been more recently reported, the striped catfish *Pangasianodon hypophthalmus* in Vietnam [30, 31]. In shrimp, bacterial infections are mostly linked to bacteria of the *Vibrio* family, in particularly to *Vibrio parahaemolyticus* which has recently been linked to an emergent disease termed acute hepatopancreatic necrosis disease [32].

Parasites

Parasitic diseases are often associated with more chronic diseases that can cause a sustained loss of productivity over the whole production cycle, and therefore the economical impact of these diseases can often be very significant. Among the most prominent parasitical diseases are the ones caused by myxozoans parasites such as *Myxobolus cerebralis* and *Tetracapsuloides bryosalmonae,* the causative agents of whirling disease and proliferative kidney diseases in salmonids, respectively [33, 34]. Ciliates are common inhabitant of both the freshwater and marine environment. Among these species, *Ichthyophthirius multifiliis* (often shortened to "Ich") is associated with high levels of mortality (up to 100%) in freshwater fish [35]. This external parasite has a life cycle comprised of three stages, including a trophonts stage during whith it feeds on the fish skin where it forms white circular lesions that leads to the disease colloquial name of "white spot disease" [35–37]. While *I. multifiliis* is limited to freshwater, another ciliated, *Cryptocaryon irritans* is found is saltwater that causes a very similar condition, sometime also referred to as "white spot disease" or "marine ich" [38].

In molluscs, two parasites are particularly noteworthy: *Marteilia refringens* and *Bonamia ostreae* which affects the European flat oyster *Ostrea edulis.* The impact of these parasites has led to the introduction of more resistant species of oyster termed *Crassostrea gigas* to replace *Ostrea edulis* as the most commonly cultivated oyster species. This manuscript will review some of the newest approaches used to study aquatic diseases, in terms of detection characterization and possible treatment strategies.

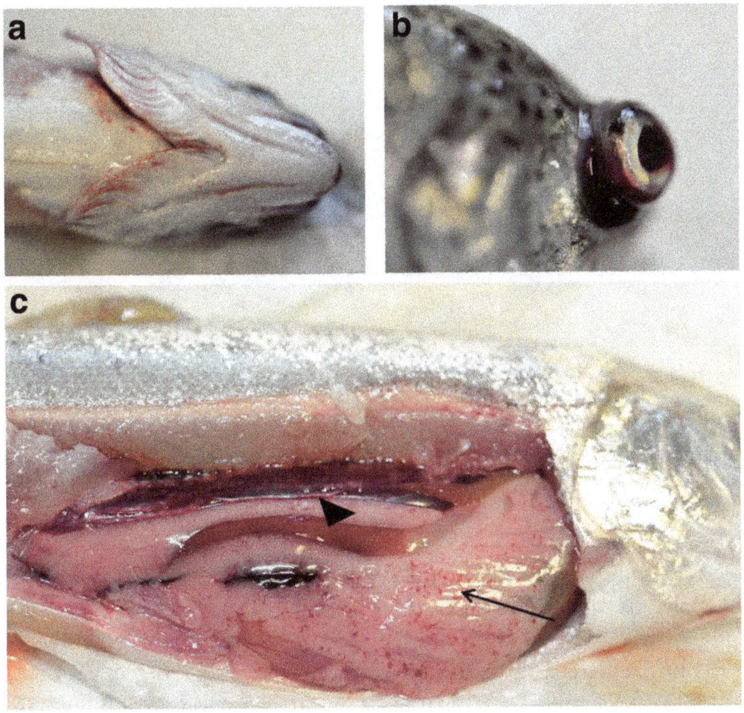

Fig. 1 Clinical signs in a rainbow trout (*Oncorhynchus mykiss*) infected with *Yersinia ruckeri* (from personal archives, previously unpublished). **a** Petechia and haemorrhages in the oral region; **b** Exophtalmia; **c** Large arrows- blood in the intestinal track and Small arrow- petechia in the visceral tissue

Bio diagnostics/characterization

Rapid detection/nanotechnology

Histological observation followed by polymerase chain reaction (PCR) [39], or cohabitation studies as performed by El-Matbouli & Soliman [40] to demonstrate transmission of CyHV-3 virus from goldfish (*Carassius auratus auratus*) to naïve carp have been the classical method of detection and demonstration of transmission of pathogen(s) to new hosts. PCR-based methods coupled to electron microscopy have also been used in categorizing aquatic pathogens, such as in the classification of the parasitic ciliate infecting shrimp [41]. However, updated methods for rapid detection is required to tackle the rapid spread of communicable pathogens in aquatic farming, especially in densely populated environment used in aquaculture. For example, preliminary differentiation of CyHV-3 from channel catfish virus was performed by restriction analysis of purified DNA extracts and led to a PCR-based method detection [42, 43]. Subsequently, a 1 step process was developed using loop-mediated isothermal amplification (LAMP) without requiring a thermal cycler for detection of CyHV-3 [44–46]. Alternatively, nested PCR or the capture of viral particles by antibodies followed by LAMP can also be used for highly sensitive detection of CyHV-3 [47–49]. PCR based methods of detection can be coupled with DNA-array technology for rapid detection of secondary infections in diseased fish [50]. For rapid and visual based detection for CyHV-3, the product of LAMP-PCR is visualized by mixing with SYBR-Green I to confirm infection [51]. Attachment of single stranded DNA molecules to gold nanoparticles allows for rapid (15 min) and sensitive detection (10^{-3} $TCID_{50}$ ml^{-1}) of SVCV RNA based on visualization (Fig. 2; reproduced from Saleh et al. [52] with permission from Springer Nature) of colloidal solution [53] and the procedure can be readily adapted for detection of aquatic viruses [54, 55]. In addition to the various molecular based methods, immunohistochemistry in terms of histological assays [56] or enzyme-linked immunosorbent assay (ELISA) are also used to detect viral infections [57–63]. Detection of viral particles in affected species and carriers is important to combat the spread of outbreaks [64]. Recently, a method described as liquid chip which combines flow cytometry, nanometer fluorescent microspheres with traditional chemical luminescence technology has been described for rapid detection of several *Rhabdoviridae* members including SVCV, IHNV and VHSV [65].

Characterization

Traditionally, pathogens of aquatic organisms have been characterized by sequence analysis [66–69], and by microscopic examination of the pathogen and/or host by differing methods that include histological staining [70] and electron microscopy [71]. Recently, deep sequencing along with microarray hybridization has been used to

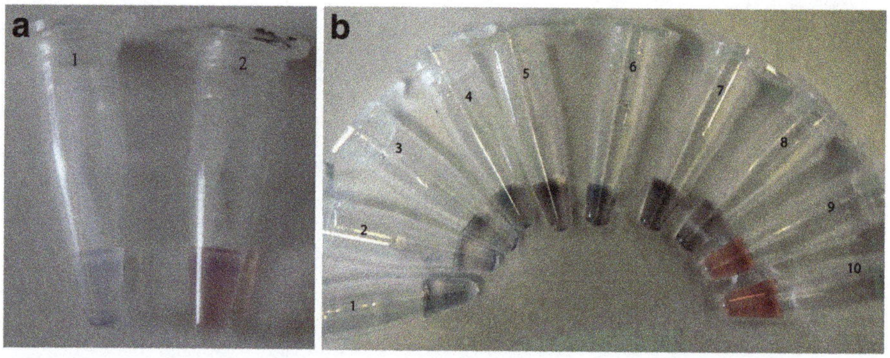

Fig. 2 Application of nanoparticles for the diagnostic of spring viraemia of carp virus. **a** Unmodified gold nanoparticles (AuNPs) for the colorimetric detection of spring viraemia of carp virus (SVCV)-RNA (from Saleh et al. [52], figure subject to copyright and *reproduced with permission* from Springer Nature). Tube 1: Positive SVCV-RNA sample (blue color). Tube 2: No template control (red color). Each tube contained 5 μl of sample, 1.8 μM of primer and 0.1 M NaCl. **b** Serial dilution of SVC-RNA (Tubes 1 to 10 contain 10^5, 10^4, 10^3, 10^2, 10, 10^{-1}, 10^{-2}, 10^{-3} 10^{-4} and 10^{-5} $TCID_{50}$ ml^{-1} SVC-RNA respectively) showing the sensitivity limit of the assay. The SVC-AuNPs assay could detect SVCV-RNA as far as the 10^{-3} $TCID_{50}$ ml^{-1} dilution (Tube 8; blue color)

identify pathogen microRNAs (miR) involved in gene regulation [72]. Similarly, real-time quantitative reverse transcription PCR (RT-qPCR) has been used to show differential expression of the host miR-10a-3p, a component of the master transcriptional regulator for spatial patterning genes termed homeobox (Hox) genes, during infections by VHSV rock bream iridovirus (RBIV) of olive flounder and rock bream [73]. Real-time quantitative PCR (qPCR) or deep RNA sequencing can be used in transcriptome analysis to characterize host-pathogen interactions [74]. Histological assays can be coupled with immunofluorescence techniques to further elaborate the ultrastructure make up of disease causing pathogens [75]. For example, indirect fluorescence immunohistochemistry was adapted to *E. ictaluri* using the monoclonal antibody Ed9 [76] as the primary antibody and a fluorescein isothiocyanate (FITC) labeled goat anti-mouse secondary antibodies [77]. This allowed identification of the bacteria with the tissue and contributed in demonstrating the role of abrasion sites as a route of infection for *E. ictaluri* in *I. punctatus* [78]. Reverse genetic experimentation in which the reading frame of various viral proteins are altered, such as the non-virion (NV) non-structural protein, G and M proteins, or recombinant viruses are produced has been used to investigate virulent factors in VHSV [79–83].

Several approaches have been applied to investigate the virulence mechanisms of bacterial pathogens. For example, in vivo induced antigen technology (IVIAT) relies on harvesting antibodies from host exposed to the pathogen of interest. The antibodies are then adsorbed against an in vitro culture of the pathogen, therefore removing the antibodies that react against antigens expressed in vitro. The only remaining antibodies, recognizing antigens specifically expressed in vivo, are then used to screen an expression library expressing random sequences from the pathogen genomes [84, 85]. Regarding aquatic species, IVIAT has been used to investigate *Edwardsiella tarda* [86], *Vibrio anguillarum* [87] as well as *A. salmonicida* subsp. *salmonicida* [88, 89] and, more recently, *Photobacterium damselae* subsp. *piscicida* [90].

Gene expression profiling has been applied to *I. multifiliis* to identify genes that are differentially regulated during the different life stages of the parasite [91, 92]. This approach has led to the discovery that gene expression in *I. multifillis* is extremely stage specific [91] and has led to a better understanding of the expression of the virulence genes in this parasite. Moreover, it has been reported that senescence of the parasite was correlated to a lower expression for the genes of its *Rickettsia* endosymbiont [92]. Similarly, Mai et al. performed an immunoproteomic analysis of *C. irritans* [93] using 2D gels and anti-*C. irritans* antibodies isolated from both rabbit and grouper (*Epinephelus coioides*). This approach allowed to identify several proteins that were differentially regulated between life stages of the parasite, including several antigenic ones with potential in vaccine development. Among the isolation were proteins of the cytoskeletal apparatus (β-tubulin and actin), as well as the enzyme enolase and the heat shock protein hsp70 [93]. Moreover, Yin et al. [94] conducted an analysis of the transcriptomes of trophont, either untreated or treated at either 12 or 25 °C. The authors described up-regulation of several genes required for the cell's survival at lower temperature and entry into dormancy [94].

Proteomics

Exogenous expression in bacteria of proteins found in aquatic pathogens followed by PAGE-Gel analysis and Western blotting with native proteins can be used to detect in vivo posttranslational modifications by differences in observed mass [95, 96]. Monoclonal antibodies against CyHV-3 have been used to measure the expression kinetics of various proteins involved in protein assembly [97]. Analyses of whole proteomes have also been carried out; for example, in *Y. ruckeri* [98], where the proteomes of four different isolates were compared under iron-replete and iron-depleted conditions. This revealed the spread of the bacterium's response to iron depletion as 61 proteins were found to be differentially expressed (35 up and 26 down-regulated). Among these were several siderophores (iron acquisition molecules that play a crucial role in the microbial infection process when iron is often the bacteria's limiting factor) that were up-regulated and catalase that were down-regulated. Interestingly, the bacteria appeared to shift from iron-based superoxide dismutase (SodB, 28.6 fold downregulated) to manganese-based using a manganese based superoxide dismutase (SodA) that was 5.6-fold upregulated.

Differential transcriptional patterns obtained from qPCR based methods [99, 100] can be coupled to protein-based studies [101] to enhance our understanding of pathogen-host interactions. For protein purification, antibodies raised against the pathogen(s) of interest can be used to capture proteins involved in host-pathogen interactions which are subsequently identified by mass spectrometry [102]. Such studies have been used to differentiate between host pathogen interactions of susceptible carp versus carrier goldfish for CyHV-3 entry and replication [103, 104]. Additionally, proteomic based approach revealed that although all 156 open reading frames (ORFs) are CyHV-3 are transcribed during viral maturation [105], only 46 proteins are incorporated into mature virions [106, 107].Whereas, exogenous expression of viral proteins can demonstrate lethal properties for those proteins [108]. Therefore, proteomic should be used to enhance and elucidate transcriptional based data.

Treatment

RNA interference (RNAi)

RNA mediated interference (RNAi) machinery is presumed to have developed as a defensive mechanism in eukaryotic organisms against viruses and transposable elements [109]. RNA-mediated interference (RNAi) by the use of short double-stranded RNA (dsRNA) was originally demonstrated in *Caenorhabditis elegans* by Fire et al. [110], and the mechanism and machinery for the function of small non-coding RNA in RNAi has since been worked out in great detail for a variety of organisms [111, 112]. During the post-transcriptional gene silencing (PTGS) of exogenous transcripts by RNAi, the RNA-induced silencing complex (RISC) converts long dsRNA transcripts into siRNA oligos (21-25 nt), which guide the complex by antisense complementation to degrade targeted genes [113]. RNAi technology has been important in understanding gene function in aquatic diseases [114] and can be used to study RNA-based viruses which are traditionally investigated by reverse genetics [115]. RNAi-based approaches are also suitable for the development of novel therapies against viral diseases of livestock and aquatic organisms and represent a promising method in developing novel therapeutics and antiviral medications [116]. A limited number of studies have reported about the treatment of viral diseases by RNAi, although RNAi based therapies for viral diseases have been in the pipeline to treat invertebrate, vertebrate and even human pathogens [117].

Studies that used RNAi technology in aquatic medicine

Viral

In a recent study, feeding shrimp with bacteria coding for dsRNA that targeted endogenous shrimp non-essential Rab7 and STAT genes caused systemic induction of the RNAi pathway against the targeted genes [118]. The technique has been applied to provide protection from an important disease in shrimp farms, termed White spot syndrome virus (WSSV), by feeding shrimp with bacteria expressing dsRNA against several important viral genes [119]. Inhibition by RNAi of WSSV was first demonstrated in a non-Shrimp cell line, termed SISK, and by intramuscular injection of live shrimp [120, 121], and the results were verified when shrimp were fed with dsRNA-transcribing bacteria [122]. Permanent *epithelioma papulosum cyprini* (EPC) and *chinook salmon embryonic* (CHSE-214) fish cell lines that express long dsRNA which target the G protein of viral hemorrhagic septicemia virus (VHSV) inhibited in vitro replication of VHSV without stimulating the interferon pathway [123]. Treatment with formaldehyde-attenuated bacterial cells that produce dsRNA targeting the hemagglutinin gene of ISAV inhibited in vitro viral replication [124]. RNAi targeting the nucleoprotein 'N' or phosphoprotein "P" has been shown to inhibit in vitro replication of SVCV [125]. Similarly, RNAi experiments targeting thymidine kinase 'TK' or DNA polymerase 'DP' of CyHV-3 inhibited in vitro replication [126]. CyHV-3 is most effectively inhibited by RNAi when multiple viral genes are targeted [126, 127].

Bacterial/parasitic

RNAi treatment has shown promising results in the treatment of parasitic infections in fish. Saleh et al. [128] demonstrated that in vitro RNAi knockdown of ATP/ADP antiporter and methionine aminopeptidase II of the *Heterosporis saurida*, parasite of the lizardfish (*Saurida undosquamis)*, reduced targeted gene transcription and spore counts in cell culture assays. Potential for RNAi-based medicine has been demonstrated in vivo by treating the oligochaete host *Tubifex tubifex* for the cnidarian myxozoan parasite (*Myxobolus cerebralis*) which causes whirling diseases in salmonid fish [129]. In subsequent trials, Sarker et al. [130] showed that *T. tubifex* soaked in solution containing dsRNA targeting the serine protease of the *M. cerebralis* inoculated the cnidarian myxozoan parasite from infecting the rainbow trout (*Oncorhynchus mykiss) host.*

Is CRISPR/Cas based medicine on the horizon?

Cre (causes recombination) and other tyrosine recombinases have traditionally been used for genomic editing. These tyrosine site-specific recombinases are typically used to reintegrate exogenous DNA flanked by palindromic into a host genome such as observed in the Cre/Lox system in which Cre is used with the accompanying Lox palindromic DNA sequence [131]. A newer genome editing tool termed CRISPR/Cas (clustered regularly interspaced short palindromic repeats/CRISPR-associated), takes advantage of the prokaryotic and archaea immune system to reintegrate foreign DNA using a Cas protein and a guide RNA (gRNA) [132]. In addition to gene editing, the nuclease activity of the CRISPR/Cas pathway can be induced to degrade foreign RNA/DNA [133]. The CRISPR/Cas gene suppression technique was recently used by Zhao et al. [134] to confirm that RNAi knockdown of CyHV-3 TK and DP genes reduced viral replication and virus titer as reported previously by our group [126].

Conclusion

Prophylactic treatments, for example aiming at strengthening or preparing the immune response such as vaccination, are always preferable to therapeutic ones [135–138]. However, preventative therapies are not always possible or practical, therapies based on small nucleotide based medicine such as siRNA or CRISPR/Cas are on the horizon. RNAi-based technology has already been suggested to be useful in aquatic and fish medicine to combat various types of diseases caused by viral and parasitic agents [116, 139]. Effectiveness of using RNAi or other nucleic based therapies rely on targeting pathogens transcripts that interfere with the hosts defensive capabilities used in viral entry or replication [140, 141]. RNAi and CRISPR/Cas mediated interference [133] along with the use small molecules to promote endogenous host response to viral infections [142, 143] are powerful emerging therapy strategies to deal with diseases in aquatic medicine. For those interesting cases where some aqua-species have become invasive, using a disease may be the methodology used to control the threat. For example, the release of CyHV-3 is seriously being considered to eradicate the invasive carp in Australia to restore populations of native fish species [144, 145] following the incidental example happening in the USA [146].

Abbreviations

CHSE-214: *Chinook salmon embryonic*; Cre: Causes recombination; CRISPR/Cas: Clustered Regularly Interspaced Short Palindromic Repeats/CRISPR associated protein 9; CyHV-3: Cyprinid herpesvirus 3; EPC: *Epithelioma papulosum cyprini*; FITC: Fluorescein isothiocyanate; gRNA: Guide RNA; Hox: Homeobox; IHNV: Infectious hematopoietic necrosis virus; ISAV: Infectious salmon anaemia virus; IVIAT: In vivo induced antigen technology; KHVD: Koi herpesvirus disease; LAMP-PCR: Loop mediated isothermal amplification PCR; NV: Non-virion protein; PAGE-Gel: Polyacrylamide gel electrophoresis gel; PCR: Polymerase chain reaction; qPCR: Real-time quantitative (RT) PCR; RBIV: Rock bream iridovirus; RNAi: RNA interference; RSIV: Red sea bream iridovirus (RSIV); siRNA: Small inhibitory Ribonucleic acid; SVCV: Spring viremia of carp virus; VHSV: Hemorrhagic septicemia virus; WSSV: White Spot Syndrome Virus

Funding

This research was supported by the Austrian Science Funds (Fonds zur Förderung der wissenschaftlichen Forschung), project P28837-B22. The funding body did not contribute to the study's design or analysis of the data.

Authors' contributions

MG, MS and SML conceived and drafted the manuscript. SMB and MEM supervised the writing and corrected the manuscript. All authors read and approved the final manuscript.

Competing interests

The authors declare that they have no competing interests.

Author details

[1]Department of Biology, New York City College of Technology of the City University of New York, Brooklyn, New York, USA. [2]Clinical Division of Fish Medicine, Department for Farm Animals and Veterinary Public Health, University of Veterinary Medicine, Veterinärplatz 1, 1210 Vienna, Austria. [3]Institute of Infectology, Friedrich-Loffler-Institut (FLI), Federal Research Institute for Animal Health, Greifswald-Insel Riems, Germany.

References

1. FAO. The state of world fisheries and aquaculture. Rome: FAO; 2016.
2. FAO. State of the world fisheries and aquaculture- 2012. Rome: FAO Fisheries and Aquaculture Department; 2012.
3. Xie J, Lü L, Deng M, Weng S, Zhu J, Wu Y, et al. Inhibition of reporter gene and Iridovirus-tiger frog virus in fish cell by RNA interference. Virology. 2005; 338:43–52.
4. Zhang QY, Gui JF. Virus genomes and virus-host interactions in aquaculture animals. Sci China Life Sci. 2015;58:156–69.
5. Fujioka H, Yamasaki K, Furusawa K, Tamura K, Oguro K, Kurihara S, et al. Prevalence and characteristics of Cyprinid herpesvirus 3 (CyHV-3) infection in common carp (*Cyprinus carpio* L.) inhabiting three rivers in Kochi Prefecture, Japan. Vet Microbiol. 2015;175:362–8.
6. Rahmati-Holasoo H, Zargar A, Ahmadivand S, Shokrpoor S, Ezhari S, Ebrahimzadeh Mousavi HA. First detection of koi herpesvirus from koi, *Cyprinus carpio* L. experiencing mass mortalities in Iran: clinical, histopathological and molecular study. J Fish Dis. 2016;39:1153–63.
7. Mayrhofer R, Pucher J, Saleh M, Menanteau-Ledouble S, Bergmann S, Focken U, et al. First detection of cyprinid herpesvirus 3 in cultured common carp in Vietnam. Fish Pathol. 2016;51:28.
8. OIE. Manual of diagnostic tests for aquatic animals. 5th ed. Paris: OIE; 2009.

9. Rakus K, Ouyang P, Boutier M, Ronsmans M, Reschner A, Vancsok C, et al. Cyprinid herpesvirus 3: an interesting virus for applied and fundamental research. Vet Res. 2013;44:85.
10. Gotesman M, Kattlun J, Bergmann SM, El-Matbouli M. CyHV-3: the third cyprinid herpesvirus. Dis Aquat Org. 2013;105:163–74.
11. Kattlun J, Gotesman M, Bergmann SM, El-Matbouli M. Die Erkrankung der Karpfen (*Cyprinus carpio*) mit dem Cypriniden Herpesvirus 3 (CyHV-3) – ein Update. Wiener Tierarztl Monatsschrift2. 2013;100:72–84.
12. Boutier M, Gao Y, Vancsok C, Suárez NM, Davison AJ, Vanderplasschen A. Identification of an essential virulence gene of cyprinid herpesvirus 3. Antivir Res. 2017;145:60–9.
13. Antychowicz J. Najnowsze badania nad etiologią, patogenezą, diagnostyką i zwalczaniem zakażenia karpi wirusem herpes karpia koi. Życie Weter. 2014;89:923–7.
14. Ashraf U, Lu Y, Lin L, Yuan J, Wang M, Liu X. Spring viraemia of carp virus: recent advances. J Gen Virol. 2016;97:1037–51.
15. Dixon P, Stone D. Spring viraemia of carp. Fish Viruses Bact. Pathobiol. Prot; 2017. p. 79–90.
16. Getchell RG, Cornwell ER, Bogdanowicz S, Andrés J, Batts WN, Kurath G, Breyta R, Choi JG, Farrell JM, Bowser PR. Complete sequences of 4 viral hemorrhagic septicemia virus IVb isolates and their virulence in northern pike fry. Dis Aquat Org. 2017;126:211–27.
17. Dixon P, Paley R, Alegria-Moran R, Oidtmann B. Epidemiological characteristics of infectious hematopoietic necrosis virus (IHNV): a review. Vet Res. 2016;47:63–89.
18. Cottet L, Rivas-Aravena A, Cortez-San Martin M, Sandino AM, Spencer E. Infectious salmon anemia virus—genetics and pathogenesis. Virus Res. 2011;155:10–9.
19. Verbruggen B, Bickley L, van Aerle R, Bateman K, Stentiford G, Santos E, et al. Molecular mechanisms of white spot syndrome virus infection and perspectives on treatments. Viruses. 2016;8:23.
20. Chinchar VG, Waltzek TB, Subramaniam K. Ranaviruses and other members of the family Iridoviridae: their place in the virosphere. Virology. 2017;511: 259–71.
21. Kurita J, Nakajima K. Megalocytiviruses. Viruses. 2012;4:521–38.
22. Duffus AL, Waltzek TB, Stöhr AC, Allender MC, Gotesman M, Whittington RJ, Hick P, Hines MK, Marschang RE. Distribution and host range of ranaviruses. In: Gray MJ, Chinchar VG, editors. Ranaviruses: lethal pathogens of ectothermic vertebrates 1. New York: Springer; 2015. p. 9–57.
23. Bonami JR, Widada JS. Viral diseases of the giant fresh water prawn Macrobrachium rosenbergii: a review. J Invertebr Pathol. 2011;106:131–42.
24. Shetty M, Maiti B, Santhosh KS, Venugopal MN, Karunasagar I. Betanodavirus of marine and freshwater fish: distribution, genomic organization, diagnosis and control measures. Indian J Virol. 2012;23:114–23.
25. Cipriano RC, Austin B. Furunculosis and other aeromonad diseases. In: Woo PT, Bruno DW, editors. Fish Dis. Disord. Vol. 3 viral, Bact. Fungal Infect. 2nd ed. Wallingford: CABI; 2011. p. 424–83. Available from: http://www.cabi.org/cabebooks/ebook/20113056419.
26. Roberts RJ. The bacteriology of teleosts. In: Roberts RJ, editor. Fish Pathol. 4th ed. London: Wiley-Blackwell; 2012. p. 339–82.
27. Barnes AC. Enteric redmouth disease (ERM) (*Yersinia ruckeri*). Fish Dis. Disord. Vol. 3 viral, Bact. fungal Infect. Wallingford: CABI; 2011. p. 484–511.
28. Austin B, Austin DA. Bacterial fish pathogens. Cham: Springer International Publishing; 2016.
29. Kumar G, Menanteau-Ledouble S, Saleh M, El-Matbouli M. *Yersinia ruckeri*, the causative agent of enteric redmouth disease in fish. Vet Res. 2015;46:103.
30. Fergusson HW, Turnbull JF, Shinn A, Thompson KD, Dung TT, Crumlish M. Bacillary necrosis in farmed *Pangasius hypophtalmus* (Sauvage) from the Mekong Delta, Vietnam. J Fish Dis. 2001;24:509–13.
31. Crumlish M, Thanh PC, Koesling J, Tung VT, Gravningen K. Experimental challenge studies in Vietnamese catfish, *Pangasianodon hypophthalmus* (Sauvage), exposed to *Edwardsiella ictaluri* and *Aeromonas hydrophila*. J Fish Dis. 2010;33:717–22. Available from: http://doi.wiley.com/10.1111/j.1365-2761.2010.01173.x
32. Lee C-T, Chen I-T, Yang Y-T, Ko T-P, Huang Y-T, Huang J-Y, et al. The opportunistic marine pathogen *Vibrio parahaemolyticus* becomes virulent by acquiring a plasmid that expresses a deadly toxin. Proc Natl Acad Sci. 2015; 112:10798–803.
33. Abd-Elfattah A, Kumar G, Soliman H, El-Matbouli M. Persistence of *Tetracapsuloides bryosalmonae* (Myxozoa) in chronically infected brown trout *Salmo trutta*. Dis Aquat Org. 2014;111:41–9.
34. Sarker S, Kallert DM, Hedrick RP, El-Matbouli M. Whirling disease revisited: pathogenesis, parasite biology and disease intervention. Dis Aquat Org. 2015;114:155–75.
35. Ruth F-F, Reed P. *Ichthyophthirius multifiliis* (White Spot) Infection in Fish. Circ. 920. 1997.
36. Matthews RA. *Ichthyophthirius multifiliis* Fouquet and Ichthyophthiriosis in Freshwater Teleosts. Adv Parasitol. 2005;59:159–241. Available from: http://linkinghub.elsevier.com/retrieve/pii/S0065308X05590031
37. Saleh M, Abdel-Baki A-A, Dkhil MA, El-Matbouli M, Al-Quraishy S. Antiprotozoal effects of metal nanoparticles against *Ichthyophthirius multifiliis*. Parasitology. 2017;144:1802–10. Available from: https://www.cambridge.org/core/product/identifier/S0031182017001184/type/journal_article
38. Wright A-DG, Colorni A. Taxonomic re-assignment of *Cryptocaryon irritans*, a marine fish parasite. Eur J Protistol. 2002;37:375–8. Available from: http://linkinghub.elsevier.com/retrieve/pii/S0932473904700358
39. Langenmayer MC, Lewisch E, Gotesman M, Hoedt W, Schneider M, El-Matbouli M, et al. Cutaneous infection with *Dermocystidium salmonis* in cardinal tetra, *Paracheirodon axelrodi* (Schultz, 1956). J Fish Dis. 2015;38:503–6.
40. El-Matbouli M, Soliman H. Transmission of *Cyprinid herpesvirus-3* (CyHV-3) from goldfish to naïve common carp by cohabitation. Res Vet Sci. 2011;90: 536–9.
41. Frischer ME, Lee RF, Price AR, Walters TL, Bassette MA, Verdiyev R, Torris MC, Bulski K, Geer PJ, Powell SA, Walker AN. Causes, diagnostics, and distribution of an ongoing penaeid shrimp black gill epidemic in the US South Atlantic Bight. J Shellfish Res. 2017;36:487–500.
42. Gilad O, Yun S, Andree K, Adkison M, Zlotkin A, Bercovier H, et al. Initial characteristics of koi herpesvirus and development of a polymerase chain reaction assay to detect the virus in koi, *Cyprinus carpio koi*. Dis Aquat Org. 2002;48:101–8.
43. Aoki T, Hirono I, Kurokawa K, Fukuda H, Nahary R, Eldar A, et al. Genome sequences of three koi herpesvirus isolates representing the expanding distribution of an emerging disease threatening koi and common carp worldwide. J Virol. 2007;81:5058–65.
44. Gunimaladevi I, Kono T, Venugopal MN, Sakai M. Detection of koi herpesvirus in common carp, *Cyprinus carpio* L., by loop-mediated isothermal amplification. J Fish Dis. 2004;27:583–9.
45. Yoshino M, Watari H, Kojima T, Ikedo M, Kurita J. Rapid, sensitive and simple detection method for koi herpesvirus using loop-mediated isothermal amplification. Microbiol Immunol. 2009;53:375–83.
46. Yoshino M, Watari H, Kojima T, Ikedo M. Sensitive and rapid detection of koi herpesvirus by LAMP method. Fish Pathol. 2006;41:19–27.
47. El-Matbouli M, Saleh M, Soliman H. Detection of cyprinid herpesvirus type 3 in goldfish cohabiting with CyHV-3-infected koi carp (*Cyprinus carpio koi*). Vet Rec. 2007;161:792–3.
48. Soliman H, El-Matbouli M. Immunocapture and direct binding loop mediated isothermal amplification simplify molecular diagnosis of Cyprinid herpesvirus-3. J Virol Methods. 2009;162:91–5.
49. Bergmann SM, Riechardt M, Fichtner D, Lee P, Kempter J. Investigation on the diagnostic sensitivity of molecular tools used for detection of koi herpesvirus. J Virol Methods. 2010;163:229.
50. Lievens B, Frans I, Heusdens C, Justé A, Jonstrup SP, Lieffrig F, et al. Rapid detection and identification of viral and bacterial fish pathogens using a DNA array-based multiplex assay. J Fish Dis. 2011;34:861–75.
51. Soliman H, El-Matbouli M. An inexpensive and rapid diagnostic method of Koi Herpesvirus (KHV) infection by loop-mediated isothermal amplification. Virol J. 2005;2:83.
52. Saleh M, Soliman H, El-Matbouli M. Gold nanoparticles as a potential tool for diagnosis of fish diseases. In: Inácio J, Cunha M V., editors. Methods Mol Biol. 2015;1247:245.
53. Saleh M, Soliman H, Schachner O, El-Matbouli M. Direct detection of unamplified spring viraemia of carp virus RNA using unmodified gold nanoparticles. Dis Aquat Org. 2012;100:3–10.
54. Saleh M, El-Matbouli M. Rapid detection of Cyprinid herpesvirus-3 (CyHV-3) using a gold nanoparticle-based hybridization assay. J Virol Methods. 2015; 217:50–4.
55. Shaalan M, Saleh M, El-Mahdy M, El-Matbouli M. Recent progress in applications of nanoparticles in fish medicine: a review. Nanomedicine. 2016;12:701–10.
56. Aoki T, Takano T, Unajak S, Takagi M, Kim YR, Bin PS, et al. Generation of monoclonal antibodies specific for ORF68 of koi herpesvirus. Comp Immunol Microbiol Infect Dis. 2011;34:209–16.

57. Adkison MA, Gilad O, Hedrick RP. An Enzyme Linked Immunosorbent Assay (ELISA) for detection of antibodies to the Koi Herpesvirus (KHV) in the Serum of Koi *Cyprinus carpio*. Fish Pathol. 2005;40:53–62.
58. Bergmann SM, Engler C, Wang Q, Zeng W, Li Y, Wang Y, et al. Investigation on antigen ELISA for detection of the envelope glycoprotein coded by ORF 149 of investigation on antigen ELISA for detection of the envelope glycoprotein coded by ORF 149 of different koi herpesvirus isolates obtained from cell cultures. J Vet Sci Med. 2017;5:1–7.
59. Cabon J, Louboutin L, Castric J, Bergmann S, Bovo G, Matras M, et al. Validation of a serum neutralization test for detection of antibodies specific to cyprinid herpesvirus 3 in infected common and koi carp (*Cyprinus carpio*). J Fish Dis. 2017;40:687–701.
60. Dishon A, Perelberg A, Bishara-Shieban J, Ilouze M, Davidovich M, Werker S, et al. Detection of carp interstitial nephritis and gill necrosis virus in fish droppings. Appl Environ Microbiol. 2005;71:7285–91.
61. St-Hilaire S, Beevers N, Joiner C, Hedrick RP, Way K. Antibody response of two populations of common carp, *Cyprinus carpio* L., exposed to koi herpesvirus. J Fish Dis. 2009;32:311–20.
62. Torrent F, Villena A, Lee PA, Fuchs W, Bergmann SM, Coll JM. The amino-terminal domain of ORF149 of koi herpesvirus is preferentially targeted by IgM from carp populations surviving infection. Arch Virol. 2016;161:2653–65.
63. Wang H, Xu L, Lu L. Detection of cyprinid herpesvirus 2 in peripheral blood cells of silver crucian carp, *Carassius auratus gibelio* (Bloch), suggests its potential in viral diagnosis. J Fish Dis. 2016;39:155–62.
64. Gaede L, Steinbrück J, Bergmann SM, Jäger K, Gräfe H, Schoon HA, et al. Koi herpesvirus infection in experimentally infected common carp *Cyprinus carpio* (Linnaeus, 1758) and three potential carrier fish species *Carassius carassius* (Linnaeus, 1758); *Rutilus rutilus* (Linnaeus, 1758); and *Tinca tinca*. J Appl Ichthyol. 2017;33:776–84.
65. Tong G, Wei X, Yin W, Liao X, Yang K, Fang Z, Sun T, Yue Z, Li X. Development of a liquid chip technique to simultaneously detect spring viremia of carp virus, infectious hematopoietic necrosis virus, and viral hemorrhagic septicemia of salmonids. J AOAC Int. 2017;100:159–64.
66. Waltzek TB, Kelley GO, Stone DM, Way K, Hanson L, Fukuda H, et al. Koi herpesvirus represents a third cyprinid herpesvirus (CyHV-3) in the family *Herpesviridae*. J Gen Virol. 2005;86:1659–67.
67. Li W, Lee X, Weng S, He J, Dong C. Whole-genome sequence of a novel Chinese cyprinid herpesvirus 3 isolate reveals the existence of a distinct European genotype in East Asia. Vet Microbiol. 2015;175:185–94.
68. Lee X, Yi Y, Weng S, Zeng J, Zhang H, He J, et al. Transcriptomic analysis of koi (Cyprinus carpio) spleen tissue upon cyprinid herpesvirus 3 (CyHV3) infection using next generation sequencing. Fish Shellfish Immunol. 2016; 49:213–24.
69. Zeng X-T, Chen Z-Y, Deng Y-S, Gui J-F, Zhang Q-Y. Complete genome sequence and architecture of crucian carp *Carassius auratus herpesvirus* (CaHV). Arch Virol. 2016;161:3577–81.
70. Monaghan SJ, Thompson KD, Adams A, Bergmann SM. Sensitivity of seven PCRs for early detection of koi herpesvirus in experimentally infected carp, *Cyprinus carpio* L., by lethal and non-lethal sampling methods. J Fish Dis. 2015;38:303–19.
71. Subramaniam K, Gotesman M, Smith CE, Steckler NK, Kelley KL, Groff JM, et al. Megalocytivirus infection in cultured Nile tilapia *Oreochromis niloticus*. Dis Aquat Org. 2016;119:253–8.
72. Donohoe OH, Henshilwood K, Way K, Hakimjavadi R, Stone DM, Walls D. Identification and Characterization of Cyprinid Herpesvirus-3 (CyHV-3) encoded MicroRNAs. Pfeffer S, editor. PLoS One. 2015;10:e0125434.
73. Jo A, Im J, Lee HE, Jang D, Nam GH, Mishra A, Kim WJ, Kim W, Cha HJ, Kim HS. Evolutionary conservation and expression of miR-10a-3p in olive flounder and rock bream. Gene. 2017;628:16–23.
74. Yuan J, Yang Y, Nie H, Li L, Gu W, Lin L, et al. Transcriptome analysis of epithelioma papulosum cyprini cells after SVCV infection. BMC Genomics. 2014;15:935.
75. Rosenkranz D, Klupp BG, Teifke JP, Granzow H, Fichtner D, Mettenleiter TC, et al. Identification of envelope protein pORF81 of koi herpesvirus. J Gen Virol. 2008;89:896–900.
76. Ainsworth J, Capley G, Waterstreet P, Munson D. Use of monoclonal antibodies in the indirect fluorescent antibody technique (IFA) for the diagnosis of *Edwardsiella ictaluri*. J Fish Dis. 1986;9:439–44.
77. Menanteau-Ledouble S, Lawrence M. Use of Fluorescent Immuno-Chemistry for the detection of *Edwardsiella ictaluri* in channel catfish(*I. punctatus*) samples. J Vis Exp. 2011;(51):e2687. https://doi.org/10.3791/2687.
78. Menanteau-Ledouble S, Karsi A, Lawrence ML. Importance of skin abrasion as a primary site of adhesion for *Edwardsiella ictaluri* and impact on invasion and systematic infection in channel catfish *Ictalurus punctatus*. Vet Microbiol. 2011;148:425–30.
79. Baillon L, Mérour E, Cabon J, Louboutin L, Quenault H, Touzain F, Morin T, Blanchard Y, Biacchesi S, Brémont M. A single amino acid change in the non-structural NV protein impacts the virulence phenotype of Viral hemorrhagic septicemia virus in trout. J Gen Virol. 2017;98:1181–4.
80. Chinchilla B, Gomez-Casado E. Identification of the functional regions of the viral haemorrhagic septicaemia virus (VHSV) NV protein: variants that improve function. Fish Shellfish Immunol. 2017;70:343–50.
81. Sun T, Yin WL, Fang BH, Wang Q, Liang CZ, Yue ZQ. Prediction of G gene epitopes of viral hemorrhagic septicemia virus and eukaryotic expression of major antigen determinant sequence. Cell Mol Biol. 2017;63:84–8.
82. Ke Q, Weaver W, Pore A, Gorgoglione B, Wildschutte JH, Xiao P, Shepherd BS, Spear A, Malathi K, Stepien CA, Vakharia VN. Role of viral hemorrhagic septicemia virus matrix (M) protein in suppressing host transcription. J Virol. 2017;91:e00279-17.
83. Kwak JS, Kim MS, Kim KH. Generation of a recombinant viral hemorrhagic septicemia virus (vhsv) expressing olive flounder (paralichthys olivaceus) interferon-γ and its effects on type I interferon response and virulence. Fish Shellfish Immunol. 2017;68:530–5.
84. Handfield M, Brady LJ, Progulske-Fox A, Hillman JD. IVIAT: a novel method to identify microbial genes expressed specifically during human infections. Trends Microbiol. 2000;8:336–9.
85. Rollins SM, Peppercorn A, Hang L, Hillman JD, Calderwood SB, Handfield M, et al. In vivo induced antigen technology (IVIAT). Cell Microbiol. 2005;7:1–9.
86. Jiao XD, Dang W, Hu YH, Sun L. Identification and immunoprotective analysis of an in vivo-induced *Edwardsiella tarda* antigen. Fish Shellfish Immunol. 2009;27:633–8.
87. Zou YX, Mo ZL, Hao B, Ye XH, Guo DS, Zhang PJ. Screening of genes expressed in vivo after infection by *Vibrio anguillarum* M3. Lett Appl Microbiol. 2010;51:564–9.
88. Menanteau-ledouble S, Soliman H, Kumar G, El-Matbouli M. Use of in vivo induced antigen technology to identify genes from *Aeromonas salmonicida* subsp. *salmonicida* that are specifically expressed during infection of the rainbow trout Oncorhynchus mykiss. BMC Vet Res. 2014;10:1–11.
89. Menanteau-Ledouble S, El-Matbouli M. Antigens of *Aeromonas salmonicida* subsp. *salmonicida* specifically induced in vivo in *Oncorhynchus mykiss*. J Fish Dis. 2016;39:1015–9.
90. Núñez-Díaz JA, Fumanal M, Viguera E, Moriñigo MA, Balebona MC. Use of in vivo induced technology to identify antigens expressed by *Photobacterium damselae* subsp. *piscicida* during infection of Senegalese sole (*Solea senegalensis*). Fish Shellfish Immunol. 2017;64:446–56.
91. Cassidy-Hanley DM, Cordonnier-Pratt M-M, Pratt LH, Devine C, Mozammal Hossain M, Dickerson HW, et al. Transcriptional profiling of stage specific gene expression in the parasitic ciliate *Ichthyophthirius multifiliis*. Mol Biochem Parasitol. 2011;178:29–39. Available from: https://doi.org/10.1016/j.molbiopara.2011.04.004
92. Abernathy J, Xu D-H, Peatman E, Kucuktas H, Klesius P, Liu Z. Gene expression profiling of a fish parasite *Ichthyophthirius multifiliis*: insights into development and senescence-associated avirulence. Comp Biochem Physiol Part D Genomics Proteomics. 2011;6:382–92. Available from: https://doi.org/10.1016/j.cbd.2011.08.003
93. Mai Y-Z, Li Y-W, Li R-J, Li W, Huang X-Z, Mo Z-Q, et al. Proteomic analysis of differentially expressed proteins in the marine fish parasitic ciliate *Cryptocaryon irritans*. Vet Parasitol. 2015;211:1–11. Available from: https://doi.org/10.1016/j.vetpar.2015.05.004
94. Yin F, Sun P, Wang J, Gao Q. Transcriptome analysis of dormant tomonts of the marine fish ectoparasitic ciliate *Cryptocaryon irritans* under low temperature. Parasit Vectors. 2016;9:280. Available from: https://doi.org/10.1186/s13071-016-1550-1
95. Fuchs W, Granzow H, Dauber M, Fichtner D, Mettenleiter TC. Identification of structural proteins of koi herpesvirus. Arch Virol. 2014;159:3257–68.
96. Reed AN. The conserved biology of herpesvirus latency: a study in cyprinid herpesvirus 3. Oregon State University; 2014.
97. Monaghan SJ, Thompson KD, Bron JE, Bergmann SM, Jung TS, Aoki T, et al. Expression of immunogenic structural proteins of cyprinid herpesvirus 3 in vitro assessed using immunofluorescence. Vet Res. 2016;47:8.
98. Kumar G, Hummel K, Ahrens M, Menanteau-Ledouble S, Welch TJ, Eisenacher M, et al. Shotgun proteomic analysis of Yersinia ruckeri strains under normal and iron-limited conditions. Vet Res. 2016;47:100.

99. Kumar G, Abd-elfattah A. Identification of differentially expressed genes of brown trout (*Salmo trutta*) and rainbow trout (*Oncorhynchus mykiss*) in response to *Tetracapsuloides bryosalmonae* (Myxozoa). Parasitol Res. 2015; 1792:929–39.
100. Kumar G, Sarker S, Menanteau-Ledouble S, El-Matbouli M. *Tetracapsuloides bryosalmonae* infection affects the expression of genes involved in cellular signal transduction and iron metabolism in the kidney of the brown trout *Salmo trutta*. Parasitol Res. 2015;114:2301–8.
101. Kumar G, Gotesman M, El-Matbouli M. Interaction of *Tetracapsuloides bryosalmonae*, the causative agent of proliferative kidney disease, with host proteins in the kidney of *Salmo trutta*. Parasitol Res. 2015;144:1721–7.
102. Gotesman M, Menanteau-Ledouble S, El-Matbouli M. Proteomic analysis of cytoskeleton proteins in fish. In: Gavin RH, editor. Cytoskelet. Methods Protoc. SE - 21. Springer New York; 2016. p. 357–72.
103. Gotesman M, Soliman H, El-Matbouli M. Antibody screening identifies 78 putative host proteins involved in Cyprinid herpesvirus 3 infection or propagation in common carp, Cyprinus carpio L. J Fish Dis. 2013;36:721–33.
104. Gotesman M, Abd-Elfattah A, Kattlun J, Soliman H, El-Matbouli M. Investigating the interactions of Cyprinid herpesvirus-3 with host proteins in goldfish *Carassius auratus*. J Fish Dis. 2014;37:835–41.
105. Ilouze M, Dishon A, Kotler M. Coordinated and sequential transcription of the cyprinid herpesvirus-3 annotated genes. Virus Res. 2012;169:98–106.
106. Michel B, Leroy B, Stalin Raj V, Lieffrig F, Mast J, Wattiez R, et al. The genome of cyprinid herpesvirus 3 encodes 40 proteins incorporated in mature virions. J Gen Virol. 2010;91:452–62.
107. Yi Y, Zhang H, Lee X, Weng S, He J, Dong C. Extracellular virion proteins of two Chinese CyHV-3/KHV isolates, and identification of two novel envelope proteins. Virus Res. 2014;191:108–16.
108. Yi Y, Qi H, Yuan J, Wang R, Weng S, He J, et al. Functional characterization of viral tumor necrosis factor receptors encoded by cyprinid herpesvirus 3 (CyHV3) genome. Fish Shellfish Immunol. 2015;45:757–70.
109. Obbard DJ, Gordon KHJ, Buck AH, Jiggins FM. The evolution of RNAi as a defence against viruses and transposable elements. Philos Trans R Soc Lond Ser B Biol Sci. 2009;364:99–115.
110. Fire A, Xu S, Montgomery MK, Kostas SA, Driver SE, Mello CC. Potent and specific genetic interference by double-stranded RNA in *Caenorhabditis elegans*. Nature. 1998;391:806–11.
111. Mochizuki K. DNA rearrangements directed by non-coding RNAs in ciliates. Wiley Interdiscip Rev RNA. 2010;1:376–87.
112. Sifuentes-Romero I, Milton SL, García-Gasca A. Post-transcriptional gene silencing by RNA interference in non-mammalian vertebrate systems: where do we stand? Mutat Res. 2011;728:158–71.
113. Kim K, Lee YS, Harris D, Nakahara K, Carthew RW. The RNAi pathway initiated by Dicer-2 in Drosophila. Cold Spring Harb Symp Quant Biol. 2006; 71:39–44.
114. Reshi ML, Wu J-L, Wang H-V, Hong J-R. RNA interference technology used for the study of aquatic virus infections. Fish Shellfish Immunol. 2014;40:14–23.
115. Biacchesi S. The reverse genetics applied to fish RNA viruses. Vet Res. 2011; 42:12.
116. Lima PC, Harris JO, Cook M. Exploring RNAi as a therapeutic strategy for controlling disease in aquaculture. Fish Shellfish Immunol. 2013;34:729–43.
117. Hammond SM. MicroRNA therapeutics: a new niche for antisense nucleic acids. Trends Mol Med. 2006;12:99–101.
118. Attasart P, Namramoon O, Kongphom U, Chimwai C, Panyim S. Ingestion of bacteria expressing dsRNA triggers specific RNA silencing in shrimp. Virus Res. 2013;171:252–6.
119. Sarathi M, Simon MC, Venkatesan C, Thomas J, Ravi M, Madan N, et al. Efficacy of bacterially expressed dsRNA specific to different structural genes of white spot syndrome virus (WSSV) in protection of shrimp from WSSV infection. J Fish Dis. 2010;33:603–7.
120. Sarathi M, Simon MC, Ahmed VPI, Kumar SR, Hameed ASS. Silencing VP28 gene of white spot syndrome virus of shrimp by bacterially expressed dsRNA. Mar Biotechnol. 2008;10:198–206.
121. Xu J, Han F, Zhang X. Silencing shrimp white spot syndrome virus (WSSV) genes by siRNA. Antivir Res. 2007;73:126–31.
122. Sarathi M, Simon MC, Venkatesan C, Hameed ASS. Oral administration of bacterially expressed VP28dsRNA to protect *Penaeus monodon* from white spot syndrome virus. Mar Biotechnol. 2008;10:242–9.
123. Kim MS, Jee BY, Cho MY, Kim JW, Do JH, Kim KH. Fugu double U6 promoter–driven long double-stranded RNA inhibits proliferation of viral hemorrhagic septicemia virus (VHSV) in fish cell lines. Arch Virol. 2012;157: 1029–38.
124. García K, Ramírez-Araya S, Díaz Ã, Reyes-Cerpa S, Espejo RT, Higuera G, et al. Inactivated E. coli transformed with plasmids that produce dsRNA against infectious salmon anemia virus hemagglutinin show antiviral activity when added to infected ASK cells. Front Microbiol. 2015;6:1–11.
125. Gotesman M, Soliman H, Besch R, El-Matbouli M. Inhibition of spring viraemia of carp virus replication in an *Epithelioma papulosum cyprini* cell line by RNAi. J Fish Dis. 2015;38:197–207.
126. Gotesman M, Soliman H, Besch R, El-Matbouli M. In vitro inhibition of cyprinid herpesvirus-3 replication by RNAi. J Virol Methods. 2014;206:63–6.
127. Adamek M, Rauch G, Brogden G, Steinhagen D. Small interfering RNA treatment can inhibit cyprinid herpesvirus 3 associated cell death in vitro. Pol J Vet Sci. 2014;17:733–5.
128. Saleh M, Kumar G, Abdel-Baki A-A, Dkhil MA, El-Matbouli M, Al-Quraishy S. In vitro gene silencing of the fish microsporidian *Heterosporis saurida* by RNA interference. Nucleic Acid Ther. 2016;26:250–6.
129. Sarker S, El-Matbouli M. Can RNAi target salmonid whirling disease in vivo ? Nucleic Acid Ther. 2015;25:285–6.
130. Sarker S, Menanteau-Ledouble S, Kotob MH, El-Matbouli MA. RNAi-based therapeutic proof of concept targets salmonid whirling disease in vivo. Vazquez-Duhalt R, editor. PLoS One. 2017;12:e0178687.
131. Meinke G, Bohm A, Hauber J, Pisabarro MT, Buchholz F. Cre recombinase and other tyrosine recombinases. Chem Rev. 2016;116:12785–820.
132. Hryhorowicz M, Lipiński D, Zeyland J, Słomski R. CRISPR/Cas9 immune system as a tool for genome engineering. Arch Immunol Ther Exp. 2017;65: 233–40.
133. Chin WX, Ang SK, Chu JJH. Recent advances in therapeutic recruitment of mammalian RNAi and bacterial CRISPR-Cas DNA interference pathways as emerging antiviral strategies. Drug Discov Today. 2017;22:17–30.
134. Zhao Y, Wang T, Yu Z, Wang H, Liu B, Wu C, et al. Inhibiting cyprinid herpesvirus-3 replication with CRISPR/Cas9. Biotechnol Lett. 2016;38:573–8.
135. Kattlun J, Menanteau-Ledouble S, El-Matbouli M. Non-structural protein pORF 12 of cyprinid herpesvirus 3 is recognized by the immune system of the common carp *Cyprinus carpio*. Dis Aquat Org. 2014;111:269–73.
136. Kattlun J, Menanteau-Ledouble S, Gotesman M, Abd-Elfattah A, Way K, Soliman H, et al. Immunogenic potential of a membrane protein encoded by the viral gene located at ORF 81 of Cyprinid Herpesvirus-3. Wien Tierarztl Monatsschr. 2016;103:3–12.
137. Monaghan SJ. Approaches to DIVA vaccination for fish using infectious salmon anaemia and koi herpesvirus disease as models. University of Stirling; 2013.
138. Monaghan SJ, Thompson KD, Smith PD, Adams A. Potential of DIVA vaccines for fish. Fish vaccines. Basel: Springer Basel; 2016. p. 143–73.
139. Samir M, Pessler F. Small non-coding RNAs associated with viral infectious diseases of veterinary importance: potential clinical applications. Front Vet Sci. 2016;3:22.
140. Feng H, Zhang Y-B, Zhang Q-M, Li Z, Zhang Q-Y, Gui J-F. Zebrafish IRF1 regulates IFN antiviral response through binding to IFNφ1 and IFNφ3 promoters downstream of MyD88 signaling. J Immunol. 2015;194:1225–38.
141. Lu L-F, Li S, Lu X-B, LaPatra SE, Zhang N, Zhang X-J, et al. Spring viremia of carp virus N protein suppresses fish IFNφ1 production by targeting the mitochondrial antiviral signaling protein. J Immunol. 2016;196:3744–53.
142. Liu L, Hu Y, Shen Y-F, Wang G-X, Zhu B. Evaluation on antiviral activity of coumarin derivatives against spring viraemia of carp virus in epithelioma papulosum cyprini cells. Antivir Res. 2017;144:173–85.
143. Liu L, Tu X, Shen YF, Chen WC, Zhu B, Wang GX. The replication of spring viraemia of carp virus can be regulated by reactive oxygen species and NF-κB pathway. Fish Shellfish Immunol. 2017;67:211–7.
144. McColl KA, Sunarto A, Williams LM, Crane MSTJ. The koi herpesvirus: dreaded pathogen or white knight? Aquac Heal Int. 2007;9:4–6.
145. McColl KA, Sunarto A, Holmes EC. Cyprinid herpesvirus 3 and its evolutionary future as a biological control agent for carp in Australia. Virol J. 2016;13:206.
146. Gibson-Reinemer DK, Chick JH, VanMiddlesworth TD, VanMiddlesworth M, Casper AF. Widespread and enduring demographic collapse of invasive common carp (*Cyprinus carpio*) in the upper Mississippi River system. Biol Invasions. 2017;19:1905–16.

Retrospective analysis of doxorubicin and prednisone as first-line therapy for canine B-cell lymphoma

Sami Al-Nadaf[1], Robert B. Rebhun[2], Kaitlin M. Curran[3], Rachel O. Venable[4], Katherine A. Skorupski[2], Jennifer L. Willcox[2] and Jenna H. Burton[2*]

Abstract

Background: A doxorubicin (DOX)-based chemotherapy protocol, CHOP, is the most effective treatment for canine high-grade B-cell lymphoma; however, the cost and time requirements associated with this protocol are not feasible for many pet owners. An alternative treatment option is the use of DOX, the most effective drug, in combination with prednisone. Prior studies with single-agent DOX included dogs with T-cell lymphoma, a known negative prognostic factor, which may have resulted in shorter reported survival times than if dogs with B-cell lymphoma were analyzed separately. The purpose of this study was to evaluate the outcome of dogs with high-grade B-cell lymphoma when treated with DOX and prednisone with or without L-asparaginase (L-ASP). Identification of prognostic factors was of secondary interest.

Results: Thirty-three dogs were included in the study; 31 dogs were evaluable for response with an overall response rate of 84%. The median progression free survival (PFS) and overall survival (OS) were 147 days and 182 days, respectively. The one-year survival fraction was 23%. No variable other than protocol completion was found to be significant for either PFS or OS including historical prognostic factors such as substage, thrombocytopenia, and body weight.

Conclusions: Dogs with high-grade B-cell lymphoma treated with DOX and prednisone with or without L-ASP have similar response rates, PFS, and OS to prior studies that did not differentiate between lymphoma immunophenotype. This protocol is not a replacement for CHOP; however, it is an alternative if time and cost are factors, while providing therapeutic benefit greater than prednisone alone.

Keywords: Adriamycin, Cancer, Canine, Chemotherapy, Immunophenotype

Background

A doxorubicin (DOX)-based chemotherapy protocol including cyclophosphamide, vincristine, and prednisone (CHOP), with or without L-asparaginase (L-ASP), is the most effective treatment for canine high-grade lymphoma. CHOP has repeatedly shown remission rates greater than 85%, with response durations of 6 to 10 months and survival times of 8 to 12 months [1–5]. However, several studies have described distinct treatment outcomes between high-grade B- and T-cell lymphoma demonstrating immunophenotype as an important prognostic factor [6–8]. When treated with a CHOP protocol, dogs with high-grade T-cell lymphoma have significantly shorter remission and survival times compared to those reported for dogs with high-grade B-cell lymphoma [9]. Multi-agent protocols report similar response rates for dogs with B- and T-cell lymphoma [10, 11]. However, response rates to a single dose of DOX for dogs with T-cell lymphoma is 50% compared to a 100% response rate for dogs B-cell lymphoma, suggesting that DOX may be a less efficacious drug for the treatment of T-cell lymphoma in dogs [12]. When deciding on a course of therapy for a dog with lymphoma, many owners consider prognosis as well as cost and time commitment of treatment. The financial burden and time

* Correspondence: jhburton@ucdavis.edu
[2]Department of Surgical and Radiological Sciences, School of Veterinary Medicine, University of California, Davis, Davis, CA, USA
Full list of author information is available at the end of the article

requirement to pursue a CHOP protocol is not feasible for many pet owners, necessitating alternative options when CHOP is declined.

DOX is the most effective single-agent drug for the treatment of canine high-grade lymphoma and DOX combined with prednisone may be offered as an alternative option to CHOP [13, 14]. This may be a more practical treatment for owners seeking to extend quality of life beyond that obtained with prednisone alone, but who are interested in a less intense protocol in terms of frequency and total number of treatments as well as cost [9]. When administered as a single-agent protocol, DOX is typically administered once every 3 weeks for 5 to 6 treatments whereas a CHOP protocol may consist of 12 to 17 chemotherapy treatments administered over 15 to 26 weeks. Outcome of dogs with lymphoma treated with a single-agent DOX protocol is inferior to CHOP, with shorter remission durations (4 to 6 months) and decreased survival times (5 to 9 months) despite relatively similar response rates (74 to 88%) [15–19]. However, previous studies evaluating DOX administered every 3 weeks for 5 to 6 treatments have not examined the association of patient outcome and immunophenotype. This raised the question as to whether prior studies that included dogs with T-cell lymphoma may underestimate survival times for dogs with B-cell lymphoma treated with single-agent DOX. The objective of this retrospective study was to investigate the outcome of dogs with high-grade B-cell lymphoma treated with DOX and prednisone with or without L-ASP. We hypothesized that these dogs would have an improved overall response rate, progression-free survival (PFS), and overall survival (OS) as compared to previous studies that included dogs with B- and T-cell lymphoma. Identification of factors associated with improved patient outcome was a secondary objective.

Results

Patient characteristics

Thirty-three dogs with high-grade B-cell lymphoma treated with at least one dose of DOX between January 2008 and December 2015 were included in the study. Information regarding signalment, weight, stage, and substage is presented in Table 1. Mixed breed dogs (27%) and golden retrievers (12%) were the most common breeds in this study.

Full staging was not performed for all dogs. Thirty-one (94%) dogs had peripheral node involvement, while one dog had thoracic and abdominal lymphadenopathy with no peripheral lymphadenopathy, and one had a colonic mass as the only site of disease. Eleven (33%) dogs were thrombocytopenic and 7 (21%) were anemic prior to first chemotherapy treatment. None of the dogs were hypercalcemic or azotemic. Sixteen (48%) dogs had thoracic radiographs, 15 (45%) dogs had an abdominal ultrasound, and 2 (6%) had a bone marrow aspirate as part of staging. Stage of disease, based on the World Health Organization criteria for canine lymphoma, was not evaluated for association with patient outcome due to the low numbers of dogs with complete staging. Additional sites of disease for the 31 dogs with peripheral node involvement included circulating blasts on initial complete blood cell count (CBC; $n = 7$), pulmonary parenchyma ($n = 1$), and nasal combined with dermal lesions (n = 1). Ten (30%) dogs were substage b and the remaining 23 were considered substage a.

Table 1 Baseline characteristics of patient population and determination of B-cell immunophenotype ($n = 33$)

Parameter		
Age (years)	Mean ± SD	8.8 ± 2.9
Sex	Male	2 (6%)
	Neutered Male	13 (39%)
	Female	1 (3%)
	Spayed Female	17 (52%)
Weight (kg)	Mean ± SD	27.6 ± 14.2
Breed	Mixed breed	9 (27%)
	Golden retriever	4 (12%)
	German shepherd	2 (6%)
	Scottish terrier	2 (6%)
	Basset Hound	2 (6%)
	Boxer	2 (6%)
	Border collie	2 (6%)
	Other (one each)	10 (31%)
Substage	a	24 (73%)
	b	9 (27%)
Immunophenotype	ICC	21 (64%)
	IHC	5 (15%)
	Flow	7 (21%)

SD standard deviation, *ICC* immunocytochemistry, *IHC* immunohistochemistry

High-grade lymphoma was diagnosed with cytology in 28 dogs (85%) and histopathology in 5 dogs (15%). B-cell phenotype was confirmed using CD79a for immunocytochemistry (ICC) for 21 dogs (64%) and immunohistochemistry (IHC) for 5 dogs (15%) [20]. Seven dogs (21%) had lymph node aspirates submitted for flow cytometric analysis to the Colorado State University Clinical Immunology Laboratory (Fort Collins, CO); B-cell phenotype was determined based on the presence of CD21 ± CD22 on an expanded population of medium to large lymphocytes.

Treatment

Twenty-one (64%) dogs received L-ASP as induction (400 kg/IU to a maximum of 10,000 units subcutaneously) prior to the first DOX treatment based on clinician preference. The median interval between L-ASP and DOX was 8 days (range, 4–21 days). All dogs received prednisone at least equivalent to 1 mg/kg every 24 h; duration of use and schedule of prednisone tapering was varied.

The median dosage of first doxorubicin was 30 mg/m^2 (range, 17.5–30 mg/m^2); 11 dogs weighed < 15 kg and treatment initiated at 1 mg/kg. Seven dogs had DOX therapy initiated at reduced dose, i.e. < 30 mg/m^2 or < 1 mg/kg for dogs weighing less than 15 kg. The median starting dose for these dogs was 27 mg/m^2 (range, 25–27 mg/m^2). The median number of doxorubicin treatments was 5 (range, 1–6 treatments); additional details regarding the number of DOX treatments administered is provided in Table 2. Eighteen (55%) dogs completed the planned treatment protocol, whereas 15 (45%) dogs did not complete their treatment protocol. Of the completed protocol group, 14 dogs completed a 5-treatment protocol, while 4 dogs completed a 6-treatment protocol. For those dogs that did not complete their planned treatment protocol, progressive disease (PD) was determined during the course of treatment in 11 dogs as recorded in their medical record. In the remaining 4 dogs, 3 dogs died either from suspected PD or treatment related toxicities, and for 1 dog the owner elected to discontinue treatment and was lost to follow-up.

Outcome

Thirty-one dogs were able to be assessed for response to treatment. One dog died the day following DOX administration and a second dog died of sepsis secondary to neutropenia 9 days after DOX administration and therefore response could not be assessed but was documented to be in a complete response (CR) at the time of death. The overall response rate (ORR) for these 31 dogs was 84% with 22 (71%) dogs experiencing a CR and 4 (13%) dogs experiencing a partial response (PR) as their best response. There was no difference in response between dogs that received a standard or reduced dose of DOX at initiation ($p = 1.0$). Two dogs had stable disease (SD) and 3 dogs had PD as their best response. The median PFS for all dogs was 147 days (range, 1–414 days; Fig. 1).

The OS for all dogs was 182 days (range, 1–556 days; Fig. 1). Of the 28 dogs able to be offered rescue treatment for progressive disease, 15 dogs received rescue chemotherapy protocols other than prednisone alone. Rescue agents included lomustine (8 dogs), mitoxantrone (6 dogs), COP (3 dogs), vincristine (3 dogs), vincristine/cytarabine/melphalan (3 dogs), dacarbazine (2 dogs), L-ASP (2 dogs), and vincristine/cyclophosphamide/B-cell monoclonal antibody (Aratana Therapuetics, Leawood, KS; 1 dog). Nine dogs continued with prednisone alone at the time of progression. Three dogs were lost to follow-up at a median of 94 days (45–102 days after treatment initiation) and censored at the date of last contact. Two dogs were humanely euthanized due to suspected DOX-induced gastrointestinal toxicity, 4 and 6 days post-infusion. The one-year survival rate for the 30 dogs with known outcomes was 23%, with 23 dogs confirmed dead within a year of treatment initiation. No dogs were alive 2 years after the start of treatment.

Historical pre-treatment prognostic factors such as substage, thrombocytopenia, and body weight were not associated with PFS (Table 3). The only variable associated with improved PFS was protocol completion. The only variables significant for OS were protocol completion and the addition of rescue chemotherapy beyond

Table 2 Doxorubicin and prednisone with or without L-asparaginase treatment and patient response

Parameter		
L-asparaginase at induction	Yes	21 (64%)
	No	12 (36%)
Number of doxorubicin treatments	1	7 (21%)
	2	3 (9%)
	3	3 (9%)
	4	1 (3%)
	5	15 (45%)
	6	4 (12%)
Completed protocol	Yes	18 (55%)
	No	15 (45%)
Best response	CR	22 (71%)
	PR	4 (13%)
	SD	2 (6%)
	PD	3 (10%)
	Not evaluated	2

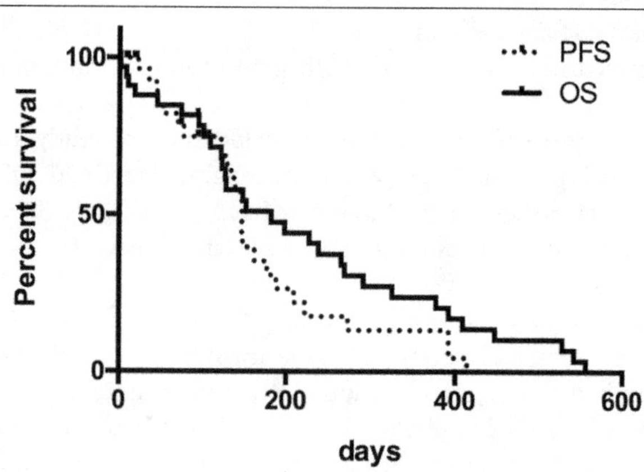

Fig. 1 Kaplan-Meier curves of progression free survival (PFS) and overall survival (OS) for 33 dogs treated with doxorubicin and prednisone with or without L-asparaginase for B-cell lymphoma

Table 3 Factors evaluated by univariate analysis for association with progression free survival (PFS) and overall survival (OS)

		n	Median PFS (days)	*p*-value	HR (95% CI)	Median OS (days)	*p*-value	HR (95% CI)
Substage	a	24	147	0.72	1.16 (0.491 to 2.92)	227	0.76	0.89 (0.379 to 2.00)
	b	9	134			148		
L-asparaginase at Induction	No	12	147	0.9	0.95 (0.417 to 2.15)	245	0.89	0.95 (0.458 to 1.96)
	Yes	21	147			152		
Thrombocytopenia	No	22	147	0.18	0.59 (0.210 to 1.30)	198	0.79	0.91 (0.416 to 1.95)
	Yes	11	127			148		
Body weight	< 15 kg	8	147	0.57	0.76 (0.302 to 1.89)	138	0.63	1.219 (0.530 to 2.90)
	> 15 kg	25	147			198		
Anemia	No	7	139	0.55	1.33 (0.540 to 3.35)	152	0.83	0.915 (0.382 to 2.17)
	Yes	26	177			227		
Protocol Completion	No	18	61	< 0.0001	5.66 (17.3 to 324)	101	< 0.0001	4.59 (7.15 to 55.3)
	Yes	15	170			291		
Protocol Duration	5 tx	15	162	0.83	1.12 (0.384 to 3.38)	308	0.87	0.91 (0.289 to 2.83)
	6 tx	4	185			226		
Rescue Chemotherapy	No	13	–	–	–	148	0.013	2.35 (1.36–7.30)
	Yes	15	–			325		

prednisone alone (Table 3). L-ASP induction was also found not to have affected the PFS ($p = 0.90$), OS ($p = 0.89$), or ORR ($p = 0.76$) between the dogs who received the induction or not. Dogs with substage b lymphoma were not more likely to receive L-ASP than substage a dogs ($p = 0.26$). There was also no difference in PFS or OS for dogs that received 5 versus 6 doses of DOX ($p = 0.82$ and $p = 0.87$, respectively).

Discussion

This study sought to determine the response rate, PFS, and OS for dogs with B-cell lymphoma when treated with a DOX and prednisone protocol with or without L-ASP induction; we hypothesized that dogs with B-cell lymphoma would have an improved response rate and outcome as compared to previous studies that included dogs with T-cell forms of lymphoma. Our hypothesis was not supported by our results as this DOX and prednisone protocol, with or without L-ASP induction, resulted in an ORR of 84%, PFS of 147 days, and OS of 182 days. While direct statistical comparison cannot be made, these findings are numerically similar to previously reported DOX protocols when immunophenotype was not assessed (ORR 74–88%; PFS 131–206 days; OS 169.5–295) [15–19]. Our study further supports that a DOX and prednisone protocol continues to result in inferior patient outcome as compared to the PFS and OS previously reported for CHOP (PFS 140–282 days; OS 257–397 days) [1–5]. Completion of protocol was the only variable that was associated with both improved PFS and OS, which is a consequence of improved response to treatment for a subset of patients. No previous historical prognostic factors were found to be associated with outcome, likely due to the evaluation of a more homogenous group of dogs by excluding T-cell immunophenotypes.

It is possible the variations in initially DOX or prednisone dosing could have altered the response rate. We feel this is unlikely, however, as the majority (79%) dogs had treatment initiated at a standard DOX dose of 30 mg/m^2 (or 1 mg/kg if less than 15 kg) and the median dose was only 10% reduced for those dogs that received a reduced DOX dose at treatment initiation. Additionally, there was no difference in response rates between those two groups. Prednisone is administered orally at home by owners and the tapering schedule was not well documented in most medical records, so the impact of this is challenging to assess. However, the role that prednisone plays in the outcome of dogs with lymphoma when they are treated with a multi-drug chemotherapy protocol without the prednisone has been called into question. There are now two prospective, controlled studies that suggest that prednisone/prednisolone may not affect the response rate, PFS, or OS for dogs with lymphoma [21, 22]. Based on this information, the authors suspect that differences in prednisone dosing and schedule likely have a negligible impact on patient outcome.

An inherent limitation by the retrospective nature of this study is the lack of standardization of response assessment. The Veterinary Cooperative Oncology Group (VCOG) consensus document, describing the evaluation criteria for the treatment response of peripheral nodal lymphoma in dogs is now the standard to measure disease response [23]. Lymph node measurements were not recorded in the medical record for all patients at all visits and therefore response to treatment was based on clinician assessment as recorded in the medical record. It is possible that based on the guidelines, some of the partial responders may have been categorized as having stable disease which could have led to an overestimation of the ORR in this study. However, the VCOG guidelines would not have altered the number of dogs that obtained a CR, as determination of a CR is based on the evaluator's judgement that lymph nodes have returned to normal size and are non-pathologic [23].

Similarly, toxicity of this protocol was not evaluated in this study due to concern that retrospective assessment of adverse events would be underestimated due to incomplete information in the medical record. However, four dogs were euthanized after their first dose of DOX. One dog with substage b lymphoma died the day following DOX administration, which could have been due to advanced stage of disease or possibly acute tumor lysis syndrome secondary to DOX administration. Two other dogs were euthanized after developing gastrointestinal toxicity 4 and 6 days after DOX treatment. However, both of these dogs were also documented to have progressive disease at this time as well, so it is challenging to elucidate retrospectively how lack of response to treatment may have played a role in the decision to euthanize when gastrointestinal signs secondary to DOX developed. Gastrointestinal toxicity is a common sequala of DOX administration, with up to 2/3 of dogs developing some degree of gastrointestinal toxicosis with < 15% of those considered severe to life-threatening [17, 24, 25]. .A fourth dog was euthanized after becoming septic after DOX-induced toxicity 9 days after treatment. Hematologic toxicities are also commonly reported after DOX administration and while most are mild in nature, they can be severe enough to cause fatal complications as others have reported as well [24, 26].

Higginbotham et al. described a single-agent DOX protocol for the treatment of high-grade B-cell lymphoma, which consisted of an initial induction of 3 treatments administered every 2 weeks with additional DOX treatment at the time of tumor progression [26]. Despite the difference in the timing of DOX administration, our continuous protocol had a comparable median number of treatments to the intermittent treatment protocol (5 treatments vs. 4.5 treatments), as well as similar outcomes (ORR of 78% and median survival time of 169.5 days) [26]. Prospective evaluation of continuous versus intermittent DOX administration could be considered to directly compare the efficacy of these two protocols.

It is possible that the findings in this study were influenced by tumor grade. A distinct biological behavior exists between histologic grades of canine lymphoma, with low-grade lymphoma characterized by slow rate of progression, incomplete responses to DOX-based chemotherapy protocols, and longer survival times [7, 9, 27, 28]. While the distinction of high- and low-grade lymphoma is ideally made based on histopathological evaluation, cytologic assessment of cell size is commonly used in practice to make this determination and has been reported to have a good correlation with histologic samples [29]. Previous studies of single-agent DOX treatment of canine lymphoma have included both high- and low-grade lymphomas when analyzing outcome. Five (12%) dogs treated with single-agent DOX in two previous studies were known to have low-grade lymphoma [15, 19]. The ORR and median survival times of these studies were 76–88% and 237–270 days respectively for all dogs treated. Although including low-grade lymphomas may have negatively impacted the treatment response rate, the median OS outcome was potentially improved. All dogs in the present study had high-grade lymphoma determined by either cytology or histopathology. High-grade B-cell lymphoma, specifically diffuse large B-cell lymphoma, in dogs has an aggressive biologic behavior and when treated with a DOX-based multi-agent chemotherapy protocol as described by Childress et al. has an ORR of 100%, but a relatively short PFI and OS of 252 and 341 days, respectively [10]. The inclusion of dogs with low-grade lymphoma in previous evaluations of single-agent DOX protocols may in part explain why dogs with B-cell phenotype in this study did not have an improved PFS or OS compared to previous studies.

In addition to determining phenotype, flow cytometry can provide cell size and level of antigen expression to further sub-classify lymphomas. A subset of high-grade B-cell lymphomas that have large cells and low MHC class II expression are known to have median survival times similar to high-grade T-cell lymphomas [30]. Only 21% of the dogs in this study were confirmed to have B-cell origin lymphoma via flow cytometry, whereas almost 66% were confirmed by ICC. ICC can be beneficial in conducting direct assessment of cell morphology in combination with its immunoreactivity. However, poor cytologic cellularity or quality can affect ICC interpretation and quantification of antigen expression [31]. Cytologic assessment of cell size is more subjective and MHC class II expression is not routinely assessed with ICC. Therefore, a subset of B-cell lymphomas with poor prognostic factors may have been within this study population, and potentially influencing the PFS and OS negatively. In the future, as additional phenotypic information becomes more readily available to subcategorize high-grade B-cell lymphoma, this could be used to further guide prognosis and treatment recommendations.

Many clinicians routinely initiate treatment for dogs with substage b lymphoma with L-ASP at induction. This practice allows time for owners to contemplate their pets' diagnosis and to decide on a treatment plan which suits their goals in terms of providing quality of life as well as logistics of finances and time. Dogs receiving L-ASP were included in this study since it has not been found to result in increased remission or survival duration when used at initiation of treatment [5, 32, 33]. Although the use of L-ASP at induction does not influence the outcome of dogs with lymphoma treated with a CHOP protocol, two studies have reported that L-ASP may be useful in the induction phase of treatment and may or may not influence remission and survival times with doxorubicin alone; however, results have been inconsistent [5, 19, 34]. In our study, dogs that did not receive L-ASP had an improved OS when compared to the population receiving L-ASP induction (245 vs. 152 days, respectively); however, this result was not statistically significant. The small sample size of this study precludes robust statistical evaluation of the impact L-ASP has when included at induction with DOX.

The limitations of this study are in part due to its retrospective nature. Inherent with all retrospective studies, some dogs were lost to follow-up and censored from OS analysis ($n = 3$), and complete staging was not performed in most dogs. Prednisone was administered in addition to the DOX and could have led to an over estimation of response rate. Many protocols incorporate prednisone in the induction period to improve patients' quality of life, and in this study the remission duration and survival exceeded the known outcomes associated with prednisone alone [9]. Inconsistent rescue therapy and choice of euthanasia have an overall impact on OS, especially if time and financial considerations are important factors. Lastly, the small sample size could have impeded relevant statistical analysis.

Conclusions

A DOX and prednisone protocol, with or without L-ASP induction, for the treatment of canine high-grade B-cell lymphoma has similar response rates, PFS, and OS to previously published protocols that did not assess for immunophenotype. While less efficacious than multi-agent protocols for lymphoma, this protocol may be suitable for owners unable to pursue a more time or financially intensive protocol and who seek therapeutic benefit greater than prednisone alone.

Methods

Study population

Dogs diagnosed with high-grade B-cell lymphoma and treated with at least one dose of DOX were retrospectively identified through the University of California, Davis Veterinary Medical Teaching Hospital, Oregon State University Lois Bates Acheson Veterinary Teaching Hospital, and Arizona Veterinary Oncology medical record databases from January 2008 to December 2015. Inclusion criteria comprised a diagnosis of high-grade lymphoma with measurable disease present at treatment initiation, confirmed B-cell phenotype, and intent to treat with DOX chemotherapy with no prior cytotoxic chemotherapy.

Signalment, body weight, age at diagnosis, clinical signs at presentation, and pretreatment diagnostics, such as CBC, serum chemistry panel, urinalysis, thoracic radiographs, abdominal imaging, and bone marrow evaluation, were abstracted from the medical record for each dog. Lymph node cytology, histopathology, and/or reports were reviewed to confirm reporting of large cell morphology and to establish the method used for immunophenotype determination.

Treatment

Dogs that had previously been treated with chemotherapy were excluded; however, oral prednisone treatment of ≤14 days and L-ASP induction ≤21 days prior to DOX administration were acceptable. Each dog received at least one dose of DOX administered intravenously (30 mg/m^2 for dogs > 15 kg or 1 mg/kg for dogs ≤15 kg). Subsequent DOX treatments were administered every 3 weeks for five to six total treatments unless progressive disease occurred prior to completion of the prescribed protocol.

Information obtained regarding the treatment protocol included use of L-ASP induction, number of treatments, and whether the DOX protocol was completed. Rescue protocols were recorded in cases where relapse occurred, and the owners elected additional therapy. Follow-up information was obtained from medical records and by phone calls to the referring veterinary hospitals. Factors evaluated for association with PFS and OS included substage, body weight, anemia, thrombocytopenia, hypercalcemia and/or azotemia at the time of diagnosis, number of total treatments (5 versus 6), protocol completion, and use of L-ASP at treatment induction. Patient outcome criteria included maximal response to therapy, PFS, and OS. A CR was considered as resolution of all clinically detectable disease. A designation of PR, SD, or PD was determined based on clinician assessment in the medical record as lymph node measurements were not recorded in all cases and standard VCOG criteria for nodal lymphoma could not be retrospectively applied to all cases. Responses and stable disease needed to be maintained for a minimum of 21 days.

Statistical analyses

Continuous data were tested for normality using the D'Agostino-Pearson test and reported using mean or median and range; categorical data were reported as frequencies and percentages. ORR were defined as the number of dogs experiencing partial or complete remission divided by the total number of dogs treated. Chi-square analysis was used to evaluate association between use of L-ASP at induction and tumor response (CR, PR or SD/PD). Fisher's exact test was used to evaluate association between substage and use of L-ASP at induction as well as association between starting DOX dosage (standard versus reduced) and response (CR/PR versus SD/PD). PFS was defined as the time of first treatment with either L-ASP or DOX until progression of disease. OS was defined as the time from first treatment with either L-ASP or DOX and death from any cause. PFS and OS analyses were performed using the Kaplan-Meier product limit method. Dogs were censored at the date of last contact if they were still alive at the time of analysis or last follow-up. A p-value of ≤0.05 was considered statistically significant. A commercially available software program was used to perform statistical analyses (Prism v 6.0b, GraphPad Software, La Jolla, CA).

Abbreviations

CBC: Complete blood count; CHOP: Cyclophosphamide, doxorubicin, vincristine, prednisone; CR: Complete response; DOX: Doxorubicin; ICC: Immunocytochemistry; IHC: Immunohistochemistry; L-ASP: L-asparaginase; ORR: Overall response rate; OS: Overall survival; PD: Progressive disease; PFS: Progression free survival; PR: Partial response; SD: Stable disease; VCOG: Veterinary Cooperative Oncology Group

Acknowledgements

Not applicable.

Funding

JB is supported by the National Cancer Institute of the National Institutes of Health under Award Number K12CA138464. The content is solely the responsibility of the authors and does not necessarily represent the official views of the National Institutes of Health. The National Institutes of Health had no role in the design of the study, collection, analysis, and interpretation of data, nor writing of the manuscript.

Authors' contributions

SA, KC, and RV abstracted data from the medical records. SA and JB analyzed and all authors interpreted the data. SA, JB, and RB drafted the manuscript and critical revision was provided by KC, RV, KS, and JW. All authors read and approved the final manuscript and agree to be accountable for all aspects of the work.

Consent for publication

Not applicable.

Competing interests

The authors declare that they have no competing interests.

Author details

[1]William R. Pritchard Veterinary Medical Teaching Hospital, School of Veterinary Medicine, University of California, Davis, Davis, CA, USA. [2]Department of Surgical and Radiological Sciences, School of Veterinary Medicine, University of California, Davis, Davis, CA, USA. [3]Department of Clinical Sciences, Carlson College of Veterinary Medicine, Oregon State University, Corvallis, OR, USA. [4]Arizona Veterinary Oncology, Gilbert, AZ, USA.

References

1. Burton JH, Garrett-Mayer E, Thamm DH. Evaluation of a 15-week CHOP protocol for the treatment of canine multicentric lymphoma. Vet Comp Oncol. 2013;11(4):306–15.
2. Chun R, Garrett LD, Vail DM. Evaluation of a high-dose chemotherapy protocol with no maintenance therapy for dogs with lymphoma. J Vet Intern Med. 2000;14(2):120–4.
3. Garrett LD, Thamm DH, Chun R, Dudley R, Vail DM. Evaluation of a 6-month chemotherapy protocol with no maintenance therapy for dogs with lymphoma. J Vet Intern Med. 2002;16(6):704–9.
4. Hosoya K, Kisseberth WC, Lord LK, Alvarez FJ, Lara-Garcia A, Kosarek CE, et al. Comparison of COAP and UW-19 protocols for dogs with multicentric lymphoma. J Vet Intern Med. 2007;21(6):1355–63.
5. MacDonald VS, Thamm DH, Kurzman ID, Turek MM, Vail DM. Does l-Asparaginase influence efficacy or toxicity when added to a standard CHOP protocol for dogs with lymphoma? J Vet Intern Med. 2005;19(5):732–6.
6. Curran K, Thamm DH. Retrospective analysis for treatment of naive canine multicentric lymphoma with a 15-week, maintenance-free CHOP protocol. Vet Comp Oncol. 2016;14:147–55.
7. Ponce F, Magnol JP, Ledieu D, Marchal T, Turinelli V, Chalvet-Monfray K, Fournel-Fleury C. Prognostic significance of morphological subtypes in canine malignant lymphomas during chemotherapy. Vet J. 2004;167(2):158–66.
8. SimonD MSN, Hirschberger J, Moritz A, Kohn B, Neumann S, et al. Efficacy of a continuous, multiagent chemotherapeutic protocol versus a short-term single-agent protocol in dogs with lymphoma. J Am Vet Med Assoc. 2008; 232(6):879–85.
9. Vail DM, Pinkerton ME, Young KM. Hematopoietic tumors. In: Withrow SJ, Vail DM, Page RL, editors. Withrow & MacEwen's small animal clinical oncology. St. Louis, MO: Elsevier; 2013. p. 608–678.
10. Childress MO, Ramos-Vara JA, Ruple A. Retrospective analysis of factors affecting clinical outcome following CHOP-based chemotherapy in dogs with primary nodal diffuse large B-cell lymphoma. Vet Comp Oncol. 2017; 16(1):E159–68.
11. Rebhun RB, Kent MS, Borrofka SA, Frazier S, Skorupski K, Rodriguez CO. CHOP chemotherapy for the treatment of canine multicentric T-cell lymphoma. Vet Comp Oncol. 2011;9(1):38–44.
12. Beaver LM, Strottner G, Klein MK. Response rate after administration of a single dose of doxorubicin in dogs with B-cell or T-cell lymphoma: 41 cases (2006-2008). J Am Vet Med Assoc. 2010;237(9):1052–5.
13. Keller ET, MacEwen EG, Rosenthal RC, Helfand SC, Fox LE. Evaluation of prognostic factors and sequential combination chemotherapy with doxorubicin for canine lymphoma. J Vet Intern Med. 1993;7(5):289–95.
14. Regan RC, Kaplan MS, Bailey DB. Diagnostic evaluation and treatment recommendations for dogs with substage-a high-grade multicentric lymphoma: results of a survey of veterinarians. Vet Comp Oncol. 2013;11(4):287–95.
15. Carter RF, Harris CK, Withrow SJ, Valli VEO, Susaneck SJ. Chemotherapy of canine lymphoma with histopathological correlation - doxorubicin alone compared to cop as 1st treatment regimen. J Am Anim Hosp Assoc. 1987; 23(6):587–98.
16. Postorino NC, Susaneck SJ, Withrow SJ. Single agent therapy with Adriamycin for canine Lymphosarcoma. J Am Anim Hosp Assoc. 1989;25(2):221–5.
17. Mutsaers AJ, Glickman NW, DeNicola DB, Widmer WR, Bonney PL, Hahn KA, et al. Evaluation of treatment with doxorubicin and piroxicam or doxorubicin alone for multicentric lymphoma in dogs. J Am Vet Med Assoc. 2002;220(12):1813–7.
18. Lori JC, Stein TJ, Thamm DH. Doxorubicin and cyclophosphamide for the treatment of canine lymphoma: a randomized, placebo-controlled study. Vet Comp Oncol. 2010;8(3):188–95.
19. Valerius KD, Ogilvie GK, Mallinckrodt CH, Getzy DM. Doxorubicin alone or in combination with asparaginase, followed by cyclophosphamide, vincristine, and prednisone for treatment of multicentric lymphoma in dogs: 121 cases (1987-1995). J Am Vet Med Assoc. 1997;210(4):512–6.

20. Vernau W, Moore PF. An immunophenotypic study of canine leukemias and preliminary assessment of clonality by polymerase chain reaction. Vet Immunol Immunopathol. 1999;69(2–4):145–64.
21. Childress MO, Ramos-Vara JA, Ruple A. A randomized controlled trial of the effect of prednisone omission from a multidrug chemotherapy protocol on treatment outcome in dogs with peripheral nodal lymphomas. J Am Vet Med Assoc. 2016;249(9):1067–78.
22. Zandvliet M, Rutteman GR, Teske E. Prednisolone inclusion in a first-line multidrug cytostatic protocol for the treatment of canine lymphoma does not affect therapy results. Vet J. 2013;197(3):656–61.
23. Vail DM, Michels GM, Khanna C, Selting KA, London CA, Veterinary cooperative oncology group. Response evaluation criteria for peripheral nodal lymphoma in dogs (v1.0)--a veterinary cooperative oncology group (VCOG) consensus document. Vet Comp Oncol. 2010;8(1):28–37.
24. Ogilvie GK, Richardson RC, Curtis CR, Withrow SJ, Reynolds HA, Norris AM, et al. Acute and short-term toxicoses associated with the administration of doxorubicin to dogs with malignant tumors. J Am Vet Med Assoc. 1989; 195(11):1584–7.
25. Withers SS, Kass PH, Rodriguez CO Jr, Skorupski KA, O'Brien D, Guerrero TA, et al. Fasting reduces the incidence of delayed-type vomiting associated with doxorubicin treatment in dogs with lymphoma. Transl Oncol. 2014;7(3):377–83.
26. Higginbotham ML, McCaw DL, Roush JK, Nietfeld JC, Wilkerson MJ, Reeds K, et al. Intermittent single-agent doxorubicin for the treatment of canine B-cell lymphoma. J Am Anim Hosp Assoc. 2013;49(6):357–62.
27. Aresu L, Martini V, Rossi F, Vignoli M, Sampaolo M, Aricò A, et al. Canine indolent and aggressive lymphoma: clinical spectrum with histologic correlation. Vet Comp Oncol. 2015;13(4):348–62.
28. Teske E, van Heerde P, Rutteman GR, Kurzman ID, Moore PF, MacEwen EG. Prognostic factors for treatment of malignant-lymphoma in dogs. J Am Vet Med Assoc. 1994;205(12):1722–8.
29. Teske E, van Heede P. Diagnostic value and reproducibility of fine-needle aspiration cytology in canine malignant lymphoma. Vet Q. 1996;18(3):112–5.
30. Rao S, Lana S, Eickhoff J, Marcus E, Avery PR, Morley PS, et al. Class II major histocompatibility complex expression and cell size independently predict survival in canine B-cell lymphoma. J Vet Intern Med. 2011;25(5):1097–105.
31. Priest HL, Hume KR, Killick D, Kozicki A, Rizzo VL, Seelig D, et al. The use, publication and future directions of immunocytochemistry in veterinary medicine: a consensus of the oncology-pathology working group. Vet Comp Oncol. 2017;15(3):868–80.
32. Piek CJ, Rutteman GR, Teske E. Evaluation of the results of a L-asparaginase-based continuous chemotherapy protocol versus a short doxorubicin-based induction chemotherapy protocol in dogs with malignant lymphoma. Vet Q. 1999;21(2):44–9.
33. Jeffreys AB, Knapp DW, Carlton WW, Thomas RM, Bonney PL, Degortari A, et al. Influence of asparaginase on a combination chemotherapy protocol for canine multicentric lymphoma. J Am Anim Hosp Assoc. 2005;41(4):221–6.
34. Valerius KD, Ogilvie GK, Fettman MJ, Walton JA, Richardson K, Powers BE, et al. Comparison of the effects of asparaginase administered subcutaneously versus intramuscularly for treatment of multicentric lymphoma in dogs receiving doxorubicin. J Am Vet Med Assoc. 1999;214(3):353–6.

Six-month safety evaluation of robenacoxib tablets (Onsior™) in dogs after daily oral administrations

Céline E. Toutain[1*], Patrick Brossard[1], Stephen B. King[2] and Rainer Helbig[1]

Abstract

Background: Robenacoxib is a non-steroidal anti-inflammatory drug available for canine and feline use for the control of pain and inflammation marketed as Onsior™. The aim of this target animal safety study was to evaluate the 6-month safety profile of oral robenacoxib administration. It was a randomized, negative-controlled, parallel group study. Thirty-two healthy, young, experimentally naïve, purebred Beagle dogs were administered 0 (sham control, Group 1), 2, 6, and 10 mg/kg robenacoxib (corresponding to the upper end of the dosage range [1X, Group 2] and multiples thereof [3X and 5X, Group 3 and 4]), orally once daily for 6 months. Assessment of safety included general health and clinical observations, physical, neurological, ophthalmological and electrocardiographic examinations, gross and histopathological examinations and clinical pathology evaluations. Blood samples were collected for toxicokinetic assessment of robenacoxib.

Results: No serious adverse events were reported. When compared with control, no treatment effect was observed for body weight, feed or water consumption, clinical pathology, urinalysis and fecal examination parameters. There were no treatment-related changes in stifle joint tissues and microscopic/histopathology examinations of all tissues/organs were normal. Salivation and soft feces were noted in all groups but observed more frequently in the treated groups as compared with control. On Day 178, increased buccal mucosal bleeding times were observed in two treated animals (Group 3 and 4) and one dog in Group 4 displayed a retinal change. Decreased hopping and conscious proprioception was noted in four treated dogs. One dog in Group 2 had ventricular premature complexes. Post-mortem changes included mild, red foci on the cecum in one dog (Group 3) and minimal duodenal discoloration in one dog (Group 4), with no corresponding histological findings in either dog. Ovarian weights were decreased in females from Group 3 and 4 with no gross or histological changes in the ovaries. Blood concentrations of robenacoxib confirmed systemic exposure of treated dogs. Exposure increased with increasing doses and there were no accumulation of robenacoxib in blood.

Conclusions: Robenacoxib was well tolerated at doses from 2 to 10 mg/kg/day and this 6-month study supports the safe use of Onsior™ (robenacoxib) tablets in dogs for the intended dosing regimen.

Keywords: Robenacoxib, Onsior™, Tablet, Target animal safety, NSAID, Dog

* Correspondence: celine.toutain@elanco.com
[1]Elanco Animal Health, a Division of Eli Lilly and Company, Mattenstrasse 24a, CH-4058 Basel, Switzerland
Full list of author information is available at the end of the article

Background

The non-steroidal anti-inflammatory (NSAID) drug robenacoxib has been developed for veterinary use in cats and dogs [1, 2]. It is highly selective for inhibition of the cyclooxygenase (COX)-2 [3–5] with a fast onset of action in cats [6] and dogs [7] and an improved safety profile as compared with non-selective NSAIDs [8–10]. It is marketed as Onsior™ and available in many countries as both injection and oral formulations for both species [11]. The oral formulation for dogs (Onsior™ tablets, Elanco Animal Health) was approved in Europe since 2008 [11] for the treatment of pain and inflammation associated with chronic osteoarthritis in dogs at a dose of 1 mg/kg (with a range 1–2 mg/kg) and more recently in the United States in 2016 [12] for the control of postoperative pain and inflammation associated with soft tissue surgery at a dose of 2 mg/kg (with a range 2–4 mg/kg).

Previous studies have demonstrated an excellent safety profile for robenacoxib when administered orally to healthy young beagle dogs at daily doses of up to 40 mg/kg for 1 month and up to 10 mg/kg for 6 months [8]. These studies were conducted with a prototype formulation of robenacoxib which necessitated a target animal safety study to be conducted with the final commercial product in order to obtain global marketing authorizations, as outlined in the guideline for evaluating the target animal safety of new veterinary products (VICH Guideline 43) [13].

The objective of the present study was therefore to investigate the long-term safety of the veterinary medicinal product (Onsior™ tablets) administered orally to dogs once daily at dosages of 0, 2, 6 and 10 mg/kg for a total duration of six consecutive months.

Methods

Objective and standards

The objective of this study was to evaluate the target animal safety of robenacoxib tablets (Onsior™, Elanco Animal Health) when administered daily to young adult dogs at 0, 2, 6 and 10 mg/kg for 6 months.

This nonclinical study was conducted in accordance with Good Laboratory Practice (GLP) [14, 15] and according to the guideline for evaluating the target animal safety of new veterinary products (VICH Guideline 43) [13]. The study was reviewed and approved by the study site Institutional Animal Care and Use Committee. It was in compliance with the U.S. Department of Agriculture's (USDA) Animal Welfare Act (9 CFR Parts 1, 2 and 3) and followed The Guide for the Care and Use of Laboratory Animals [16, 17]. This manuscript was prepared in compliance with the ARRIVE guidelines for reporting animal in vivo experiments [18].

Animals and maintenance

A total of 40 (20 males and 20 females; approximately 5 months of age) healthy, experimentally naïve, vaccinated Beagle dogs were obtained commercially from a laboratory animal supplier. All animals were acclimatized for 50 days before study initiation. Following clinical pathology evaluations and a detailed physical and neurological examination before study start, 32 animals (16 males and 16 females) were considered suitable for the study and enrolled.

All dogs were housed individually in approximately 1.2 sq.m runs on raised floor caging that provided adequate room for exercise and under climate controlled conditions (temperature, 18 to 29 °C; humidity, 30% to 70%). Fluorescent lighting was provided for approximately 12 h per day. Animals were fed ad libitum with a certified commercial canine diet for approximately 6 h daily and water was available ad libitum.

Allocation to groups

This was a randomized, controlled, blinded, 6-month study with a parallel design. Using a block randomization procedure stratified by sex and weight, 32 animals (16 males weighing 8.28 to 13.79 kg and 16 females weighing 6.61 to 9.20 kg) were randomized on Day – 1 to one of the following four groups (4 males and 4 females per group): Group 1, placebo (sham); Group 2, 2 mg/kg robenacoxib; Group 3, 6 mg/kg robenacoxib; and Group 4, 10 mg/kg robenacoxib.

The animals were identified by a microchip implant and vendor tattoo. The cage number of the animal was identified by the study number, animal number, and sex, but did not include the treatment to blind personnel responsible for any data collection.

Investigational veterinary product and administration

The investigational veterinary products (i.e. the pharmaceutical form being evaluated) were supplied as commercial Onsior™ tablets containing 5, 10, 20 or 40 mg of robenacoxib. The number and size of the tablets administered orally depended on the most recent body weights and the target dose level required (either 2, 6 or 10 mg/kg). The control animals were sham dosed. Tablets were administered after overnight fasting once daily for a total of 26 weeks, from Day 1 to 181 (the day before study completion). After each dose, approximately 5 mL tap water was administered orally with a syringe. Feed was offered 1 to 2 h following dosing. The tablets were administered without feed in order to maximize systemic exposure since robenacoxib oral bioavailabilty is decreased with co-administration with feed [19].

Measurements and variables recorded

Throughout the study, all animals were observed at least twice daily for general health, morbidity, mortality, injury, and availability of feed and water. On days of treatment, detailed clinical observations were conducted twice per day, at least 6 h apart, once in the morning at 1 h post-dose

(±15 min) and once in the evening. The observations included, but were not limited to, eyes, mucus membranes, respiratory system, circulatory system, autonomic and central nervous systems, somatomotor activity and behavior pattern.

Body weights were measured at least weekly throughout the study. Feed and water consumption were measured daily. A veterinarian conducted physical and neurological examinations 2 days before and 7, 30, 91, 150, and 178 days after the first dose. General physical examinations included general condition and behavior, general ocular without ophthalmoscope, integument, musculoskeletal, gastrointestinal, body temperature, cardiovascular and respiratory including assessment by auscultation, and reproductive system by external examination.

Electrocardiography and ophthalmoscopic examinations were conducted once during acclimatization and within 1 week before the scheduled study completion. Evaluations were performed by a board-certified veterinary cardiologist and ophthalmologist, respectively.

The complete panel of clinical pathology endpoints (hematology, blood chemistry and urinalysis) according to VICH GL43 [13] was analyzed during acclimatization and 30, 91, and 181 days after the first dose. Buccal mucosal bleeding time (BMBT) was evaluated during acclimatization and 31, 92, and 178 days after the first dose.

Fecal and urine samples were collected for analysis once during acclimatization and 30, 91, and 181 days after the first dose. Feces were weighed and were then observed for color, consistency, size, parasites, and other abnormalities.

Blood samples for toxicokinetics

Blood samples (2 mL) were collected from all animals via the jugular vein for determination of the blood concentrations of robenacoxib. Samples were collected pre-dose and at 15 and 30 min, 1, 2, 5, 8, 12, and 24 h post-dosing on the day of the first dose and 30 and 150 days after the first dose. Samples were placed in tubes containing K_2 EDTA and stored frozen until analyzed.

Determination of robenacoxib blood concentrations has been described previously [19]. Briefly, following an initial solid phase extraction, robenacoxib was quantified by high pressure liquid chromatography – ultra violet (HPLC-UV) for concentrations > 500 ng/mL and by liquid chromatography – mass spectrometry (LC-MS) for concentrations < 500 ng/mL. The analytical method was validated using quality control spiked matrix specimens run with each sequence of unknown samples, and independent of calibration standards. The lower limit of quantitation (LLOQ) of the analytical method was 2 ng/mL.

The analytical data were processed as individual time versus blood concentration profiles using the validated pharmacokinetic evaluation software DEBA (Data Evaluation in BioAnalytics; release 4.0, Copyright Dr. C.N. Thumm-Kraus, Software und Beratung, 1999) and the following parameters were estimated: AUClast, Tmax and Cmax.

Pathological examination

Euthanasia was performed by sodium pentobarbital solution administration. A board-certified veterinary pathologist conducted complete post-mortem examinations on all animals at the necropsy 182 days after the first dose. Macroscopic examinations were conducted for external or internal abnormalities. A full complement of organs and tissues, including tibial cartilage, was collected from all animals and fixed in neutral buffered formalin. Tibia specimens were placed into 5% formic acid and decalcified for 5 weeks prior to histological processing.

Body and organ weights were recorded for all animals and organ weight ratios were calculated (relative to body and brain weights). Histopathology examination of fixed hematoxylin and eosin-stained paraffin sections was performed by a blinded board-certified veterinary pathologist and any observed lesions were graded using a 4-step grading system (minimal, mild, moderate and severe) to enable comparison between the dose groups.

Statistical analysis of data

Statistical analyses were conducted using SAS® (Statistical analysis system, Version 8.2, Cary, North Carolina: SAS Institute Inc.). For each endpoint, data from the treatment groups (Groups 2, 3, or 4) were compared with data from the control group (Group 1). The experimental unit was the individual animal.

Endpoints measured one time post-treatment that did not include a pre-treatment measurement (absolute organ weights and organ weight relative to body and brain weights) were analyzed using an analysis of variance (ANOVA) with classification variables 'treatment', 'sex', and the two-way interaction term 'treatment by sex'. The treatment main effect was evaluated only if the 'treatment by sex' was not significant ($p > 0.05$). If the treatment effect was significant ($p \leq 0.10$), pair-wise comparisons of treatment groups with the control group were tested.

Endpoints measured multiple times post-treatment that included a pre-treatment measurement (body weights, feed consumption, and clinical pathology) were analyzed using repeated measures analysis of covariance (RMANCOVA) with classification variables 'treatment', 'time', and 'sex'; the two-way interactions 'treatment by time', 'treatment by sex', and 'sex by time'; the three-way interaction 'treatment by time by sex'; and the pre-treatment value closest to dosing was used as a covariate. If the 'treatment by time' interaction was significant ($p \leq 0.10$), each treatment group was compared to the control through the simple effect of 'treatment' for each time point. The treatment main effect was evaluated only if all the two-way and three-way interactions were not significant. If the treatment effect was significant ($p \leq 0.10$), pair-wise comparisons of treatment groups with the control group were tested.

Results

Investigational veterinary product doses

The actual mean dose levels for males and females for the groups receiving 2, 6 and 10 mg/kg of robenacoxib was 2.24, 6.26, and 10.24 mg/kg/day, respectively. Individual robenacoxib doses reached or exceeded the intended oral dose levels in all treatment groups.

Clinical assessments

There was no mortality and no serious adverse events in any animal until scheduled termination on Day 182. All dogs were healthy through study termination. Dogs gained approximately 20% weight during the study. Body weights and feed consumption changes were similar between controls and treated groups throughout the study (Table 1). There were no statistically significant differences between control and treated animals ($P = 0.4147$) for feed consumption (Table 1). No relevant variations in water consumption were observed.

During animal observations, salivation was noted in all groups, but most frequently in Group 3 (6 mg/kg). Similarly soft/mucoid/watery feces were noted in all groups, but more frequently in the treated groups as compared to control group. On Day 178, unilateral or bilateral decreased hopping was noted in three treated animals (two dogs in Group 2; 2 mg/kg and one dog in Group 4; 10 mg/kg). One of these dogs (Group 2) had abnormalities noted on neurological examination (absence of panniculus reflex) prior to treatment. Unilateral decreased conscious proprioception was also noted on Day 178 in one treated dog in Group 4.

Increased BMBTs were observed in one female (Group 3; 6 mg/kg) and one male (Group 4; 10 mg/kg) on Day 178 (5 min 55 s and 5 min 10 s, respectively). Both dogs had values within normal limits (i.e. between 1 to 5 min) prior to treatment (1 min 55 s and 3 min 51 s, respectively). Mean BMBT values were similar between the control and the treated groups.

One female (Group 4; 10 mg/kg) had a single retinal fold in the tapetal fundus of the left eye noted on Day 177.

Cardiovascular auscultation was normal in all dogs. Three ventricular premature complexes (VPCs) were noted in the terminal ECG on Day 178 of one male (Group 2; 2 mg/kg).

Examination of the reproductive system was normal in all dogs. Urinalysis parameters and fecal analysis findings were comparable between control and treated groups at all time points.

Clinical pathology

Summary data for selected hematology and clinical chemistry parameters are presented in Tables 2 and 3. The hematology values were in general comparable between control and treated animals with a few exceptions. A treatment by time effect was identified for hemoglobin (increased in Group 2 on Day 91; $P = 0.0283$) and a treatment effect on reticulocytes (increased in Group 3; $P = 0.0215$) and eosinophils (increased in Group 4; $P = 0.0003$).

Similarly, clinical chemistry parameters were comparable between control and treated animals, with the exception of a treatment by time effect on albumin ($P = 0.0254$), direct bilirubin ($P = 0.0717$) and cholesterol ($P = 0.0913$) and a treatment effect on calcium ($P = 0.0423$).

All coagulation parameters were comparable between control and treated groups at all time points.

Gross and microscopic evaluation

Two dogs had gastrointestinal tract lesions on gross examination: one male in Group 3 (6 mg/kg) had mild, red foci on the cecum and one female in Group 4 (10 mg/kg) had minimal, red mucosal discoloration of the duodenum. The gross lesions did neither correspond to any histological changes nor correlate to clinical findings in either dog. In addition, there were no relevant microscopic observations present in male or female dogs (summary data for histology are presented in Table 4).

Summary data for organ weights are presented in Table 5. Mean ovarian weights were statistically significantly decreased in females in Group 3 and 4 (1.3 and 1.1 g, respectively) when compared to controls (1.9 g); however, there were no gross or histopathologic changes

Table 1 Summary of body weight and feed consumption; mean (SD), $N = 8$

Variable (units)		Group 1 (sham)	Group 2 (2 mg/kg)	Group 3 (6 mg/kg)	Group 4 (10 mg/kg)	*P*-value Treatment
Body weight (kg)	Pretest	9.32 (2.17)	9.27 (2.00)	9.18 (1.52)	9.12 (1.51)	0.2736
	Week 26	11.24 (2.40)	11.29 (2.25)	11.19 (1.71)	10.84 (1.59)	
Feed consumption (g/animal/day)	Pretest	230.3 (44.2)	227.1 (36.8)	211.9 (45.4)	238.7 (41.9)	0.4147
	Week 26	283.5 (66.2)	311.9 (40.4)	277.7 (54.2)	360.8 (224.7)	

Table 2 Summary of hematology data; mean (SD), N = 8

Variable (reference range and units)[a]	Day	Group 1 (sham)	Group 2 (2 mg/kg)	Group 3 (6 mg/kg)	Group 4 (10 mg/kg)	P-value[2] Treatment
White blood cell count (5.0–14.1 × 10^3/μL)	Pretest	12.25 (2.10)	12.81 (2.53)	15.81 (5.14)	13.88 (4.39)	0.2703
	30	9.91 (0.95)	12.29 (2.72)	11.74 (2.51)	11.31 (1.71)	
	91	10.15 (1.80)	10.45 (1.36)	12.83 (2.69)	12.46 (3.96)	
	181	9.34 (2.25)	11.03 (4.63)	11.30 (1.81)	10.59 (1.99)	
Red blood cell count (4.95–7.87 × 10^6/μL)	Pretest	7.079 (0.396)	7.344 (0.407)	6.994 (0.582)	6.935 (0.597)	0.7588
	30	7.124 (0.570)	7.169 (0.677)	6.940 (0.492)	6.910 (0.357)	
	91	7.103 (0.411)	7.590 (0.701)	6.995 (0.448)	6.984 (0.534)	
	181	6.835 (0.380)	6.880 (0.538)	6.633 (0.389)	6.948 (0.289)	
Reticulocytes (< 80 × 10^3/μL)	Pretest	42.70 (14.25)	51.36 (35.09)	45.20 (13.76)	42.90 (13.09)	**0.0962**
	30	32.89 (14.74)	40.03 (16.68)	47.28 (16.49)	35.43 (12.29)	
	91	13.73 (8.39)	22.65 (9.31)	26.43 (15.38)	22.76 (8.48)	
	181	28.48 (24.78)	21.51 (8.90)	41.43 (18.70)	30.53 (15.87)	
Eosinophils (0.0–1.3 × 10^3/μL)	Pretest	0.226 (0.062)	0.278 (0.179)	0.270 (0.097)	0.358 (0.102)	**0.0005**
	30	0.248 (0.122)	0.265 (0.137)	0.291 (0.095)	0.453 (0.141)	
	91	0.228 (0.057)	0.274 (0.115)	0.288 (0.089)	0.465 (0.207)	
	181	0.276 (0.073)	0.301 (0.112)	0.340 (0.109)	0.598 (0.176)	
Platelets (211–621 × 10^3/μL)	Pretest	333.5 (52.7)	311.9 (49.7)	269.3 (63.1)	300.3 (46.4)	0.8921
	30	346.8 (81.4)	333.9 (36.1)	295.9 (90.0)	315.8 (37.3)	
	91	313.9 (62.7)	313.3 (61.6)	301.5 (68.4)	306.4 (54.4)	
	181	301.3 (84.0)	298.6 (63.8)	269.0 (90.2)	277.1 (41.5)	
Hemoglobin (11.9–18.9 g/dL)	Pretest	15.54 (0.73)	15.70 (0.85)	15.49 (1.28)	15.04 (1.30)	0.8821
	30	16.09 (1.00)	15.90 (1.02)	15.88 (1.13)	15.49 (1.20)	
	91	15.60 (0.66)	16.68 (1.35)	15.69 (1.00)	15.45 (1.26)	
	181	15.76 (0.79)	15.53 (1.21)	15.45 (0.92)	15.93 (0.61)	
Hematocrit (35–57%)	Pretest	43.94 (2.12)	44.86 (2.46)	43.63 (3.66)	42.56 (3.51)	0.8776
	30	45.11 (3.16)	44.45 (2.98)	44.31 (3.31)	43.20 (2.89)	
	91	44.05 (2.95)	46.68 (4.00)	43.66 (2.86)	42.63 (4.16)	
	181	42.65 (2.40)	42.53 (3.36)	41.71 (2.28)	43.19 (1.57)	

Footnote:
[a] These reference ranges are to be used for information only and the pretest values collected before the dosing period during acclimatization should be used for interpretation in the context of this study
[2] *P*-values in bold denote significance

noted in the ovaries of any dog. Mean pooled spleen weights were statistically significantly higher in Group 2 and 4 (69 and 72 g, respectively) when compared to controls (51 g). Microscopically, all spleens were within normal limits. There were no statistically significant differences in individual male or female mean spleen weights when compared to controls. Mean pooled thyroid/parathyroid gland weight (relative to body weight) was statistically increased in Group 4 when compared to controls. The organ weight increase was minimal (15%) and there were no corresponding microscopic findings present. No other organ weight parameter showed statistical significance of interest.

Gross evaluation of tibial plateaus did not reveal any alterations in any animals. Histopathologic evaluation of medial and lateral tibial articular cartilage revealed minimal superficial collagen fibrillation, chondrocyte and proteoglycan loss in two male animals (one control and one in Group 3 [6 mg/kg]). This minimal, spontaneous change was seen in the inner half of the medial tibia (area not protected by meniscus) in both cases.

Toxicokinetics

The Cmax and AUClast data following dosing on Days 1, 30, and 150 demonstrated consistent and adequate exposure of all treated dogs and reached comparable levels

Table 3 Summary of clinical chemistry data; mean (SD), N = 8

Variable (reference range and units)[a]	Day	Group 1 (sham)	Group 2 (2 mg/kg)	Group 3 (6 mg/kg)	Group 4 (10 mg/kg)	*P*-value[2] Treatment
Alkaline phosphatase (1–114 U/L)	Pretest	89.3 (25.9)	101.5 (21.9)	86.4 (11.5)	94.4 (16.1)	0.8687
	30	76.8 (28.7)	82.9 (16.8)	70.0 (10.6)	79.3 (15.0)	
	91	47.9 (17.6)	53.5 (14.2)	45.1 (10.9)	50.6 (8.5)	
	181	36.6 (17.1)	41.8 (15.3)	36.1 (6.0)	42.1 (8.6)	
Aspartate aminotransferase (28–60 U/L)	Pretest	35.1 (5.3)	35.5 (5.3)	38.1 (8.3)	36.1 (9.5)	0.7180
	30	31.1 (6.8)	30.3 (6.2)	30.1 (4.0)	30.4 (3.8)	
	91	30.4 (5.5)	34.8 (3.8)	31.3 (5.4)	26.8 (3.5)	
	181	27.9 (8.6)	27.1 (5.3)	27.8 (4.7)	28.8 (3.7)	
Alanine aminotransferase (10–109 U/L)	Pretest	27.6 (5.0)	28.8 (4.1)	28.4 (7.8)	28.6 (7.2)	0.8099
	30	30.6 (7.1)	29.4 (5.6)	32.6 (5.8)	29.3 (3.5)	
	91	30.5 (6.6)	36.0 (10.1)	31.9 (5.1)	34.1 (12.9)	
	181	32.3 (12.8)	29.0 (7.0)	33.6 (9.5)	37.6 (12.8)	
Creatine kinase (52–368 U/L)	Pretest	312.1 (153.0)	261.8 (98.7)	278.8 (52.5)	324.4 (228.5)	0.7749
	30	216.5 (57.9)	186.8 (56.5)	182.1 (26.6)	211.4 (40.8)	
	91	185.8 (38.8)	248.3 (153.8)	182.3 (44.3)	163.8 (41.6)	
	181	197.1 (81.3)	174.4 (55.3)	180.9 (59.0)	179.1 (45.8)	
Urea nitrogen (8–28 mg/dL)	Pretest	11.0 (2.6)	11.5 (1.6)	11.4 (2.1)	11.1 (1.9)	0.5554
	30	13.8 (2.8)	13.3 (1.6)	13.4 (2.3)	13.8 (1.8)	
	91	15.3 (1.9)	15.0 (2.8)	14.1 (2.9)	13.0 (2.4)	
	181	15.1 (2.4)	15.5 (2.5)	14.3 (2.8)	15.6 (1.8)	
Creatinine (0.5–1.7 mg/dL)	Pretest	0.59 (0.08)	0.60 (0.05)	0.59 (0.04)	0.58 (0.07)	0.8214
	30	0.70 (0.14)	0.69 (0.06)	0.66 (0.07)	0.68 (0.07)	
	91	0.73 (0.10)	0.74 (0.07)	0.69 (0.08)	0.69 (0.10)	
	181	0.76 (0.14)	0.74 (0.09)	0.74 (0.05)	0.74 (0.07)	
Total Protein (5.4–7.5 g/dL)	Pretest	5.83 (0.20)	5.56 (0.17)	5.75 (0.31)	5.68 (0.27)	0.6166
	30	5.90 (0.26)	5.61 (0.11)	5.76 (0.36)	5.75 (0.25)	
	91	5.69 (0.16)	5.46 (0.15)	5.55 (0.40)	5.60 (0.23)	
	181	6.46 (0.14)	6.19 (0.14)	6.23 (0.38)	6.25 (0.30)	
Albumin (2.9–3.9 g/dL)	Pretest	3.34 (0.16)	3.18 (0.12)	3.20 (0.15)	3.21 (0.10)	0.0631
	30	3.24 (0.17)	3.08 (0.15)	3.09 (0.16)	3.19 (0.16)	
	91	3.48 (0.15)	3.35 (0.12)	3.24 (0.19)	3.36 (0.11)	
	181	3.64 (0.12)	3.31 (0.12)	3.31 (0.22)	3.45 (0.13)	
Direct bilirubin (0.0–0.3 mg/dL)	Pretest	(–)	(–)	(–)	(–)	0.4098
	30	0.00 (0.00)	0.01 (0.04)	0.00 (0.00)	0.04 (0.05)	
	91	0.04 (0.05)	0.00 (0.00)	0.03 (0.05)	0.00 (0.00)	
	181	0.01 (0.04)	0.00 (0.00)	0.01 (0.04)	0.01 (0.04)	
Cholesterol (135–278 mg/dL)	Pretest	164.3 (30.1)	145.8 (24.3)	155.5 (22.5)	158.6 (23.1)	0.1893
	30	156.6 (26.6)	136.5 (19.2)	142.4 (14.7)	146.0 (18.0)	
	91	153.1 (41.3)	131.1 (18.6)	133.9 (12.1)	147.4 (24.8)	
	181	194.4 (54.2)	186.1 (55.0)	177.1 (37.6)	158.0 (30.4)	
Calcium (9.1–11.7 mg/dL)	Pretest	11.01 (0.33)	10.73 (0.21)	10.86 (0.26)	10.91 (0.26)	**0.0423**
	30	11.03 (0.28)	10.93 (0.18)	10.85 (0.26)	10.99 (0.27)	
	91	10.54 (0.15)	10.46 (0.09)	10.30 (0.20)	10.46 (0.31)	

Table 3 Summary of clinical chemistry data; mean (SD), N = 8 *(Continued)*

Variable (reference range and units)[a]	Day	Group 1 (sham)	Group 2 (2 mg/kg)	Group 3 (6 mg/kg)	Group 4 (10 mg/kg)	*P*-value[2] Treatment
	181	10.86 (0.37)	10.74 (0.11)	10.69 (0.18)	10.88 (0.23)	

Footnote:
[a] These reference ranges are to be used for information only and the pretest values collected before the dosing period during acclimatization should be used for interpretation in the context of this study
[2] P-values in bold denote significance
(–) Direct bilirubin was not analyzed for the pretest interval due to a protocol deviation

during study treatment (Table 6). There was one exception in Group 2 (2 mg/kg) where there was a marked increase (approximately 3–4 folds) in the mean Cmax and AUClast at Day 150. The mean Cmax were observed between 0.5 and 2 h post-dose for the three dose levels throughout the study duration. Blood concentrations were below the limit of quantitation (< 2 ng/mL) within 24 h post-dose in the Group 2 (2 mg/kg) and 3 (6 mg/kg) for all animals at all time points. For Group 4 (10 mg/kg), three animals on Day 30 and Day 150 had low but detectable blood levels (≤ 3 ng/mL) at 24 h post-dose, with a majority of the animals exhibiting blood concentrations below the limit of quantification. In general, the Cmax and AUClast showed a dose-related increase between the three dose groups and did not markedly change as a function of duration of administration, indicating absence of accumulation.

Discussion

The objective of this study was to evaluate the safety of repeated oral administrations of robenacoxib in dogs and to identify adverse effects associated with overdoses and chronic administration. This pivotal study is the only 6-month target animal safety study performed with the commercial tablets of robenacoxib for dogs and was a mandatory component of the safety data package required for registration [20]. The dose levels and multiples thereof were chosen in accordance with the VICH GL43 [13] to identify a margin of safety.

Onsior™ tablets for dogs were first approved in Europe for chronic osteoarthritis at a dose of 1 mg/kg, with a 1–2 mg/kg range. The upper end of the dosage range (i.e. 2 mg/kg) was chosen for the 1X dosage and the classical 3X (6 mg/kg) and 5X (10 mg/kg) dosages were applied. Onsior™ tablets were later submitted in the United States for surgical indications at a dose of 2 mg/kg, with a 2–4 mg/kg range. For this indication, the dosages used in this study correspond to 0.5, 1.5 and 2.5 times the maximum targeted exposure. The investigational veterinary products were administered without feed in order to maximize systemic exposure since robenacoxib oral bioavailabilty is decreased (by approximately 25%) with co-administration with feed [19]. Lower exposure and a corresponding higher safety margin should occur if Onsior™ tablets are administered with feed.

To date, five NSAIDs of the coxib class are available for dogs (deracoxib, robenacoxib, cimicoxib, firocoxib and mavacoxib) and only robenacoxib is licensed for cats. To the author's knowledge, there is no other disclosure of safety data generated with the other coxibs and with overdoses with the exception of deracoxib [21], which is also marketed by Elanco Animal Health. For cimicoxib, firocoxib and mavacoxib, only clinical safety data at the therapeutic doses are published [22–26].

No serious adverse events were reported during this study. All treated animals were in good general health throughout the study duration. It was therefore concluded that administration of robenacoxib was well tolerated at oral doses of 2 to 10 mg/kg once daily for up to 6 months and supports the safe use of Onsior™ tablets at the recommended doses.

Clinical findings (salivation and soft feces) were observed in all groups but more frequently in the treated animals. These observations were reported infrequently in a small number of dogs and commonly seen in dogs under laboratory conditions as well as in the normal dog population [27]. Thus, they were considered incidental. With the exception of minor neurological findings (decreased hopping and proprioception) in four treated animals and a minor ophthalmoscopic finding (single retinal fold) in one treated dog, at the end of the study, all animals appeared healthy. No explanation was provided to the observation of decreased hopping and causality to the treatment is unknown. Since the observation was made at the end of the study only, it is also unknown whether this condition was transient.

In the ECG, three ventricular premature complexes were noted on the terminal ECG of a dog in Group 2 (2 mg/kg). Rare ventricular premature complexes can be a normal variant in Beagles, occurring with a prevalence of 0.6% to 1.0% of control animals [28] during routine electrocardiography and 18.8% (males) to 26.1% (females) of normal animals in 18–24 h Holter studies [29]. The affected animal belonged to the low dose group, therefore the arrhythmia was unlikely to represent a treatment effect. The potential of COX-2 inhibitors to cause increased risks of cardiovascular diseases, including thromboembolic stroke and myocardial infarction, has been described after long-term use in humans with drugs like rofecoxib or celecoxib [30–33]. Since then, the cardiovascular toxicity of COX-2 inhibitors, as well as other

Table 4 Summary data of histology

Tissue Observation, severity (localization)	Group 1 (sham)	Group 2 (2 mg/kg)	Group 3 (6 mg/kg)	Group 4 (10 mg/kg)
Adrenal glands				
Normal	8	8	8	8
Aorta				
Normal	8	8	8	8
Bone marrow				
Normal (femur)	8	8	8	8
Normal (rib)	8	8	8	8
Normal (sternum)	8	8	8	8
Bone				
Normal (femur)	7	7	8	8
Cartilage degeneration, minimal (femur)	1	1	0	0
Normal (rib)	8	8	8	8
Normal (sternum)	8	8	8	8
Brain				
Normal	7	8	8	8
Gliosis, minimal	1	0	0	0
Eyes, optic nerves				
Normal	8	8	8	8
Gallbladder				
Normal	8	8	8	8
Gastronintestinal tract				
Normal (esophagus)	8	8	8	8
Normal (stomach)	8	8	8	7
Focal mineralization, minimal (stomach, cardia)	0	0	0	1
Normal (duodenum)	8	8	8	8
Normal (ileum)	8	8	7	8
Mucosal atrophy, minimal (ileum)	0	0	1	0
Normal (jejunum)	8	8	8	8
Normal (cecum)	8	8	8	8
Normal (colon)	7	8	8	8
Cyst, mild (colon)	1	0	0	0
Normal (rectum)	8	8	8	8
Gonads				
Normal (ovaries)	4	4	4	4
Normal (testis)	2	4	3	3
Seminiferous tubules hypoplasia, minimal (testis)	2	0	1	1
Hypospermatogenesis, moderate (testis)	1	0	0	0
Heart				
Normal	7	8	8	8
Hematocyst, minimal (valvular)	1	0	0	0
Kidneys				
Normal	0	1	0	0
Lymphocytic infiltration, minimal	0	1	1	0

Table 4 Summary data of histology *(Continued)*

Tissue Observation, severity (localization)	Group 1 (sham)	Group 2 (2 mg/kg)	Group 3 (6 mg/kg)	Group 4 (10 mg/kg)
Tubular mineralization, minimal	8	7	8	8
Tubular regeneration, minimal	1	0	0	0
Liver				
Normal	8	7	7	4
Mononuclear infiltrate, minimal	0	1	1	4
Lung				
Normal	0	1	2	1
Hemorrhage, minimal	0	0	0	1
Alveolar histiocytosis, minimal or mild	6	6	4	5
Lymphocytic infiltration, minimal	6	3	3	3
Subacture inflammation, minimal	0	0	2	0
Lymph nodes				
Normal (mandibular)	8	8	8	8
Normal (mesenteric)	8	8	8	8
Normal (tracheobronchial)	8	8	8	8
Pancreas				
Normal	7	8	8	8
Lymphocytic infiltration, minimal	1	8	8	8
Pituitary				
Normal	6	8	6	7
Cyst, minimal or mild	2	0	2	1
Prostate				
Normal	4	4	1	4
Lymphocitic infiltration, minimal or mild	0	0	3	0
Salivary gland				
Normal	6	7	6	8
Lymphocytic infiltration, minimal	2	1	2	0
Skeletal muscle				
Normal	8	8	8	8
Skin				
Normal	8	8	8	8
Spinal cord (cervical, thoracic and lumbar)				
Normal	8	8	8	8
Spleen				
Normal	8	8	8	8
Thymus				
Normal	0	0	1	1
Cyst, minimal or mild	2	4	0	3
Lymphoid depletion, minimal to moderate	8	8	7	6
Thyroid				
Normal	8	8	8	8
Trachea				
Normal	8	8	8	8

Table 4 Summary data of histology *(Continued)*

Tissue Observation, severity (localization)	Group 1 (sham)	Group 2 (2 mg/kg)	Group 3 (6 mg/kg)	Group 4 (10 mg/kg)
Urinary bladder				
Normal	8	8	8	8
Uterus with cervix				
Normal	3	3	4	4
Cyst, mild	1	0	0	0
Pseudocyesis, mild	0	1	0	0
Vagina				
Normal	8	8	8	8

Data are the number of dogs with presence of normal histology or detected abnormalities
N = 8 per group (4 males and 4 females)

non-selective NSAIDs, has been the subject of concerns and controversy in human medicine [34, 35]. However, to the author's knowledge, cardiovascular effects during coxib therapy have not been reported in animals, including dogs [1]. It is unlikely that COX-2 selective inhibition poses a thrombogenic risk to dogs. Indeed, dogs do not develop atherosclerosis and are not pre-disposed to occlusion-induced arrhythmias. As compared to humans, they have many more branching vessels in the heart, hence have exceptional myocardial vascular collateralization capability. Moreover, published safety data on robenacoxib [8, 36] or other coxibs [10, 21, 25, 37, 38] did not highlight any cardiovascular risks in dogs.

A few hematology and clinical chemistry values (displayed in Tables 2 and 3) were statistically different from the controls in some treated groups. These differences were all of small magnitude and within the normal reference and/or pretest values. In addition, there were no dose dependency or correlative findings, thus considered incidental and neither toxicologically relevant nor related to treatment. The coagulation parameters and BMBTs were comparable between control and treated groups, despite an increase in BMBT in two treated dogs, that were marginally higher than normal (i.e. slightly above 5 min). No effect of treatment on urine or fecal analysis parameters was observed.

The weight variation in the spleens was most likely due to differences in contraction rates and removal of blood prior to being weighed. Although weight changes in the ovaries in the higher treatment groups were statistically significant, there were no histopathologic changes. The thyroid/parathyroid gland weight increase in Group 4 was

Table 5 Summary of body (kg) and organ (g) weights; mean (SD), N = 8 unless stated

Organ	Group 1 (sham)	Group 2 (2 mg/kg)	Group 3 (6 mg/kg)	Group 4 (10 mg/kg)	P-value[1] Treatment
Body weight	11.23 (2.43)	11.31 (2.28)	11.18 (1.69)	10.78 (1.68)	0.8599
Adrenal glands	1.05 (0.15)	1.10 (0.21)	1.09 (0.17)	1.09 (0.16)	0.9364
Brain	75.69 (6.15)	77.12 (4.93)	78.50 (7.30)	74.62 (4.03)	0.4629
Epididymides (*N* = 4)	3.70 (0.92)	3.82 (0.42)	4.35 (0.63)	3.90 (0.30)	0.4915
Heart	86.57 (19.57)	84.26 (13.63)	85.48 (18.00)	84.51 (17.31)	0.9714
Kidneys	54.25 (13.40)	50.60 (8.81)	49.37 (11.02)	53.59 (14.19)	0.5232
Liver	316.83 (58.45)	323.03 (37.76)	303.03 (55.02)	298.05 (60.58)	0.6478
Lung	90.49 (16.43)	87.50 (12.44)	87.09 (14.23)	90.07 (13.05)	0.7920
Ovaries (N = 4)	1.86 (0.51)	1.88 (0.22)	1.29 (0.30)	1.14 (0.41)	**0.0319**
Pituitary glands	0.07 (0.01)	0.07 (0.02)	0.07 (0.01)	0.08 (0.02)	0.3945
Salivary gland	5.45 (1.43)	5.36 (0.99)	5.69 (1.08)	5.14 (1.16)	0.8261
Spleen	50.93 (15.95)	69.04 (15.92)	52.13 (20.22)	71.59 (20.26)	**0.0131**
Testes (N = 4)	13.35 (4.02)	17.37 (3.19)	16.36 (4.48)	17.91 (2.86)	0.3470
Thymus gland	6.39 (3.49)	7.47 (3.34)	7.72 (3.62)	5.43 (1.77)	0.4936
Thyroid/parathyroid glands	0.87 (0.20)	0.88 (0.19)	0.89 (0.18)	1.00 (0.16)	**0.4457**

Footnote:
[1] P-values in bold denote significance

Table 6 Mean (CV%) pharmacokinetic parameters by group for robenacoxib administered orally once daily for 6 months at 3 dose levels

Group (Dose)	Day	Cmax (ng/mL)	AUClast (h x ng/mL)	Tmax (h)
2 (2 mg/kg)	1	1888 (55)	2091 (23)	1.03 (64)
	30	1384 (51)	2042 (32)	1.06 (58)
	150	5277 (45)	6629 (45)	0.94 (19)
3 (6 mg/kg)	1	4255 (51)	8626 (53)	1.28 (63)
	30	5940 (55)	9700 (24)	1.13 (51)
	150	4146 (64)	7602 (44)	0.81 (32)
4 (10 mg/kg)	1	6612 (44)	15,246 (35)	1.88 (19)
	30	5877 (39)	13,803 (22)	1.25 (52)
	150	4777 (36)	11,077 (32)	1.25 (52)

minimal without any correlative histologic findings and was thus considered clinically irrelevant. No other effects on organ weights were observed.

There were no macroscopic changes at post-mortem examination and no histologic changes in the kidney or liver. Creatinine, urea concentration and urine analysis were normal and not different to controls in the treated dogs. The clinical pathology evaluations did not reveal abnormalities in the liver enzymes (alkaline phosphatase, alanine and aspartate aminotransferases). Overall, there were no signs of toxicity on kidney and liver. The gastrointestinal lesions on gross examination (cecal red foci and duodenum discoloration) were mild or minimal and not associated with any microscopic observations, changes in bodyweight, feed consumption, or serum total protein. The sporadic changes in albumin and feces consistency were considered as not relevant.

The histopathologic evaluation of tibial cartilage did not reveal any tissue damage. The minimal histologic change of the tibia was considered as non-treatment-related.

The observed inter-individual variability (in Group 2, coefficient of variations are ranging from 19 to 64%, 45–54% and 23–45% for Tmax, Cmax and AUClast, respectively) of the pharmacokinetic parameters is probably over-estimated in this study. The blood sampling schedule was established in order to monitor drug exposure, rather than document the full pharmacokinetic concentration-time profile of robenacoxib. Hence, a limited sampling schedule was selected not to interfere with the primary safety endpoints evaluation. Inter-individual varibility for Tmax is moderately elevated. More time points around the expected Tmax would be required for more accurate determination of the Tmax and Cmax. In addition, uncertainty on Cmax is closely correlated with uncertainty on AUC parameters.

In Group 2, while AUC and Cmax values from study day 1 to day 30 were comparable, results from day 30 to day 150 revealed a marked increase in mean Cmax and AUC. As all concentrations pre-dose and 24 h post-dose were below the limit of quantification, no accumulation occurred as expected by the short terminal half-life (approximately 1 h) [19] of robenacoxib. This increase was not observed in the other dose-groups, and thus considered as incidental. This is supported by the repeat-dose kinetics in a previous study of the same design but using non-final formulation [8], which showed no evidence of accumulation or changes in the pharmacokinetics of robenacoxib during repeated administration for 6 months. Altogether, there is no evidence of accumulation of robenacoxib with repeated treatment.

Conclusion

This 6-month laboratory target animal safety study was required for the registration of the veterinary product Onsior™. Clinical findings in the study included salivation and soft feces observed both in control and treated animal, but more frequently in the treated groups. Sporadic abnormalities that were observed only in treated animals were: slight increased BMBTs in two animals, a single retinal change, minor neurological observations in four animals, ventricular premature complexes in one animal, minimal or mild gastrointestinal tract lesions on gross examination in two animals and mean ovarian weight decrease. The gross lesions or organ weight changes did not correspond to any histological changes and there were no other relevant microscopic observations. There were no indications of toxicity to the liver or kidney.

There were no serious adverse events during the study and all dogs were in good health until study completion. Robenacoxib also had no detrimental effects on cartilage or joints. No systemic accumulation of robenacoxib was observed. Altogether, this study supports the safe daily long-term use of Onsior™ tablets at the recommended labeled doses and a margin of safety up to 10 mg/kg when assessed in healthy beagle dogs.

Abbreviations

ANOVA: Analysis of variance; APPT: Activated partial thromboplastin time; AUC: Area under the curve; BMBT: Buccal mucosal bleed times; Cmax: Maximum blood drug concentration; COX: Cyclooxygenase; ECG: Electrocardiogram; FDA-CVM: Food and Drug Administration's Center for Veterinary Medicine; GLP: Good Laboratory Practice; GMP: Good Manufacturing practice; HPLC: High-Performance Liquid Chromatography; K2-EDTA: Ethylenediaminetetraacetic acid dipotassium; LC-MS/MS: Liquid chromatography tandem mass spectrometry; LLOQ: Lower limit of quantification; NSAID: Non-steroidal anti-inflammatory drug; RMANCOVA: Repeated measures analysis of covariance; Tmax: Time to maximum blood concentration following drug administration; VICH: Veterinary International Conference on Harmonization

Acknowledgements

The authors thank the study staff for their valuable assistance with the conduct of the study. The authors also thank Parag Shah (Lilly Capability Center India) for providing medical writing assistance with this manuscript.

Funding

The study was funded by the Sponsor i.e. Novartis Animal Health which is now owned by Elanco Animal Health.

Authors' contributions
CET prepared the manuscript; PB, SBK and RH revised it critically. SBK and RH were responsible for the conception and design of the study, CET and PB were responsible for the pharmacokinetic analysis and interpretation, RH supervised the safety data analysis and interpretation. All the authors have read and approved the final version.

Consent for publication
Not applicable.

Competing interests
All authors are employees of Elanco Animal Health, a Division of Eli Lilly and Company.

Author details
[1]Elanco Animal Health, a Division of Eli Lilly and Company, Mattenstrasse 24a, CH-4058 Basel, Switzerland. [2]Elanco Animal Health, a Division of Eli Lilly and Company, 2500 Innovation Way, Greenfield, IN 64140, USA.

References
1. Kim TW, Giorgi M. A brief overview of the coxib drugs in the veterinary field. Am J Anim Vet Sci. 2013;8(2):89–97.
2. European Medicines Agency. Onsior: European Public Assessment Report, Scientific discussion. 2008. http://www.ema.europa.eu/docs/en_GB/document_library/EPAR_-_Scientific_Discussion/veterinary/000127/WC500067756.pdf. Accessed 06 Mar 2018.
3. King JN, Dawson J, Esser RE, Fujimoto R, Kimble EF, Maniara W, et al. Preclinical pharmacology of robenacoxib: a novel selective inhibitor of cyclooxygenase-2. J Vet Pharmacol Ther. 2009;32(1):1–17.
4. King JN, Rudaz C, Borer L, Jung M, Seewald W, Lees P. In vitro and ex vivo inhibition of canine cyclooxygenase isoforms by robenacoxib: a comparative study. Res Vet Sci. 2010;88(3):497–506.
5. Giraudel JM, Toutain PL, King JN, Lees P. Differential inhibition of cyclooxygenase isoenzymes in the cat by the NSAID robenacoxib. J Vet Pharmacol Ther. 2009;32(1):31–40.
6. Giraudel JM, King JN, Jeunesse EC, Lees P, Toutain PL. Use of a pharmacokinetic/pharmacodynamic approach in the cat to determine a dosage regimen for the COX-2 selective drug robenacoxib. J Vet Pharmacol Ther. 2009;32(1):18–30.
7. Schmid VB, Spreng DE, Seewald W, Jung M, Lees P, King JN. Analgesic and anti-inflammatory actions of robenacoxib in acute joint inflammation in dog. J Vet Pharmacol Ther. 2010;33(2):118–31.
8. King JN, Arnaud JP, Goldenthal EI, Gruet P, Jung M, Seewald W, et al. Robenacoxib in the dog: target species safety in relation to extent and duration of inhibition of COX-1 and COX-2. J Vet Pharmacol Ther. 2011; 34(3):298–311.
9. King JN, Hotz R, Reagan EL, Roth DR, Seewald W, Lees P. Safety of oral robenacoxib in the cat. J Vet Pharmacol Ther. 2012;35(3):290–300.
10. Monteiro-Steagall BP, Steagall PV, Lascelles BD. Systematic review of nonsteroidal anti-inflammatory drug-induced adverse effects in dogs. J Vet Intern Med. 2013;27(5):1011–9.
11. European Medicines Agency. European Public Assessment Report, Onsior Summary of Product Characteristics. 2008. http://www.ema.europa.eu/docs/en_GB/document_library/EPAR_-_Product_Information/veterinary/000127/WC500067759.pdf. . Accessed 06 Mar 2018.
12. Food and Drug Administration Freedom of Information Summary: Original New Animal Drug Application NADA 141–463 (Onsior Robenacoxib Tablets Dogs). 2016. https://www.regulations.gov/document?D=FDA-2016-N-0002-0026. Accessed 14 Aug 2018.
13. Veterinary International Conference on Harmonization (VICH) Guideline 43: Target Animal Safety for Veterinary Pharmaceutical Products. 2008. http://www.vichsec.org/guidelines/pharmaceuticals/pharma-safety/pharma-target-animal-safety.html. Accessed 06 Mar 2018.
14. United States Food and Drug Administration, Code of Federal Regulations Title 21, Part 58, Good Laboratory Practice for nonclinical laboratory studies. https://www.accessdata.fda.gov/scripts/cdrh/cfdocs/cfcfr/CFRSearch.cfm?CFRPart=58. Accessed 06 Mar 2018.
15. Organisation for Economic Cooperation and Development (OECD) Series on Principles of Good Laboratory Practice (GLP) and Compliance Monitoring. http://www.oecd.org/chemicalsafety/testing/oecdseriesonprinciplesofgoodlaboratorypracticeglpandcompliancemonitoring.htm. Accessed 06 Mar 2018.
16. U.S. Department of Agriculture's Animal Welfare Act, 9 CFR Parts 1, 2 and 3. 1989. https://www.federalregister.gov/topics/animal-welfare. Accessed 06 Mar 2018.
17. Guide for the Care and Use of Laboratory Animals. Institute of Laboratory Animal Resources. Washington, D.C: National Academy Press; 1996.
18. Kilkenny C, Browne WJ, Cuthill IC, Emerson M, Altman DG. Improving bioscience research reporting: the ARRIVE guidelines for reporting animal research. Osteoarthr Cartil. 2012;20(4):256–60.
19. Jung M, Lees P, Seewald W, King JN. Analytical determination and pharmacokinetics of robenacoxib in the dog. J Vet Pharmacol Ther. 2009; 32(1):41–8.
20. European Medicines Agency: Evaluation of the safety of veterinary medicinal products for the target animals, Directive 81/852/EEC. . http://www.ema.europa.eu/docs/en_GB/document_library/Scientific_guideline/2009/10/WC500004360.pdf Accessed 06 Mar 2018.
21. Roberts ES, Van Lare KA, Marable BR, Salminen WF. Safety and tolerability of 3-week and 6-month dosing of Deramaxx (deracoxib) chewable tablets in dogs. J Vet Pharmacol Ther. 2009;32(4):329–37.
22. Grandemange E, Fournel S, Woehrle F. Efficacy and safety of cimicoxib in the control of perioperative pain in dogs. J Small Anim Pract. 2013; 54(6):304–12.
23. Hanson PD, Brooks KC, Case J, Conzemius M, Gordon W, Schuessler J, et al. Efficacy and safety of firocoxib in the management of canine osteoarthritis under field conditions. Vet Ther. 2006;7(2):127–40.
24. Kondo Y, Takashima K, Matsumoto S, Shiba M, Otsuki T, Kinoshita G, et al. Efficacy and safety of firocoxib for the treatment of pain associated with soft tissue surgery in dogs under field conditions in Japan. J Vet Med Sci. 2012;74(10):1283–9.
25. Lees P, Pelligand L, Elliott J, Toutain PL, Michels G, Stegemann M. Pharmacokinetics, pharmacodynamics, toxicology and therapeutics of mavacoxib in the dog: a review. J Vet Pharmacol Ther. 2015;38(1):1–14.
26. Payne-Johnson M, Becskei C, Chaudhry Y, Stegemann MR. Comparative efficacy and safety of mavacoxib and carprofen in the treatment of canine osteoarthritis. Vet Rec. 2015;176(11):284.
27. Hubbard K, Skelly BJ, McKelvie J, Wood JL. Risk of vomiting and diarrhoea in dogs. Vet Rec. 2007;161(22):755–7.
28. Detweiler DK. Electrocardiographic monitoring in toxicological studies: principles and interpretations. Adv Exp Med Biol. 1983;161:579–607.
29. Ulloa HM, Houston BJ, Altrogge DM. Arrhythmia prevalence during ambulatory electrocardiographic monitoring of beagles. Am J Vet Res. 1995;56(3):275–81.
30. Caporali R, Montecucco C. Cardiovascular effects of coxibs. Lupus. 2005; 14(9):785–8.
31. Funk CD, FitzGerald GA. COX-2 inhibitors and cardiovascular risk. J Cardiovasc Pharmacol. 2007;50(5):470–9.
32. Salvo F, Fourrier-Reglat A, Bazin F, Robinson P, Riera-Guardia N, Haag M, et al. Cardiovascular and gastrointestinal safety of NSAIDs: a systematic review of meta-analyses of randomized clinical trials. Clin Pharmacol Ther. 2011; 89(6):855–66.
33. Farkouh ME, Kirshner H, Harrington RA, Ruland S, Verheugt FW, Schnitzer TJ, et al. Comparison of lumiracoxib with naproxen and ibuprofen in the therapeutic arthritis research and gastrointestinal event trial (TARGET), cardiovascular outcomes: randomised controlled trial. Lancet. 2004; 364(9435):675–84.
34. Sanghi S, MacLaughlin EJ, Jewell CW, Chaffer S, Naus PJ, Watson LE, et al. Cyclooxygenase-2 inhibitors: a painful lesson. Cardiovasc Hematol Disord Drug Targets. 2006;6(2):85–100.
35. Bombardier C, Laine L, Reicin A, Shapiro D, Burgos-Vargas R, Davis B, et al. Comparison of upper gastrointestinal toxicity of rofecoxib and naproxen in patients with rheumatoid arthritis. VIGOR Study Group. N Engl J Med. 2000; 343(21):1520–8, 2. following 8
36. Toutain CE, Heit MC, King SB, Helbig R. Safety evaluation of the interchangeable use of robenacoxib (Onsior) tablets and solution for injection in dogs. BMC Vet Res. 2017;13(1):359.

Retrospective evaluation of toceranib phosphate (Palladia®) use in the treatment of inoperable, metastatic, or recurrent canine pheochromocytomas

Margaret L. Musser[1,2*], Kathryn L. Taikowski[1,3], Chad M. Johannes[2] and Philip J. Bergman[4]

Abstract

Background: Effective treatment options for inoperable, metastatic, or recurrent canine pheochromocytomas are lacking. In humans, specific germline mutations exist that drive the development of pheochromocytomas. Pharmaceutical blockade of these abnormalities with small molecule inhibitors are an effective treatment strategy. Similar mutations may exist in the dog, and thus, treatment with similar small molecule inhibitors may provide a survival advantage. The purpose of this study was to assess the role of toceranib phosphate in the treatment of inoperable, metastatic, or recurrent canine pheochromocytomas.

Results: Retrospectively, medical records of dogs that had a diagnosis or suspect diagnosis of a pheochromocytoma were reviewed for information regarding response to toceranib phosphate and overall outcome. Five dogs were identified that fit the inclusion criteria. All five experienced clinical benefit (1 partial response, 4 stable disease). Progression-free interval (PFI) for the dog with the partial response was 61 weeks. PFI for the two dogs with stable measurable disease were 36 weeks and 28 weeks. PFI in the two dogs with stable metastatic disease were at least 11 weeks and 18 weeks.

Conclusions: Based on this limited series of dogs, the results suggest that toceranib may have biological activity in dogs with primary and metastatic pheochromocytomas. Larger studies are needed to define the use and response to toceranib in dogs with gross, microscopic, and metastatic pheochromocytoma.

Keywords: Pheochromocytoma, Toceranib, Canine, Metastasis, Recurrent

Background

Pheochromocytomas (PCs) are tumors comprised of neoplastic chromaffin cells of the adrenal medulla. Pheochromocytomas overproduce catecholamines, specifically epinephrine and norepinephrine, in an episodic manner, leading to intermittent clinical signs, including weakness, collapse, hypertension, panting, polyuria and polydipsia, and decreased appetite [1, 2]. Pheochromocytomas are uncommon in the dog, but must be considered malignant as severe consequences including invasion into the caudal vena cava, retroperitoneal hemorrhage, and metastatic spread can occur [2, 3].

Definitive treatment of a PC requires adrenalectomy [2]. However, anesthesia and surgical removal of an adrenal tumor is a high-risk procedure, carrying an overall 51% postoperative complication rate, which increases to 60% in dogs with PC [4]. These complications can include significant blood pressure variations, tachyarrhythmias, intraoperative hemorrhage, and intraoperative death [3, 4]. Vascular invasion into the caudal vena cava, reported in up to 82% of cases, [4, 5] complicates the surgical approach, but the impact on survival in these cases is unclear [4–6].

* Correspondence: mmusser@iastate.edu
[1]VCA Veterinary Referral and Emergency Center, Norwalk, CT, USA
[2]Present address: Iowa State University College of Veterinary Medicine, Ames, IA, USA
Full list of author information is available at the end of the article

A median survival time of 53 weeks has been reported in dogs following surgical removal of a PC [7], with some living for 2–3 years [8, 9]. However, some PCs are not amenable to surgical removal or surgery is contraindicated due to the presence of widespread metastatic disease [6]. The benefit of medical treatment in these cases is unknown.

Pheochromocytomas affect 2 to 8 per million people per year [10, 11] and are biologically similar to those that affect dogs [1]. Standard of care is surgical removal, which often results in a normal lifespan for those individuals with local disease. However, 10–30% will develop distant metastatic disease, and in the 6.5 to 16.5% of patients that develop recurrence after surgical removal [12–14], 50% develop distant metastasis [14]. In the case of any distant metastasis, only 40–60% of patients survive an additional 5 years [1, 15]. These advanced-stage malignant PCs are resistant to chemotherapy and radiation therapy, and the side effects of treatment often outweigh the benefits [16].

In humans, hereditary germline mutations, and abnormally regulated angiogenesis and oxygen metabolism pathways, drive the pathogenesis of many metastatic PCs [17]. Therefore, recent PC research and clinical trials have focused on drugs that target these specific abnormalities. Sunitinib malate is a small molecule inhibitor that targets multiple tyrosine kinase receptors, including c-KIT, FLT3 and RET, and those that help to drive angiogenesis including vascular endothelial growth factor receptors (VEGFR) 1 and 2, and platelet-derived growth factor receptor-β (PDGFRβ) [12, 17, 18]. Recent research suggests that use of sunitinib in human patients with advanced PCs will result in tumor size reduction, disease stabilization, and improvement of hypertension [16, 17, 19, 20].

Toceranib phosphate is a tyrosine kinase inhibitor (TKI) available in veterinary medicine that is molecularly similar to sunitinib, and blocks the same key receptors associated with angiogenesis: VEGFR and PDGFR [21, 22]. Thus, it may be a good treatment option for canine patients suffering from advanced PCs that are biologically similar to human PCs, or in those patients where surgical removal is not a viable treatment option. This study aimed to determine if a response to toceranib is present in dogs with advanced inoperable, recurrent, or metastatic PCs. Based on the human literature, we hypothesized that dogs with a measurable PC or metastatic disease would have a biological response to treatment with toceranib.

Methods

Medical records of dogs diagnosed with a PC and treated with toceranib were collected and reviewed via solicitation through the American College of Veterinary Internal Medicine Oncology Listserv, an e-mail based forum for oncology diplomates. Only dogs with complete records regarding signalment, history, initial complaint, physical examination findings, abdominal and thoracic imaging, treatment with toceranib for at least 10 weeks, and with adequate follow-up including records of side effects, were included in the study. The diagnosis of a PC was based on histopathology of the surgically removed tumor, or suspicion of a PC based on elevated plasma or urine metanephrine or normetanephrine levels as previously described [3, 23–27].

Data collected included breed, weight, clinical signs at diagnosis and duration of clinical signs, findings of thoracic and abdominal imaging, histopathology results, blood pressure, results of fundic examinations, urine metanephrine/normetanephrine levels if available, evidence of cardiac arrhythmias, therapy prior to the start of toceranib, reason for toceranib use (inoperable measurable disease, microscopic disease, treatment of recurrent disease, metastatic disease, or maintenance after completion of other therapy), toceranib dose and dose schedule, duration of toceranib treatment, best response to treatment using previously defined criteria [28], side effects induced by toceranib using the veterinary cooperative oncology group-defined criteria [29], concurrent chemotherapy and supportive medications, concurrent diseases, and patient outcome.

Progression-free interval (PFI) was calculated for all dogs and defined as the time from the day of first toceranib treatment to the time of disease progression (defined as either local regrowth, local progression, and/or metastasis), to the time of toceranib discontinuation due to adverse effects, or to the time of data submission. For dogs with measurable disease, as in previous publications describing the use of toceranib in dogs, clinical benefit (CB) was determined by best response to therapy and was defined as a complete response (CR) or partial response (PR) of any duration, or stable disease (SD) of at least ten weeks in duration [30].

Response to therapy was evaluated via serial abdominal ultrasounds, thoracic radiographs, and in one case urine catecholamine measurements. Animals experiencing SD less than 10 weeks in duration or progressive disease (PD) as their best response to toceranib were not classified as achieving CB.

Results

Data for 6 dogs from 5 different sites were received. Five dogs were identified that fit the inclusion criteria (Table 1).

The sixth dog did not have adequate evidence of a PC diagnosis, and so was excluded from analysis. There were four spayed females and one castrated male. Breeds included one of each: Shih Tzu, Australian Terrier, Pomeranian, Dachshund, and Pit Bull. Mean weight was 12.1 kg (range 2.6–29 kg) with a mean age of 11.5 years (range 9.5–14 years). Clinical signs at diagnosis were varied, but included prolonged gastrointestinal signs (vomiting,

Table 1 Summary of patient characteristics and response to toceranib

Patient	Breed	Treatment of Measurable Disease or Metastatic Disease	Response	PFI (weeks)	Reason for Toceranib Discontinuation	Alive?
1	Shih Tzu	Measurable	SD	36	Diarrhea	Y
2	Aus. Terrier	Microscopic/Metastatic	SD	18	Ongoing	Y
3	Pomeranian	Measurable	SD	28	Ongoing	Y
4	Dachshund	Measurable	PR	61	Ongoing	Y
5	Pit Bull	Metastatic	SD	11	Lameness	N

PFI: Progression free interval

diarrhea, decreased appetite, and weight loss) in three dogs, and exercise intolerance, heavy panting, and polyuria/polydipsia in two dogs. One dog was non-clinical and the PC was an incidental finding during work-up of a concurrent disease. Excluding this dog, clinical signs for the other four dogs were present for a mean of 22 weeks (range 1–52 weeks).

Physical examinations were unremarkable in all dogs. No cardiac arrhythmias were noted in any dogs at any time. A fundic examination was performed in four dogs, which was normal in all patients evaluated.

Abdominal radiographs were taken in one dog, which revealed mild hepatomegaly and a small liver mass. An abdominal ultrasound was completed in all dogs; all were diagnosed with a right-sided unilateral adrenal mass. Three of the dogs had evidence of caudal vena caval invasion. One additional dog developed a recurrent adrenal mass with invasion of the caudal vena cava one year after initial PC diagnosis and surgical treatment. Additional ultrasonographic findings included mesenteric lymphadnopathy concerning for metastatic disease ($n = 1$), an incidental splenic mass ($n = 1$), an incidental caudal abdominal mass ($n = 1$), mild hepatomegaly consistent with vacuolar hepatopathy ($n = 3$), renal cortical hyperechogenicity consistent with degenerative renal changes ($n = 3$), mild pancreatic enlargement and hyperechogenicity consistent with chronic pancreatitis ($n = 1$), scant peritoneal effusion ($n = 1$), mild urinary bladder wall thickening ($n = 1$), and one patient with multiple ventral caudal abdominal subcutaneous nodules suspected to be metastasis from a previously diagnosed mammary carcinoma (given location and the reported subcutaneous metastatic rate of 30% for canine mammary carcinomas [31]; diagnostic sampling was not pursued).

An abdominal CT scan was completed in two dogs for further evaluation of the adrenal mass. This confirmed the presence of the suspected adrenal mass in both dogs. In addition, in one patient invasion of the adrenal mass into the phrenicoabdominal vein and right liver was identified, which was not clear on the abdominal ultrasound completed prior to the CT scan.

Two dogs were diagnosed with adrenal PC based on elevated urine catecholamine levels evaluated through Marshfield Labs. One dog had an elevated normetanephrine/creatinine ratio (2268 μg/g creatinine; reference interval [RI] 28–380 μg/g creatinine). The other had an elevated norepinephrine/creatinine ratio (0.152 μg/mg creatinine; RI 0.001–0.037 μg/mg creatinine) and an elevated dopamine/creatinine ratio (0.1 μg/mg creatinine; RI 0.00–0.031 μg/mg creatinine). The remaining three dogs did not have urine or plasma catecholamine levels evaluated.

Full staging (thoracic and abdominal imaging) was completed for all dogs, which revealed that at diagnosis three dogs had evidence of suspect metastatic disease. One dog had pulmonary metastatic disease based on CT (thoracic radiographs were not completed). The remaining four dogs were free of pulmonary metastatic disease based on thoracic radiographs. One dog had evidence of several enlarged mesenteric lymph nodes on ultrasound concerning for early metastatic disease (as mentioned above). CT scan identified a suspect bony lesion in L1 of one additional dog which was concerning for metastatic disease. No dogs had evidence of multiple endocrine neoplasia syndromes type 1 or 2.

Three dogs underwent surgical removal of their adrenal tumors and had a histologic diagnosis of PC. Additional surgical findings included a caudal abdominal lipoma, a splenic hematoma, and chronic hepatopathy (abnormalities noted previously on ultrasound, as described above). One dog that was treated surgically had evidence of caudal vena cava invasion at surgery, but not during the planning abdominal ultrasound. A CT scan was not completed in this dog. The three dogs that received surgical treatment also had blood pressure readings taken prior to and after surgical removal of the pheochromocytoma. Mean blood pressure prior to surgery was 135 mmHg (range 72–204 mmHg). Mean blood pressure after surgery was 113 mmHg (range 80–151 mmHg).

In the three dogs that had surgical removal of their PC, toceranib therapy was started at the time of recurrent, inoperable disease in one dog, for adjuvant treatment of incomplete surgical margins and the development of pulmonary metastatic disease in the second, and for treatment of pulmonary metastatic disease in the third. In the remaining two dogs, toceranib was given to treat inoperable measurable disease.

All dogs received toceranib at a starting target dose of 2.75 mg/kg orally, rounded up to the nearest available tablet size, every other day ($n = 1$) or Monday, Wednesday, and Friday ($n = 4$). At the time of data submission, three dogs were still receiving toceranib; two had treatment discontinued due to adverse side effects (one due to grade 2–3 lameness; one due to grade 2 diarrhea, grade 2 anorexia, grade 2 lethargy, and grade 3 liver enzyme elevations). Two of the three still receiving treatment had been on continuous toceranib for seven and eight months. The third had been on toceranib for a total of 17 months, including a one-month treatment break following the development of an elevated urine protein/creatinine ratio, which resolved after the treatment break. The two patients no longer on toceranib had been treated for a total of six and nine months. One patient was treated concurrently with metronomic cyclophosphamide (dog 5). Additional supportive medications included enalapril ($n = 3$), metronidazole ($n = 2$), maropitant ($n = 1$), famotidine ($n = 1$), s-adenosylmethionine and silybin A + B ($n = 1$), amlodipine ($n = 1$), carprofen ($n = 1$), gabapentin ($n = 1$), tramadol ($n = 1$), and omeprazole ($n = 1$).

Four dogs had a normal blood pressure prior to starting toceranib (one dog was not evaluated). During toceranib treatment, two dogs developed hypertension (defined as a mean systolic blood pressure of > 160 mmHg as previously described [32]) greater than 220 mmHg. Enalapril was started in both dogs which resulted in the normalization of the blood pressure. In both dogs enalapril was continued for the duration of toceranib therapy.

Three dogs required a treatment break, discontinuation, or decreased dose due to adverse side effects. One dog developed grade 2 diarrhea, grade 2 anorexia, grade 2 lethargy, and grade 3 liver enzyme elevations that progressed while on toceranib. Several drug holidays were pursued, which resulted in temporary control of adverse effects, but even at a lower dose the gastrointestinal signs returned and toceranib was ultimately discontinued after nine months of treatment. One dog developed grade 1 diarrhea and grade 3 proteinuria. Enalapril was started for the proteinuria and a one-month break was given. This resolved the proteinuria and toceranib was restarted at a lower dose (1.9 mg/kg PO Monday, Wednesday, Friday). One dog experienced grade 2–3 lameness which resulted in toceranib discontinuation (Table 1).

Clinical benefit (CR, PR, SD) was noted for all five dogs (Table 1). Four of the dogs treated with toceranib had SD. For these four dogs, PFI was determined to be at least 11, 18, 28, and 36 weeks. In one of these dogs, response was evaluated via an additional urine normetanephrine/creatinine ratio which showed normalization of the ratio following the start of toceranib treatment (levels decreased from 2268 μg/g creatinine to 326 μg/g creatinine; RI 28–380 μg/g creatinine). The fifth dog had a PR with a PFI of 61 weeks that as of data submission is on-going.

At the time of data submission, four dogs were still alive. One dog (dog 5) had been humanely euthanized due to progressive metastatic pulmonary disease 23 months after surgery to remove the primary PC, and 11 months after starting toceranib therapy for metastatic disease. The dog was on a total of six months of toceranib which was discontinued five months prior to euthanasia due to lameness and negative impact on quality of life.

Discussion

The aim of this retrospective study was to evaluate the biologic response of dogs with inoperable, metastatic, or recurrent PCs to standard toceranib treatment. Beyond surgical removal, which is the treatment of choice, information about adjuvant therapy is lacking. The best treatment practices for inoperable, recurrent, or metastatic tumors is also unknown. Based on this limited case series, it appears that toceranib may have biological activity in dogs with microscopic and macroscopic PCs (primary or metastatic disease), and that toceranib might be a reasonable treatment option for owners who are hesitant to pursue surgery, for tumors that are not amenable to surgical removal, and for dogs with distant metastatic disease.

Pheochromocytomas in humans and dogs are clinically similar. Optimal treatment centers on surgical removal, with limited treatment options for inoperable tumors, those that are metastatic, and those that are recurrent. In humans, intensive chemotherapy, radiation therapy, and radiopharmaceutical agents (^{131}I-metaiodobenzylguanidine) result in palliation of symptoms, but do not have an impact on survival [16]. Tyrosine kinase inhibitors that target c-KIT, FLT3, RET, VEGFR 1 and 2, or PDGFRβ appear to have the best biological response, reported to be around 60% [16, 17, 19, 20].

In humans, hereditary germline mutations and mutations in the von Hippel-Lindau (VHL) gene lead to the development of multiple neuroendocrine tumors including PCs [17]. An abnormally functioning VHL gene allows the activation of hypoxia-inducible transcription factors (HIF) which in turn promotes cell growth, angiogenesis, cell survival, and activation of VEGF and PDGF [33]. Similarly, mutations in succinate dehydrogenase (SDH) subunits B and D lead to the activation of HIF and the development of aggressive PCs [1]. Blockade of these mutations with small molecule inhibitors such as sunitinib via the VEGFR cell signaling pathway have led to improved quality of life, tumor size reduction, and control of PC-induced clinical signs such as hypertension [17].

One study has evaluated canine PCs, and the related paraganglioma, for SDH mutations. In that study 50% of PCs (3/6) had germline mutations in SDH, indicating that the disease may have some genetic similarities to humans [34]. Canine VHL mutations have been evaluated in canine renal carcinoma [35], but not yet in PCs, to the authors' knowledge. However, due to the evidence of SDH mutations and similar pathogenesis, it seems reasonable to conclude that human and canine PCs may be similar in their development, and thus treatment with similar TKIs blocking the VEGFR pathway may offer a therapeutic advantage for our canine patients.

Despite these similarities, the reported treatment of PCs in dogs has been largely limited to surgical removal. One case report describes the use of the radiopharmaceutical ^{131}I-metaiodobenzylguanidine for an inoperable PC in a Yorkshire terrier [36]. ^{131}I-metaiodobenzylguanidine is an alkyl-guanidine derivative with a molecular structure similar to norepinephrine. Selective uptake by a PC will occur after intravenous administration. The dog experienced stable disease for one and a half months after the first injection, but five months later developed progressive disease. A second injection was administered but the patient died three weeks later, likely due to compression-induced bowel ischemia [32]. To the authors' knowledge, there are no reported studies of chemotherapy or toceranib for the treatment of canine PCs.

Toceranib phosphate is an oral TKI approved for the use in dogs with Patnaik grade II or III, recurrent, cutaneous mast cell tumors with or without regional lymph node involvement. However, it appears to have efficacy against multiple tumors types, including various neuroendocrine tumors [30]. It is known to block multiple receptors including VEGFR and PDGFR [21] that stimulate angiogenesis, a known driver of human PCs.

Three dogs developed grade 1 or 2 clinical toxicities, which is in keeping with the previously reported toxicity rate for toceranib of 77.6% [30]. In addition, the toxicities observed, such as diarrhea, decreased appetite, lameness/muscle weakness, proteinuria, and hypertension, were those previously associated with toceranib [30, 32]. Neutropenia was not reported in this group of dogs. Two dogs had effects that were severe enough to warrant discontinuation of toceranib, and an additional patient required a significant dose reduction due to grade 3 proteinuria. In a recent study evaluating the use of toceranib in solid tumors, 20% of patients required a drug holiday or dose reduction, although this reduction did not appear to affect efficacy [37]. The number of dogs in this study that required discontinuation of treatment was much higher, but that is likely due to low patient numbers and lack of statistical power.

Two dogs developed hypertension, one of which was the same dog that developed grade 3 proteinuria. Hypertension is a known side effect of toceranib and has previously been reported to occur in 37% of treated dogs [32]. Hypertension is also a well-known side effect in humans treated with sunitinib. In a systematic review of the side effects associated with TKIs for the treatment of gastrointestinal stromal tumors, which inherently should not cause hypertension like PCs, 36% of human patients developed hypertension while on sunitinib [38]. In addition, in a study of humans with PC and paragangliomas treated with sunitinib, 82% had hypertension at presentation, and 35% had exacerbation of their hypertension while on sunitinib [17]. The underlying pathogenesis of TKI-induced hypertension is unknown. Prevailing theories include: (1) VEGF blockade, which prevents nitric oxide synthetase production of nitric oxide, allowing endothelin driven vasoconstriction; (2) decreased VEGF which may remodel capillaries and lead to endothelial dysfunction; or perhaps (3) TKIs may induce tumor cell apoptosis, leading to release of stored catecholamines and thus hypertension [39]. Recently, it has been determined that the development of hypertension while on a TKI is a biomarker of efficacy in some human patients treated with sunitinib [40]. In the current study, the two dogs that developed hypertension after starting treatment with toceranib both had a prolonged PFI (28 weeks and 61 weeks, respectively), and include the one dog that had a PR. One could make the argument that the development of hypertension may infer a more robust and durable response to toceranib.

There are many limitations to the current study due to its retrospective nature and small patient numbers. Histopathologic confirmation of a PC diagnosis was not obtained in all dogs. However, this is often the case in practice as a presurgical presumptive diagnosis of PC is frequently based on clinical signs and abdominal imaging alone [1, 2, 8]. The addition of urine normetanephrine/creatinine ratio measurement may aid in the diagnosis of pheochromocytoma, allowing for appropriate targeted therapy. However, sensitive and specific reference ranges have not been established to confirm the diagnosis of a PC in all clinical situations [23–27]. In addition, this diagnostic is not readily available at most laboratories (available, to the authors' knowledge, through Marshfield Labs, ARUP Labs, and some local human hospitals). Similarly, metastatic disease, although suspected in several dogs, was not confirmed at the time of development or on necropsy. In addition, the natural course of this cancer in these dogs prior to diagnosis and the impact of toceranib on that natural progression, is unknown.

One dog received metronomic cyclophosphamide in addition to the toceranib. Although cyclophosphamide is used to treat humans with PC in a combination protocol with vincristine and dacarbazine, use as a single agent has not been reported [41]. In addition, low-dose metronomic cyclophosphamide (used in the dog reported herein), has not been evaluated for efficacy in human or canine PC. The impact of the addition of cyclophosphamide on this dog's outcome is unknown, but may have positively contributed to the stable disease observed (dog 5). Therefore, given these caveats, it is impossible to definitively conclude that toceranib has clinical benefit for canine PCs.

Conclusions

Despite the aforementioned limitations, this study suggests that toceranib may offer clinical benefit to dogs with PCs. Additional studies investigating the presence of germline mutations similar to those identified in humans could help to support this conclusion. Furthermore, prospective studies are needed to better elucidate the potential role of toceranib in the treatment of both macroscopic and microscopic PCs.

Abbreviations

CB: Clinical benefit; CR: Complete response; HIF: Hypoxia-inducible transcription factors; PCs: Pheochromocytomas; PD: Progressive disease; PDGFRβ: Platelet-derived growth factor receptor-β; PFI: Progression-free interval; PR: Partial response; RI: Reference interval; SD: Stable disease; SDH: Succinate dehydrogenase; TKI: Tyrosine kinase inhibitor; VEGFRs: Vascular endothelial growth factor receptors; VHL: von Hippel-Lindau gene

Acknowledgements

The authors would like to thank doctors Antony Moore, Karen Oberthaler, Sharon Shor, and Carrissa Wood, for contributing dogs to this study.

Funding

No third-party support or funding was received in connection with this study.

Authors' contributions

MLM, KLT, and PJB designed this retrospective study. MLM and KLT supervised case information collection and data analysis. MLM and KLT wrote the manuscript. MLM, KLT, CMJ, and PJB assisted in writing and final editing of the manuscript. All authors read and approved the final manuscript.

Consent for publication

Not applicable

Competing interests

CMJ is a former employee of Pfizer Animal Health and has served as a member of the Zoetis Inc. (formerly Pfizer Animal Health) Oncology Advisory Board and occasionally received honoraria for these activities. PJB is a Palladia Advisory Board member and has ongoing studies sponsored by Zoetis. The remaining authors declare no potential conflicts of interest with respect to the research, authorship, and/or publication of this article.

Author details

[1]VCA Veterinary Referral and Emergency Center, Norwalk, CT, USA. [2]Present address: Iowa State University College of Veterinary Medicine, Ames, IA, USA. [3]Present address: Ohio State University College of Veterinary Medicine, Columbus, OH, USA. [4]VCA Clinical Studies, Los Angeles, CA, USA.

References

1. Galac S, Korpershoek E. Pheochromocytomas and paragangliomas in humans and dogs. Vet comp Oncol, Epub. 2017;
2. Lunn KF, Page RL. Tumors of the endocrine system. In: Withrow SJ, Vail DM, Page RL, editors. Withrow and MacEwan's small animal clinical oncology. 5th ed. St. Louis: Elsevier; 2013. p. 512–3.
3. Gostelow R, Bridger N, Syme HM. Plasma-free metanephrine and free normetanephrine measurement for the diagnosis of pheochromocytoma in dogs. J Vet Intern Med. 2013;27:83–90.
4. Kyles AE, Feldman EC, De Cock HEV, et al. Surgical management of adrenal gland tumors with and without associated tumor thrombi in dogs: 40 cases (1994-2001). J Am Vet Med Assoc. 2003;223:654–62.
5. Herrera MA, Mehl ML, Kass PH, et al. Predictive factors and the effect of phenoxybenzamine on outcome in dogs undergoing adrenalectomy for pheochromocytoma. J Vet Intern Med. 2008;22:1333–9.
6. Massari F, Nicoli S, Romanelli G, et al. Adrenalectomy in dogs with adrenal gland tumors: 52 cases (2002-2008). J Am Vet Med Assoc. 2011;239:216–21.
7. Schwartz P, Kovak JR, Koprowski A, et al. Evaluation of prognostic factors in the surgical treatment of adrenal gland tumors in dogs: 41 cases (1999-2005). J Am Vet Med Assoc. 2008;232:77–84.
8. Barthez PY, Marks SL, Woo J, et al. Pheochromocytoma in dogs: 61 cases (1984-1995). J Vet Intern Med. 1997;11:272–8.
9. Gilson SD, Withrow SJ, Orton EC. Surgical treatment of pheochromocytoma: technique, complications, and results in six dogs. Vet Surg. 1994;23:195–200.
10. Beard CM, Sheps SG, Kurland LT, et al. Occurrence of pheochromocytoma in Rochester, Minnesota, 1950 though 1979. Mayo Clin Proc. 1983;12:802–4.
11. Stenström G, Svärdsudd K. Pheochromocytoma in Sweden 1958-1981. An analysis of the national Cancer registry data. Acta Med Scand. 1986;220(3): 225–32.
12. Plouin PF, Chatellier G, Fofol I, et al. Tumor recurrence and hypertension persistence after successful pheochromocytoma operation. Hypertension. 1997;29(5):1133–9.
13. van Heerden JA, Roland CF, Carney JA, et al. Long-term evaluation following resection of apparently benign pheochromocytoma(s)/ paraganglioma(s). World J Surg. 1990;14(3):325–9.
14. Amar L, Servais A, Gimenez-Roqueplo AP, et al. Year of diagnosis, features at presentation, and risk of recurrence in patients with pheochromocytoma or secreting paraganglioma. J Clin Endocrinol Metab. 2005;90(4):2110–6.
15. Averbuch SD, Steakley CS, Young RC, et al. Malignant pheochromocytoma: effective treatment with a combination of cyclophosphamide, vincristine, and dacarbazine. Ann Intern Med. 1988;109(4):267–73.
16. Jimenez C, Cabanillas ME, Santarpia L, et al. Use of the tyrosine kinase inhibitor sunitinib in a patient with von Hippel-Lindau disease: targeting angiogenic factors in pheochromocytoma and other von Hippel-Lindau disease-related tumors. J Clin Endocrinol Metab. 2009;94(2):386–91.
17. Ayala-Ramirez M, Chougnet CN, Habra MA, et al. Treatment with sunitinib for patients with progressive metastatic pheochromocytomas and sympathetic paragangliomas. J Clin Endocrinol Metab. 2012;97(11):4040–50.
18. Chow LQ, Eckhardt SG. Sunitinib: from rational design to clinical efficacy. J Clin Oncol. 2007;25(7):884–96.
19. Saito Y, Tanaka Y, Aita Y, et al. Sunitinib induces apoptosis in pheochromocytoma tumor cells by inhibiting VEGFR2/Akt/mTOR/S6K1 pathways through modulation of Bcl-2 and BAD. Am J Physiol Endocrinol Metab. 2012;302:E615–25.
20. Joshua AM, Ezzat S, Asa SL, et al. Rationale and evidence for sunitinib in the treatment of malignant paraganglioma/pheochromocytoma. J Clin Endocrinol Metab. 2009;94(1):5–9.
21. London CA, Hannah AL, Zadovoskya R, et al. Phase I dose-escalating study of SU11654, a small molecule receptor tyrosine kinase inhibitor, in dogs with spontaneous malignancies. Clin Cancer Res. 2003;9:2755–68.
22. London CA. Tyrosine kinase inhibitors in veterinary medicine. Top Companion Anim Med. 2009;24(3):106–12.
23. Kook PH, Boretti FS. Hersberger, et al. urinary catecholamine and metanephrine to creatinine ratios in healthy dogs at home and in a hospital environment and in 2 dogs with pheochromocytoma. J Vet Intern Med. 2007;21:388–93.
24. Kook PH, Grest P, Quante S, et al. Urinary catecholamine and metadrenaline to creatinine ratios in dogs with a pheochromocytoma. Vet Rec. 2010; 166(6):169–74.
25. Quante S, Boretti FS, Kook PH, et al. Urinary catecholamine and metanephrine to creatinine ratios in dogs with hyperadrenocorticism or pheochromocytoma, and in healthy dogs. J Vet Intern Med. 2010;24(5):1093–7.
26. Green BA, Frank EL. Comparison of plasma free metanephrines between healthy dogs and 3 dogs with pheochromocytoma. Vet Clin Pathol. 2013;42(4):499–503.

27. Salesov E, Boretti FS, Sieber-Ruckstuhl NS, et al. Urinary and plasma catecholamines and metanephrines in dogs with pheochromocytoma, hypercortisolism, nonadrenal disease and in healthy dogs. J Vet Intern Med. 2015;29(2):597–602.
28. Nguyen SM, Thamm DH, Vail DM, et al. Response evaluation criteria for solid tumors in dogs (v1.0): a veterinary cooperative oncology group (VCOG) consensus document. Vet Comp Oncol. 2015;13(3):176–83.
29. Veterinary cooperative oncology group – common terminology criteria for adverse events (VCOG-CTCAE) following chemotherapy or biological antineoplastic therapy in dogs and cats v1.1. Vet Comp Oncol. 2016;14(4): 417–46.
30. London C, Mathie T, Stingle N, et al. Preliminary evidence for biologic activity of toceranib phosphate (palladia®) in solid tumours. Vet Comp Oncol. 2012;10(3):194–205.
31. Moulton JE, Taylor DON, Doran CR, et al. Canine mammary tumors. Vet Path. 1971;7:289–320.
32. Tjostheim SS, Stepien RL, Markovic LE, et al. Effects of toceranib phosphate in systolic blood pressure and proteinuria in dogs. J Vet Intern Med. 2016;30(4):951–7.
33. Dahia PLM. Pheochromocytoma and paraganglioma pathogenesis: learning from genetic heterogeneity. Nat Rev Cancer. 2014;14(2):108–19.
34. Holt DE, Henthorn P, Howell VM, et al. Succinate dehydrogenase subunit D and succinate dehydrogenase subunit B mutation analysis in canine phaeochromocytoma and paraganglioma. J Comp Pathol. 2014;151(1):25–34.
35. Pressler BM, Williams LE, Ramos-Vara JA, et al. Sequencing of the von Hippel-Lindau gene in canine renal carcinoma. J Vet Intern Med. 2009;23(3):592–7.
36. Bommarito DA, Lattimer JC, Selting KA, et al. Treatment of a malignant pheochromocytoma in a dog using 131I metaiodobenzylguanidine. J Am Anim Hosp Assoc. 2011;47(6):e188–94.
37. Bernabe LF, Portela R, Nguyen S, et al. Evaluation of the adverse event profile and pharmacodynamics of toceranib phosphate administered to dogs with solid tumors at doses below the maximum tolerated dose. BMC Vet Res. 2013;9:190.
38. Sodergren SC, White A, Efficace F, et al. Systematic review of the side effects associated with tyrosine kinase inhibitors used in the treatment of gastrointestinal stromal tumors of behalf of the EORTC quality of life group. Crit Rec Oncol Hematol. 2014;91(1):35–46.
39. Aparicio-Gallego G, Afonso-Afonso FJ, León-Mateos L, et al. Molecular basis of hypertension side effects induced by sunitinib. Anti-Cancer Drugs. 2011;22(1):1–8.
40. George S, Reichardt P, Lechner T, et al. Hypertension as a potential biomarker of efficacy in patients with gastrointestinal stromal tumor treated with sunitinib. Ann Oncol. 2012;23(12):3180–7.
41. Scholz T, Eisenhofer G, Pacak K, et al. Clinical review: current treatment of malignant pheochromocytoma. J Clin Endocrinol Metab. 2007;92(4):1217–25.

Permissions

All chapters in this book were first published in VR, by BioMed Central; hereby published with permission under the Creative Commons Attribution License or equivalent. Every chapter published in this book has been scrutinized by our experts. Their significance has been extensively debated. The topics covered herein carry significant findings which will fuel the growth of the discipline. They may even be implemented as practical applications or may be referred to as a beginning point for another development.

The contributors of this book come from diverse backgrounds, making this book a truly international effort. This book will bring forth new frontiers with its revolutionizing research information and detailed analysis of the nascent developments around the world.

We would like to thank all the contributing authors for lending their expertise to make the book truly unique. They have played a crucial role in the development of this book. Without their invaluable contributions this book wouldn't have been possible. They have made vital efforts to compile up to date information on the varied aspects of this subject to make this book a valuable addition to the collection of many professionals and students.

This book was conceptualized with the vision of imparting up-to-date information and advanced data in this field. To ensure the same, a matchless editorial board was set up. Every individual on the board went through rigorous rounds of assessment to prove their worth. After which they invested a large part of their time researching and compiling the most relevant data for our readers.

The editorial board has been involved in producing this book since its inception. They have spent rigorous hours researching and exploring the diverse topics which have resulted in the successful publishing of this book. They have passed on their knowledge of decades through this book. To expedite this challenging task, the publisher supported the team at every step. A small team of assistant editors was also appointed to further simplify the editing procedure and attain best results for the readers.

Apart from the editorial board, the designing team has also invested a significant amount of their time in understanding the subject and creating the most relevant covers. They scrutinized every image to scout for the most suitable representation of the subject and create an appropriate cover for the book.

The publishing team has been an ardent support to the editorial, designing and production team. Their endless efforts to recruit the best for this project, has resulted in the accomplishment of this book. They are a veteran in the field of academics and their pool of knowledge is as vast as their experience in printing. Their expertise and guidance has proved useful at every step. Their uncompromising quality standards have made this book an exceptional effort. Their encouragement from time to time has been an inspiration for everyone.

The publisher and the editorial board hope that this book will prove to be a valuable piece of knowledge for researchers, students, practitioners and scholars across the globe.

List of Contributors

Nicole Rose
Western Veterinary Specialist and Emergency Centre, Calgary, AB, Canada

Lorraine Toews
Health Sciences Library, University of Calgary, Calgary, AB, Canada

Daniel S. J. Pang
Veterinary Clinical and Diagnostic Sciences, Faculty of Veterinary Medicine, University of Calgary, Calgary, AB, Canada
Hotchkiss Brain Institute, University of Calgary, Calgary, AB, Canada

Carmela Valastro, Debora Campanile, Delia Franchini and Antonio Di Bello
Department of Veterinary Medicine, University of Bari "Aldo Moro", SP. Casamassima km 3, 70010 Bari, Valenzano, Italy

Mariarosaria Marinaro
Department of Infectious Diseases, Istituto Superiore di Sanità, Viale Regina Elena 299, 00161 Rome, Italy

Fabiana Piscitelli, Roberta Verde and Vincenzo Di Marzo
Endocannabinoid Research Group (ERG), Institute of Biomolecular Chemistry (ICB), Consiglio Nazionale delle Ricerche (CNR), Via Campi Flegrei 34, 80078 Pozzuoli, Napoli, Italy

Flavia Bruna and Paulette Conget
Centro de Medicina Regenerativa, Facultad de Medicina, Clínica Alemana - Universidad del Desarrollo, Av. Las Condes 12, 438, Lo Barnechea, Santiago 7710162, Chile

Francisca Bahamondes
Centro de Medicina Regenerativa, Facultad de Medicina, Clínica Alemana - Universidad del Desarrollo, Av. Las Condes 12, 438, Lo Barnechea, Santiago 7710162, Chile
Departamento de Ciencias Clínicas, Facultad de Ciencias Veterinarias y Pecuarias, Universidad de Chile, Av. Santa Rosa 11, 735, Santiago, Chile

Estefania Flores and Gino Cattaneo
Departamento de Ciencias Clínicas, Facultad de Ciencias Veterinarias y Pecuarias, Universidad de Chile, Av. Santa Rosa 11, 735, Santiago, Chile

Gabriele Friton and Jonathan N. King
Elanco Animal Health Inc., Companion Animal Development, CH-4058 Basel, Switzerland

Caryn Marie Thompson and Stephen King
Elanco Animal Health Inc., Companion Animal Development, Greenfield, IN 46140, USA

Daniela Karadzovska
Elanco Australasia Pty Limited, Food Animal Development, Kemps Creek, NSW 2178, Australia

Daniel Nenene Qekwana and Dikeledi Sebola
University of Pretoria, Faculty of Veterinary Science, Department of Paraclinical Sciences, Section Veterinary Public Health, Pretoria, Gauteng, South Africa

Agricola Odoi
University of Pretoria, Faculty of Veterinary Science, Department of Paraclinical Sciences, Section Veterinary Public Health, Pretoria, Gauteng, South Africa
University of Tennessee, College of Veterinary Medicine, Department of Biomedical and Diagnostic Sciences, Knoxville, TN, USA

James Wabwire Oguttu
University of South Africa, College of Agriculture and Environmental Sciences, Department of Agriculture and Animal Health, Johannesburg, South Africa

Hein Imberechts
Operational Directorate Bacterial Diseases, CODA-CERVA (Veterinary and Agrochemical Research Centre), 1180 Brussels, Belgium

Laura E. J. Peeters
Operational Directorate Bacterial Diseases, CODA-CERVA (Veterinary and Agrochemical Research Centre), 1180 Brussels, Belgium
Department of Pathology, Bacteriology and Avian Diseases, Faculty of Veterinary Medicine, Ghent University, 9820 Merelbeke, Belgium

Annemieke Smet and Freddy Haesebrouck
Department of Pathology, Bacteriology and Avian Diseases, Faculty of Veterinary Medicine, Ghent University, 9820 Merelbeke, Belgium

Marc Heyndrickx
Department of Pathology, Bacteriology and Avian Diseases, Faculty of Veterinary Medicine, Ghent University, 9820 Merelbeke, Belgium
Technology and Food Science Unit, Institute for Agricultural and Fisheries Research, 9090 Melle, Belgium

Patrick Butaye
Department of Pathology, Bacteriology and Avian Diseases, Faculty of Veterinary Medicine, Ghent University, 9820 Merelbeke, Belgium
Department of Biosciences, School of Veterinary Medicine, Ross University, Basseterre, Saint Kitts and Nevis

Geertrui Rasschaert and Els Daeseleire
Technology and Food Science Unit, Institute for Agricultural and Fisheries Research, 9090 Melle, Belgium

Siska Croubels and Mathias Devreese
Department of Phamacology, Toxicology and Biochemistry, Faculty of Veterinary Medicine, Ghent University, 9820 Merelbeke, Belgium

Jeroen Dewulf
Veterinary Epidemiology Unit, Department of Reproduction, Obstetrics and Herd health, Faculty of Veterinary Medicine, Ghent University, 9820 Merelbeke, Belgium

Céline E. Toutain and Rainer Helbig
Elanco Animal Health, a Division of Eli Lilly and Company, Mattenstrasse 24A, CH-4058 Basel, Switzerland

Mark C. Heit and Stephen B. King
Elanco Animal Health, a Division of Eli Lilly and Company, 2500 Innovation Way, Greenfield, IN 64140, USA

Hyeok-Soo Shin, Heung-Myong Woo and Byung-Jae Kang
College of Veterinary Medicine and Institute of Veterinary Science, Kangwon National University, Chuncheon 24341, Republic of Korea

Franz Josef Söbbeler and Sabine Beate Rita Kästner
Small Animal Clinic (Söbbeler, Kästner), University of Veterinary Medicine Hanover Foundation, Bünteweg 9, 30559 Hannover, Germany

Inés Carrera and Patrick Kircher
Clinic of Diagnostic Imaging (Carrera, Kircher), Vetsuisse Faculty, University of Zurich, Winterthurestrasse 258c, 8057 Zurich, Switzerland

Kirby Pasloske, Millagahamada and Gedara Ranasinghe
Jurox Pty Ltd. (Pasloske, Ranasinghe), 85 Gardiner St, Rutherford, NSW 2320, Australia

Xuerong Zhou, Qian Rong, Min Xu, Yuanli Zhang, Qi Dong, Yuanling Xiao, Qiji Liu, Helin Chen, Xiaoyu Yang, Kaisheng Yu, Yinglun Li, Ling Zhao, Gang Ye, Fei Shi and Cheng Lv
College of Veterinary Medicine, Sichuan Agricultural University, Chengdu, Sichuan 611130, People's Republic of China

Marios Charalambous
Faculty of Brain Sciences, UCL Institute of Neurology, University College London, London WC1E 6BT, UK

Sara K. Shivapour
College of Veterinary Medicine, Iowa State University, Ames, Iowa 50011, USA

David C. Brodbelt
Department of Production and Population Health, Royal Veterinary College, Hawkshead Lane, Hatfield, Herts AL9 7TA, UK

Holger A. Volk
Department of Clinical Science and Services, Royal Veterinary College, Hawkshead Lane, Hatfield, Herts AL9 7TA, UK

Lidia Pitti and Maria L. Díaz-Bertrana
Departamento de Patología Animal, Universidad de Las Palmas de Gran Canaria, Las Palmas de Gran Canaria, Spain

Maarten Oosterlinck
Department of Surgery and Anaesthesiology of Domestic Animals, Faculty of Veterinary Medicine, Ghent University, Ghent, Belgium

Joaquin Sopena, José M. Carrillo and Mónica Rubio
Departamento Medicina y Cirugía Animal, Cátedra García Cugat, Universidad CEU Cardenal Herrera, Valencia, Spain

Angelo Santana
Departamento de Matemáticas, Universidad de las Palmas de Gran Canaria, Las Palmas, Spain

José M. Vilar
Departamento de Patología Animal, Instituto Universitario de Investigaciones Biomédicas Y Sanitarias, Universidad de Las Palmas de Gran Canaria, Arucas, Spain

Kevin J. Mc Peake and Daniel S. Mills
Animal Behaviour, Cognition and Welfare Group, School of Life Sciences, University of Lincoln, Lincoln, Lincolnshire, UK

Alessandro Menozzi, Fausto Quintavalla and Simone Bertini
Department of Veterinary Science, University of Parma, Strada Del Taglio 10, 43126 Parma, Italy

Manuel Dall'Aglio
Veterinary Practitioner, Parma, Italy

Luca Dallavalle
ATI Pets Srl, Fatro Group SpA, Ozzano dell'Emilia, Bologna, Italy

Valentina Meucci
Department of Veterinary Science, University of Pisa, Pisa, Italy

Cheryl A. London
College of Veterinary Medicine, The Ohio State University, Columbus OH AND Cummings School of Veterinary Medicine, Tufts University, North Grafton, MA, USA

Roberta Portela
Premier Veterinary Group, 3927 W. Belmont Ave, Chicago, IL 60618, USA

Christian Schoen
Nanopartz Inc., 146 Barberry Place, Loveland, CO 80537, USA

Elizabeth M. Schuh
Veterinary Cancer Group, 2887 Edinger Ave, Tustin, CA 92780, USA

Heather L. Gardner
Sackler School at Tufts University, Boston, MA, USA

Rowena M. A. Packer and Holger A. Volk
Department of Clinical Science and Services, Royal Veterinary College, Hatfield, Hertfordshire AL9 7TA, UK

Luisa De Risio
Animal Health Trust, Newmarket, Suffolk CB8 7UU, UK

Michael Gotesman
Department of Biology, New York City College of Technology of the City University of New York, Brooklyn, New York, USA

Simon Menanteau-Ledouble, Mona Saleh and Mansour El-Matbouli
Clinical Division of Fish Medicine, Department for Farm Animals and Veterinary Public Health, University of Veterinary Medicine, Veterinärplatz 1, 1210 Vienna, Austria

Sven M. Bergmann
Institute of Infectology, Friedrich-Loffler-Institut (FLI), Federal Research Institute for Animal Health, Greifswald-Insel Riems, Germany

Sami Al-Nadaf
William R. Pritchard Veterinary Medical Teaching Hospital, School of Veterinary Medicine, University of California, Davis, Davis, CA, USA

Robert B. Rebhun, Katherine A. Skorupski, Jennifer L. Willcox and Jenna H. Burton
Department of Surgical and Radiological Sciences, School of Veterinary Medicine, University of California, Davis, Davis, CA, USA

Kaitlin M. Curran
Department of Clinical Sciences, Carlson College of Veterinary Medicine, Oregon State University, Corvallis, OR, USA

Rachel O. Venable
Arizona Veterinary Oncology, Gilbert, AZ, USA

Margaret L. Musser
VCA Veterinary Referral and Emergency Center, Norwalk, CT, USA
Iowa State University College of Veterinary Medicine, Ames, IA, USA

Kathryn L. Taikowski
VCA Veterinary Referral and Emergency Center, Norwalk, CT, USA
Ohio State University College of Veterinary Medicine, Columbus, OH, USA

Chad M. Johannes
Iowa State University College of Veterinary Medicine, Ames, IA, USA

Philip J. Bergman
VCA Clinical Studies, Los Angeles, CA, USA

Index

CPSIA information can be obtained
at www.ICGtesting.com
Printed in the USA
LVHW061754140222
711000LV00009B/58

9 781639 890071